Investing in Texas:

Financing Health Coverage Expansion

Conference Background Papers
March 22, 2002

by the Policy Research Project directed by
David C. Warner
Kenneth S. Apfel
Jacqueline L. Angel

Center for Health and Social Policy
Policy Paper No. 2

Lyndon B. Johnson School of Public Affairs
The University of Texas at Austin

The LBJ School of Public Affairs publishes a wide range of public policy issue titles. For order information and book availability call 512/471-4218 or write to: Office of Communications, Lyndon B. Johnson School of Public Affairs, The University of Texas at Austin, Box Y, Austin, TX 78713-8925. Information is also available online at <www.utexas.edu/lbj/pubs/>.

ISBN: 0-89940-594-0

Policy Research Project Participants

Project Directors:

David C. Warner, M.P.A., Ph.D., Professor (Wilbur Cohen Professorship), Lyndon B. Johnson School of Public Affairs, The University of Texas at Austin

Kenneth S. Apfel, M.A., M.P.Aff., Professor (Sid Richardson Chair in Public Affairs), Lyndon B. Johnson School of Public Affairs, The University of Texas at Austin

Jacqueline L. Angel, M.A., Ph.D., Associate Professor, Lyndon B. Johnson School of Public Affairs, The University of Texas at Austin

2001-2002 Student Members:

Scott Atnip, B.S., Political Science, Sam Houston State University

Kate Brodsky, B.A., Sociology and Environmental Studies, University of California-Santa Cruz

Chester E. Brooks Jr. (Former Texas State Senator), B.A., Government and Business, University of Texas

Karla Vanessa Buitrago, B.A., History, Loyola University/New Orleans

Evan Christman, B.A., Economics, St. Mary's College of Maryland

Yolanda Davila-Hernandez, B.A., Political Science, Williams College

Tony De Lawyer, B.A., Public Justice, St. Mary's University

Jamie Dudensing, B.S., Nursing, Texas Tech University Health Science Center

Jennifer Allen Eldridge, B.A., Zoology, University of Wisconsin-Madison

Lisa Ewart, B.A., History, Wake Forest University

Victor Fabrega, B.A., Public Administration/Political Science, University of Cuyo, Argentina

Laura G. Garcia, B.A., Public Policy Studies, University of Chicago

Elizabeth C. Kaufman, B.A., Sociology/International Relations, Colorado College

Leah Kegler, B.A., Political Science and Interpersonal Communication, Purdue University

Kristie Kimbell, B.S., Sociology, Texas A&M University; M.S.W., University of Texas-Arlington

Laura Hawley Koenig, B.A., Plan II, University of Texas at Austin

Kristen Lindberg, B.A., Economics, Smith College

Jed Perry, B.A., Political Science, American University

Daniel B. Starr, B.A., Public Research/Communication, Evergreen State College

Sarah Stout, B.A., Political Science and Spanish, University of Wisconsin-Madison

Jie Zhou, B.A., English, Beijing Foreign Studies University, China

Table of Contents

Foreword

The Lyndon B. Johnson School of Public Affairs has established interdisciplinary research on policy problems as the core of its educational program. A major part of this program is the nine-month policy research project, in the course of which two or more faculty members from different disciplines direct the research of ten to thirty graduate students of diverse backgrounds on a policy issue of concern to a government or nonprofit agency. This "client orientation" brings the students face to face with administrators, legislators, and other officials active in the policy process and demonstrates that research in a policy environment demands special talents. It also illuminates the occasional difficulties of relating research findings to the world of political realities.

This volume and its companion entitled "Investing in Texas: Financing Health Coverage Expansion: Conference Proceedings, March 22, 2002," are the first in a new series of publications produced by the Center for Health and Social Policy (CHASP). CHASP, established in 2002 and located at the LBJ School, was created to conduct groundbreaking research, educate students and practitioners to become future leaders, and provide a forum for today's foremost policymakers and scholars to debate pressing issues in the realm of health and social policy.

This volume contains background papers that were produced during the 2001-2002 academic year, and presented at a March 2002 conference entitled "Investing in Texas: Financing Health Coverage Expansion." This conference was the culmination of a two-year policy research project, funded by the Foundation for Insurance Regulatory Studies in Texas (FIRST), to study the uninsured and to propose alternatives for increasing and improving health insurance coverage in Texas. It is our intention that the findings of this research will assist policymakers and other stakeholders to evaluate various policy options available for expanding and improving health coverage in the State of Texas.

The curriculum of the LBJ School is intended not only to develop effective public servants but also to produce research that will enlighten and inform those already engaged in the policy process. The project that resulted in this report has helped to accomplish the first task; it is our hope that the report itself will contribute to the second.

Finally, it should be noted that neither the LBJ School nor The University of Texas at Austin necessarily endorses the views or findings of this report.

Edwin Dorn
Dean

Acknowledgements

The background papers herein benefited from the assistance of a number of observers, experts, and interested persons who are cited in the appropriate papers. The project also benefited from presentations by experts and stakeholders who came to class and presented their perspectives. Those presenters included:

- Edli Colberg, Demographer/Program Specialist, Research, Planning and Evaluation, Texas Health and Human Services Commission
- Anne Dunkelberg, Senior Analyst, Center for Public Policy Priorities
- Caton Fenz, Aide to Representative Garnet Coleman
- DeAnn Friedholm, Executive Director, Children's Defense Fund of Texas
- Dianne Longley, Director of the State Planning Grant on the Uninsured at the Texas Department of Insurance
- Jose Marrero, JAM Creative
- Christopher Sharman, Sherry Mathews Advertising – SCHIP outreach and public relations

Our faculty assistants Camille Hossner, Debra Moore, and Sharon Tutchings have performed above and beyond the call of duty on the policy research project, related research, and organizing many meetings.

Lauren Jahnke provided editorial assistance for each of these papers, and Jennifer Eldridge prepared them for publication. In addition, Jennifer Eldridge developed and maintained the website for the project, which can be found at http://www.insuretexans.org.

We give special acknowledgement to the Foundation for Insurance Regulatory Studies in Texas (FIRST) for the financing provided over the two years of this research project. Funding was also provided by the Wilbur Cohen Professorship and the Sid Richardson Chair.

David Warner
Kenneth Apfel
Jacqueline Angel

Executive Summary

This volume contains nine background papers that were produced during the 2001-2002 academic year, and presented at a March 2002 conference entitled "Investing in Texas: Financing Health Coverage Expansion." The conference proceedings are available in a companion volume entitled "Investing in Texas: Financing Health Coverage Expansion: Conference Proceedings, March 22, 2002." Both are available on the website http://www.insuretexans.org.

The first paper, "Demographic Profile of the Uninsured in Texas," by Victor Fabrega and Tony de Lawyer, provides crucial background information on both the uninsured and the insured populations in the State. The data cover several different categories of the uninsured in Texas: age, race, income, employment status, educational attainment, citizenship status, and type of family. General findings and limitations of the data are also provided.

"Expansion Through Waivers," by Leah Kegler and Laura G. Garcia, offers a compelling option for developing a Section 1931 state plan amendment to insure low-income parents and then using this expansion to leverage funds to create a budget neutral Section 1115 waiver to extend coverage to low-income childless adults in Texas. A model for a HIFA waiver detailing the cost of expansion is presented. Also included is a discussion of approaches in various states to expanding access using waivers and amendments to Medicaid and SCHIP plans, along with lessons learned from each state's experience.

The third paper, "Health Care Access for Immigrants in Texas," by Jennifer Eldridge, examines important issues concerning Texas' uninsured immigrants, and discusses the possibility of using Community Health Center expansions to reach these individuals.

The piece, "Premium Assistance Programs: Reducing the Number of Uninsured Working Texans with Low to Moderate Incomes," by Lisa Ewart, explores the impact of premium assistance programs and the programmatic considerations that policy makers should address when implementing them.

"SCHIP Full-Cost Buy-In Programs," by Jie Zhou, describes how an SCHIP full-cost buy-in program could work in Texas to increase access to insurance to children with family incomes too high to qualify for subsidized public programs, but who may not have access to employer-based coverage and who cannot afford the premiums charged in the individual market.

The sixth paper, "Assessing the Impact of Medicaid and SCHIP Reimbursement Rates on Access to Care in Texas," by Yolanda Davila, Elizabeth Kaufman, and Sarah Stout, examines the longstanding debate over the adequacy of Medicaid and SCHIP reimbursement to health care providers around the State, and the resulting impact on provider participation in public programs.

Next, “Expanding Health Insurance Coverage with the Texas Health Insurance Risk Pool,” by Jed MacKay Perry, addresses different policy options for using the State’s risk pool to expand health insurance coverage. Different options addressed include altering cost-sharing requirements, using more restrictive managed care, subsidizing individuals with lower incomes, allowing small employers to buy into the pool, and increasing the level of financing for the pool.

The eighth paper, “Education Needs and Health Insurance Options: Critical Gaps and Potential Solutions for Texas,” by Scott Atnip, Karla Buitrago, Kristen Lindberg, and Dan Starr, addresses the lack of awareness among businesses and consumers of the health insurance options available to them, and the costs and benefits of these options.

Finally, “Investing in Texas: Financing Health Coverage Expansion,” by Kate Brodsky, Evan Christman, Jamie Dudensing, Kristie Kimbell, and Laura Koenig, examines financing options available for expanding health coverage in Texas given the current constrained financial forecast. The paper focuses on ways to maximize funds under the current health care funding systems, as well as the examination of new revenue-generation mechanisms, such as implementation of new taxes or new tax structures.

This volume and its companion are the first in a new series of publications produced by the Center for Health and Social Policy (CHASP). CHASP, established in 2002 and located at the LBJ School, was created to conduct groundbreaking research, educate students and practitioners to become future leaders, and provide a forum for today's foremost policymakers and scholars to debate pressing issues in the realm of health and social policy.

We believe that the findings of this research will assist policymakers and other stakeholders to evaluate various policy options available for expanding and improving health coverage in the State of Texas.

List of Tables

List of Figures

List of Acronyms

AABD	Aged, Blind and Disabled
AAHP	American Association of Health Plans
AAP	American Academy of Pediatrics
AARP	American Association of Retired Persons
AFDC	Aid to Families with Dependent Children
AHRQ	Agency for Healthcare Research and Quality
ATTC	Advocacy Training Technical Assistance Center
BAT	Business Activity Tax
BBA	Balanced Budget Act
BMI	Body Mass Index
BS	Blue Shield
CBO	Community Based Organization
CC	Contra Costa Health Plan (California)
CHAMPUS	Civilian Health and Medical Program of the Uniformed Services
CHC	Community Health Center
CHIP	Children's Health Insurance Program
CIHCP	County Indigent Health Care Programs
CMS	Centers for Medicare and Medicaid Services
COB	Coordination of Benefits
COBRA	Consolidated Omnibus Budget Reconciliation Act of 1986
CPS	Current Population Survey
CPT	Current Procedural Terminology
CSA	CHIP Service Areas

CTS	Community Tracking Study
DHHS	U.S. Department of Health and Human Services
DHS	Department of Human Services
DOBI	Department of Banking and Insurance (New Jersey)
DRG	Diagnosis Related Grouping
DSH	Disproportionate Share Hospital
DSHS	Department of Social and Health Services (Washington)
EPO	Exclusive Provider Organization
EPSDT	Early and Periodic Screening, Diagnosis and Treatment
ER	Emergency Room
ERISA	Employee Retirement Income Security Act
ESI	Employer-Sponsored Insurance
FAMIS	Family Access to Medical Insurance Security Plan
FFS	Fee-for-Service
FFY	Federal Fiscal Year
FHIAP	Family Health Insurance Assistance Program (Oregon)
FMAP	Federal Medical Assistance Percentage
FPL	Federal Poverty Level
FQHC	Federally-Qualified Health Center
FUUSA	Families Under Urban and Social Attack
FY	Fiscal Year
GME	Graduate Medical Education
GR	General Revenue
GRTL	General Revenue Tax Levy
HB	House Bill

HCAF	Health Care Access Fund
HCFA	Health Care Financing Administration
HCO	Health Care Orientation
HD	Hospital District
HHS	U.S. Department of Health and Human Services
HHSC	Health and Human Services Commission (Texas)
HIAA	Health Insurance Association of America
HICAP	Health Information, Counseling and Advocacy Program
HIFA	Health Insurance Flexibility and Accountability
HIPAA	Health Insurance Portability and Accountability Act
HIPP	Health Insurance Premium Payment
HIRSP	Health Insurance Risk Sharing Plan (Wisconsin)
HMO	Health Maintenance Organization
HRSA	Health Resources and Services Administration
HSC	Health Science Center
ICF/MRs	Intermediate Care Facilities For The Mentally Retarded
IGI	Intergovernmental Initiative
IHC	Indigent Health Care
IHCD	Indigent Health Care Division
IHCP	Indigent Health Care Program
IMD	Institutes for Mental Diseases
INS	Immigration and Naturalization Service
IRO	Independent Review Organization
KPNC	Kaiser Permanente Northern California
LHP	Louisiana Health Plan

MAO	Medical Assistance Only
MCCA	Medicare Catastrophic Coverage Act
MCHB	Maternal and Child Health Bureau
MCO	Managed Care Organization
MCPI	Medical Consumer Price Index
MEPS	Medical Expenditure Panel Survey
MEWA	Multiple Employer Welfare Association
MHC	Migrant Health Center
MHMR	Mental Health Mental Retardation
MMC	Medicaid Managed Care
MRMIB	Major Risk Medical Insurance Program (California)
NACHC	National Association of Community Health Centers
NAIC	National Association of Insurance Commissioners
NCHS	National Center for Health Statistics
NFIB	National Federation of Independent Business
NGA	National Governors Association
NHIC	National Heritage Insurance Company
NHIS	National Health Interview Survey
NMCHIP	Comprehensive Health Insurance Pool (New Mexico)
NSAF	National Survey of America's Families
OBRA	Omnibus Budget Reconciliation Act
OCHI	Office of Consumer Health Insurance (Illinois)
OMB	Office of Management and Budget
OPIC	Office of Public Insurance Council
P&A	Protection and Advocacy (Programs)

PCCM	Primary Care Case Management
PCP	Primary Care Provider
PHP	Preferred Health Plan
PMPM	Per-Member Per-Month
PPO	Preferred Provider Organization
PPRI	Public Policy Research Institute at Texas A&M University
PRWORA	Personal Responsibility and Work Opportunity Reconciliation Act
RBRVS	Resource Based Relative Value Scale
RHCS	Rural Health Care System
RVU	Relative Value Unit
SB	Senate Bill
SCHIP	State Children's Health Insurance Program
SDA	Service Delivery Areas
SDA	Standard Dollar Amount
SEH	Small Employer Health Benefits Program
SFY	State Fiscal Year
SHARS	School Health and Related Services
SHIBA	Senior Health Insurance Benefits Advisors
SHINE	Serving Health Insurance Needs of Elders
SHIP	State Health Insurance Assistance Programs
SIPP	Survey of Income and Program Participation
SOAH	State Office of Administrative Hearings
SPG	State Planning Grant
SSA	Social Security Act
SSI	Supplemental Security Income

SSN	Social Security Number
STAR	State of Texas Access Reform
TAC	Texas Association of Counties
TACHC	Texas Association of Community Health Centers
TAMU	Texas A&M University
TANF	Temporary Assistance to Needy Families
TANPH	Texas Association of Public and Nonprofit Hospitals
TCADA	Texas Commission on Alcohol and Drug Abuse
TCC	Temporary Continuation of Coverage
TCHP	Texas Children's Health Plan
TCP	TexCare Partnership
TDH	Texas Department of Health
TDHS	Texas Department of Human Services
TDI	Texas Department of Insurance
TDMHMR	Texas Department of Mental Health and Mental Retardation
TEA	Texas Education Agency
Texas HEART	Texas Health Education Assistance Resources and Training Organization
THA	Texas Hospital Association
THCIC	Texas Health Care Information Council
THIRP	Texas Health Insurance Risk Pool
THQA	Texas Health Quality Alliance
THSteps	Texas Healthy Steps
TMA	Texas Medical Association
TORCH	Texas Organization of Rural and Community Hospitals

UPL	Upper Payment Limit
UPPP	University Physician Practice Plan
UTHSC-SA	University of Texas Health Science Center at San Antonio
UTHSC-Tyler	University of Texas Health Science Center at Tyler
UTMB	University of Texas Medical Branch at Galveston
UT-Tyler	University of Texas at Tyler
VHAP	Vermont Health Access Plan (Vermont)
VLA	Vermont Legal Aid, Inc. (Vermont)

Chapter 1. Demographic Profile of the Uninsured in Texas

by Victor Fabrega and Tony De Lawyer

Introduction

The Lone Star State is proud of its size and likes to declare that it is the home of the biggest and the best in America. Unfortunately, the superlative could also be applied in qualifying the state in terms of the level to which its large and ethnically varied population enjoys access to health coverage. State-to-state comparisons show that Texas exhibits the second highest rate of uninsured population in the country, and also falls behind other states with similar characteristics in size and population composition.

Regardless of the philosophical discussion about the way in which health coverage should be promoted and provided—such as through public programs versus private sector options—a serious discussion of the issue should begin with a basic knowledge and understanding of the population at stake. This paper provides current counts and demographic characteristics of the uninsured in Texas. It also aims to define different segments of the population that share unique characteristics which make them distinct targets of public policies or market-oriented strategies.

This report also provides a state-to-state comparison showing where Texas stands relative to other states, especially to those that seem to be comparable. We show areas in which other states face similar challenges or, on the contrary, have already found effective ways to reduce the lack of health insurance for their population.

The generation of information about specific aspects of the uninsured population, such as poverty level, citizenship status, family size, and labor status among others, is limited by the fact that a collection of different sources and agencies provide fractional data that should be pulled together in order to estimate of the total number of individuals that lack health access. The deeper the detail provided, the greater the risk is of producing inaccurate figures that may lead to inadequate policy decisions. The assumptions and limitations of the following figures are described, and short descriptions of the major sources of information on the uninsured for Texas and for the nation are provided.

Demographic Profile

Nearly one in five Texans lacked health insurance coverage in 2000.[1] These figures place Texas at the very top of the ranking of states with the highest percentage of population not covered by health insurance.[2] Nevertheless, the lack of insurance coverage does not affect all Texas residents equally. Analysis of the insured population in terms of its demographic characteristics and geographic location shows a different likelihood of being insured, depending upon factors such as poverty level, age, work-status, and race and ethnicity, among others. These factors constitute relevant elements that should be taken into account when designing public policies aimed at improving the health access of Texas families.

The total population in Texas was nearly 21 million in April 2000 as measured by the U.S. 2000 Census.[3] Estimates derived from the March 2001 Current Population Survey (CPS) indicate that about 16.5 million Texan residents had insurance coverage and about 4.5 million people lacked health insurance in 2000.[4] The almost 80 percent of the total state population with health insurance obtains coverage through different means: approximately 60 percent of the total state population has private insurance, 10 percent receives Medicare, and the remaining 9 percent are Medicaid or SCHIP beneficiaries.

Age

The age breakdown of the uninsured population clearly shows the positive effects of government programs such as Medicaid, Medicare, and SCHIP, within certain age groups, especially among the elderly. However, the age breakdown of the uninsured may also indicate that a considerable number of children had not yet been reached. Overall, the uninsured population was made up of 68.4 percent adults and 31.6 percent children aged 0-18 years. A remarkable proportion of the young adult population lacks insurance coverage. For example, among Texans aged 18 to 24, almost 40 percent did not have insurance, a figure that decreases for older populations, 26 percent in the age group 25-34; 23 percent in the age group 35-44; and 19 percent in the age group 45-64. Among those aged 65 and over, only one percent were uninsured, which reflects the impact of Medicare.

Table 1.1
Uninsured Population in Texas by Age Group, 2000

Age Group	Number	Percentage	Percentage within the same category
Ages 6 and Younger	470,240	10.4	18.1
Ages 7 – 17	878,244	19.5	23.2
Ages 18 – 24	743,264	16.5	38.7
Ages 25 – 34	779,066	17.3	26.7
Ages 35 – 44	752,655	16.7	22.7
Ages 45 - 64	854,618	19.0	19.3
Ages 65 +	22,566	0.5	1.1
Total	4,500,653	100.0	21.4
Under Age 18	1,348,484	30.0	21.2
Under Age 65	4,478,087	99.5	23.6
Ages 18 – 64	3,129,602	69.5	24.9

Adapted from: U.S. Department of Labor, Bureau of Labor Statistics, ***2001 March Current Population Survey.*** Online. Available: http://www.bls.census.gov/cps/cpsmain.htm. Accessed: April 8, 2002.

Figure 1.1
Percent Distribution of Uninsured Population in Texas by Age Group, 2000

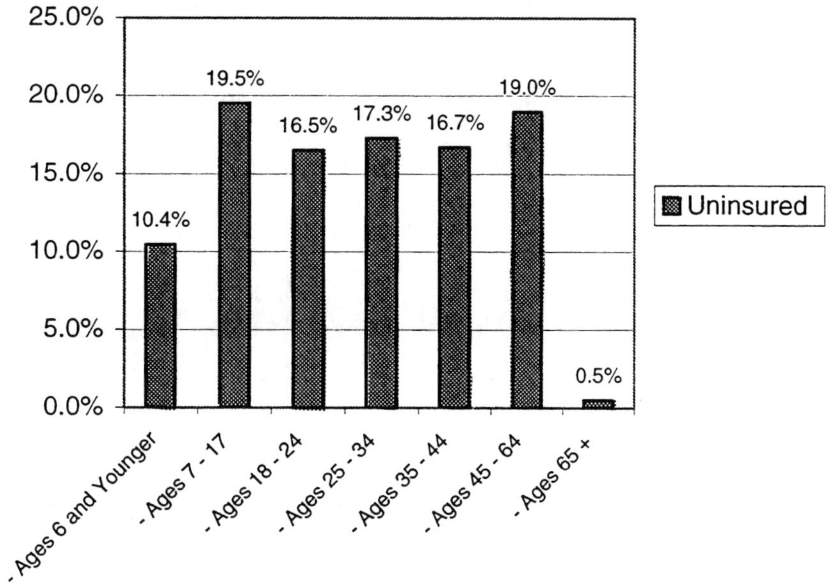

Adapted from: U.S. Department of Labor, Bureau of Labor Statistics, *2001 March Current Population Survey*. Online. Available: http://www.bls.census.gov/cps/cpsmain.htm. Accessed: April 8, 2002.

Gender and Area of Residence

Although females slightly outnumbered males in the total population, men of all ages are 3.6 percent more likely to go without any kind of health insurance coverage. Eighty-five percent of the uninsured population lives in metropolitan areas (see Table 1.2 and Table 1.3).

Table 1.2
Uninsured Population in Texas by Sex, 2000

Sex	Number	Percentage	Percentage within the same category
Male	2,330,622	51.8	22.5
Female	2,170,031	48.2	20.3
Total	4,500,653	100.0	21.4

Adapted from: U.S. Department of Labor, Bureau of Labor Statistics, *2001 March Current Population Survey*. Online. Available: http://www.bls.census.gov/cps/cpsmain.htm. Accessed: April 8, 2002.

Table 1.3
Uninsured Population in Texas by Size of Place, 2000

Area of Residence	Number	Percentage	Percentage within the same category
In Metropolitan Area	3,860,897	85.8	21.7
Outside Metropolitan Area	639,756	14.2	19.8
Total	4,500,653	100.0	21.4

Adapted from: U.S. Department of Labor, Bureau of Labor Statistics, *2001 March Current Population Survey*. Online. Available: http://www.bls.census.gov/cps/cpsmain.htm. Accessed: April 8, 2002.

Race and Hispanic Ethnicity

Although the lack of access to health coverage deeply affects Texans across all demographic categories, the Hispanic population faces a greater risk of being uninsured than do other groups. While Hispanics comprised 32 percent of the total Texas population they made up 57.6 percent of the total number of individuals without health insurance in 2000. On the other hand, the non-Hispanic white population comprised 52.4 percent of the state population, but its share of the uninsured population was 31.6 percent for the same year. The African-American population constitutes 12 percent of the state population and accounts for 10.8 percent of the uninsured (see Table 1.4 and Figure 1.2).

Table 1.4
Uninsured Population in Texas by Race/Hispanic Ethnicity, 2000

Race / Hispanic Ethnicity	Number	Percentage	Percentage within the same category
Anglo and other	1,420,140	31.6	12.2
Black	487,617	10.8	21.2
Hispanic	2,592,896	57.6	36.7
Total	4,500,653	100.0	21.4

Adapted from: U.S. Department of Labor, Bureau of Labor Statistics, *2001 March Current Population Survey*. Online. Available: http://www.bls.census.gov/cps/cpsmain.htm. Accessed: April 8, 2002.

The uninsured rates among racial and ethnic groups also shows the higher likelihood of lacking coverage among Hispanics. Within the same race and ethnicity category, Hispanics go without insurance at a disproportionate rate 36.7 percent when compared to African-Americans at 21.2 percent, and Anglo and other non Hispanics 12.2 percent (see Table 1.4 and Figure 1.2).

Figure 1.2
Percent Distribution of Uninsured Population within same Racial/Ethnic Category, Texas, 2000

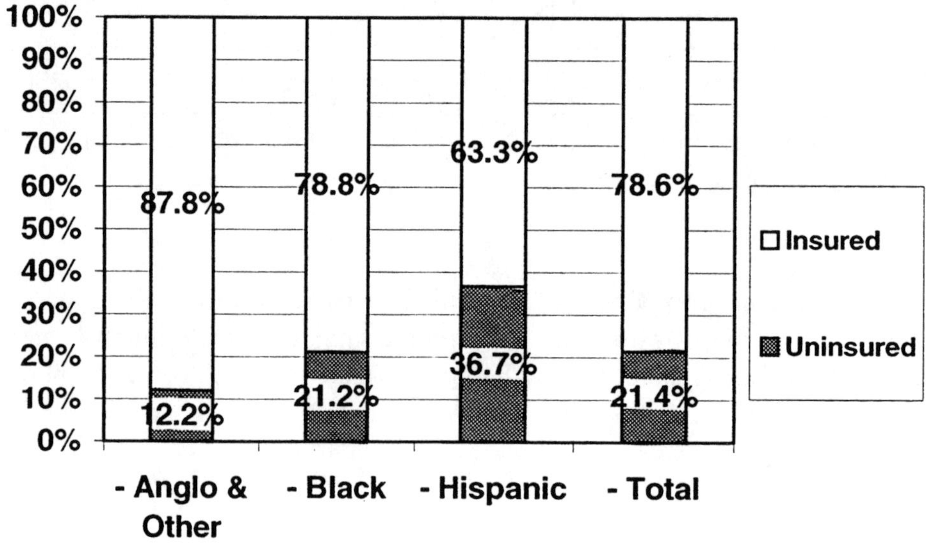

Adapted from: U.S. Department of Labor, Bureau of Labor Statistics, *2001 March Current Population Survey*. Online. Available: http://www.bls.census.gov/cps/cpsmain.htm. Accessed: April 8, 2002.

Educational Attainment

Almost half of the total uninsured aged 18 and older have not completed high school (42.5 percent), while almost a third of them have obtained a high school diploma (as their highest level of formal education). On the contrary, only 8 percent of the uninsured have attained a college or higher degree and 21 percent have some college education or have earned an associate degree (see Table 1.5).

Table 1.5
Uninsured Population 18 Years and Older by Educational Attainment, Texas, 2000

Educational Attainment	Number	Percentage	Percentage within the same category
Less than High School	1,339,727	42.5	41.0
High School	896,686	28.4	21.9
Some College or Associate Degree	669,208	21.2	16.6
College or Higher	246,548	7.8	7.5
Total	3,152,169	100.0	21.5

Adapted from: U.S. Department of Labor, Bureau of Labor Statistics, *2001 March Current Population Survey*. Online. Available: http://www.bls.census.gov/cps/cpsmain.htm. Accessed: April 8, 2002.

Type of Family

More than one half of Texas' uninsured adults were non-married—47.9 percent—and a third of them were single in 2000 (including single-parents). Married people with children made up nearly a quarter of the uninsured, while couples with no children represented an additional 14 percent (see Table 1.6). Finally, single-parent families made up the remaining 12 percent of the state's uninsured residents (see Table 1.7).

Table 1.6
Uninsured Population 18 years and Older by Marital Status, Texas, 2000

Marital Status	Number	Percentage	Percentage within the same category
Married	1,511,249	47.9	17.2
Widowed	63,325	2.0	6.7
Divorced or Separated	519,443	16.5	28.9
Single, Never Married	1,058,152	33.6	33.8
Total	3,152,169	100.0	21.5

Adapted from: U.S. Department of Labor, Bureau of Labor Statistics, *2001 March Current Population Survey*. Online. Available: http://www.bls.census.gov/cps/cpsmain.htm. Accessed: April 8, 2002.

Table 1.7
Uninsured Parents at Home, Texas, 2000

Presence of Parent(s) at Home	Number	Percentage	Percentage within the same category
Both Parents Present	805,523	61.8	17.8
Only Mother Present	326,364	25.1	24.0
Only Father Present	49,984	3.8	24.8
Neither Parent Present	120,867	9.3	58.1
Total	1,302,738	100.0	20.7

Adapted from: U.S. Department of Labor, Bureau of Labor Statistics, 2001 March Current Population Survey. Online. Available: http://www.bls.census.gov/cps/cpsmain.htm. Accessed: April 8, 2002.

Family Income and the Federal Poverty Level (FPL)

The categorization of uninsured individuals according to their family income as a percentage of the federal poverty level makes clear that 41 percent, or about 1.8 million persons, falls right above the 200 percent federal poverty level (FPL). On the contrary, 27 percent, or about 1.2 million, are under the 100 percent FP level and 32 percent (1.4 million) earn a family income that is between 100 and 199 percent of the federal poverty level (see Table 1.8 and Figure 1.3).

Table 1.8
Uninsured Population in Texas by Federal Poverty Levels, 2000

Percent of Poverty Category	Number	Percentage	Percentage within the same category
Under 50	466,670	10.4	38.7
51 to 99	744,113	16.6	39.6
100 to 149	787,617	17.6	37.3
150 to 199	647,229	14.4	29.7
200 to 249	551,402	12.3	26.0
250 or higher	1,289,019	28.7	11.2
Total	4,486,051	100.0	21.4
Under 100	1,210,783	27.0	39.2
100 – 199	1,434,846	32.0	33.4
200 or higher	1,840,422	41.0	13.5
Total	4,486,051	100.0	21.4

Adapted from: U.S. Department of Labor, Bureau of Labor Statistics, *2001 March Current Population Survey*. Online. Available: http://www.bls.census.gov/cps/cpsmain.htm. Accessed: April 8, 2002.

Figure 1.3
Percent Share of Total Population Without Health Insurance in 2000 by Poverty Category (FPL)

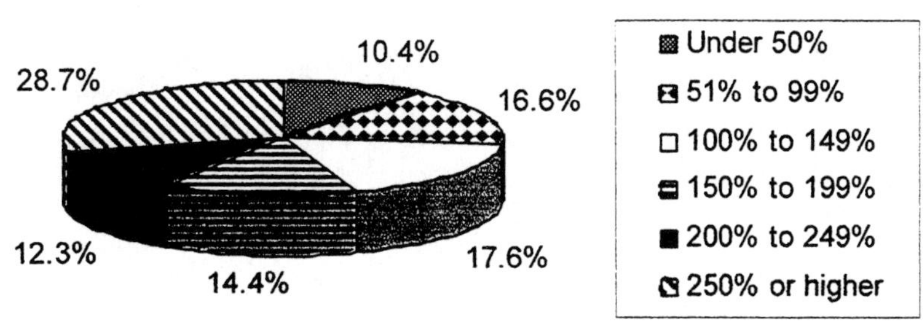

Adapted from: U.S. Department of Labor, Bureau of Labor Statistics, *2001 March Current Population Survey*. Online. Available: http://www.bls.census.gov/cps/cpsmain.htm. Accessed: April 8, 2002.

Among the population with family incomes below 200 percent of the FPL, children deserve special attention since age and family income makes them eligible for public programs provided that they meet other criteria such as citizenship status. Almost 68 percent of the 1.4 million uninsured children under 19 years old are also under the 200 percent federal poverty level that qualifies them for either Medicaid or SCHIP. More precisely, 33 percent of these children population (466,093 persons) live in families with incomes under the 100 percent FPL. About one-third of the uninsured children in Texas live in families that earn between 100 and 199 percent FPL. In contrast, another third of the uninsured children under 19 years old without health insurance are above the 200 percent FPL (see Table 1.9 and Figure 1.4).

Table 1.9
Dependent/Related Uninsured Children Under Age 18 by Percent of Poverty Category, Texas, 2000

Percent of Poverty Category	Number	Percentage	Percentage within the same category
Under 50	123,714	9.5	24.7
51 to 99	290,690	22.3	37.6
100 to 149	260,891	20.0	34.9
150 to 199	207,641	15.9	26.6
200 to 249	147,401	11.3	22.4
250 or Higher	272,400	20.9	9.6
Total	1,302,738	100.0	20.7
Under 100	414,404	31.8	32.5
100 – 199	468,532	36.0	30.6
Under 200	882,936	67.8	31.5
200 or Higher	419,802	32.2	12.0
Total	1,302,738	100.0	20.7

Adapted from: U.S. Department of Labor, Bureau of Labor Statistics, *2001 March Current Population Survey*. Online. Available: http://www.bls.census.gov/cps/cpsmain.htm. Accessed: April 8, 2002.

Figure 1.4
Percentage of Children under Age 19 without Health Insurance, by Federal Poverty Level, 2000

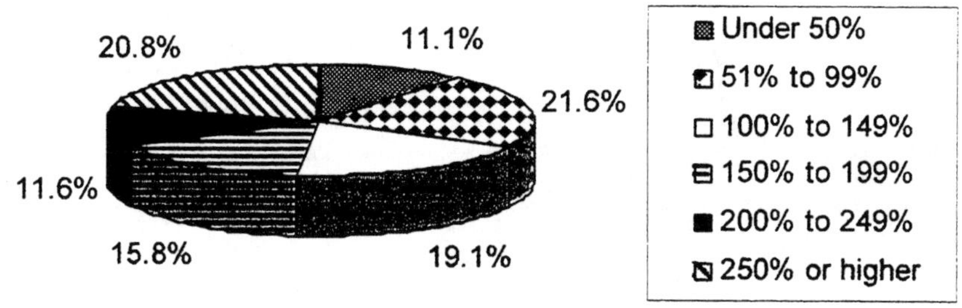

Adapted from: U.S. Department of Labor, Bureau of Labor Statistics, *2001 March Current Population Survey*. Online. Available: http://www.bls.census.gov/cps/cpsmain.htm. Accessed: April 8, 2002.

Employment Status

Out of the 4.5 million Texans lacking health coverage, almost half of them were not retired working adults aged 18 to 64. This number represents 69 percent of the uninsured population aged 18-64. Twenty-four percent of working adults are not in the labor force, and the remaining 7 percent are unemployed individuals. In other words, if dependent children were added, it is evident that the vast majority of the uninsured in Texas are from working families (See Table 1.10 and Figure 1.5).

Table 1.10
Working Uninsured Population in Texas by Labor Force Status, 2000

Labor Force Status	Number	Percentage	Percentage within the same category
Non retired persons 18 and older			
Employed	2,089,800	68.7	21.5
Unemployed	225,793	7.4	49.5
Not in Labor Force	726,241	23.9	30.4
Total	3,041,833	100.0	23.8

Adapted from: U.S. Department of Labor, Bureau of Labor Statistics, *2001 March Current Population Survey*. Online. Available: http://www.bls.census.gov/cps/cpsmain.htm. Accessed: April 8, 2002.

Figure 1.5
Percentage of Total Population Without Health Insurance by Labor Force Status, 2000

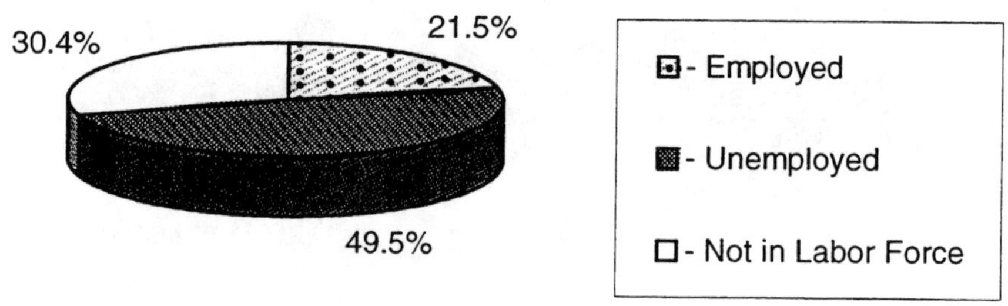

Adapted from: U.S. Department of Labor, Bureau of Labor Statistics, *2001 March Current Population Survey*. Online. Available: http://www.bls.census.gov/cps/cpsmain.htm. Accessed: April 8, 2002.

Firms with fewer than 10 employees provided jobs to one third of the working uninsured, while companies with 1,000 or more employees employed almost another quarter of the same population. Between both extremes, it is found that medium size companies also employed a considerable percentage of workers without health insurance: 13 percent were working for firms with 10 to 24 employees and 14 percent or all working uninsured had jobs in companies with 100 to 499 employees. The percentage noticeably decreases among workers of companies with 100 to 499 employees—8 percent—and even more those working for firms with 500 to 999 employees—5 percent (see Table 1.11 and Figure 1.6

Table 1.11
Uninsured Workers by Number of Employees in Company, Texas, 2000

Company Size (by number of employees company-wide)	Uninsured Workers	Percentage	Percentage within the same category
Fewer than 10 employees	688,227	32.9	36.0
10 through 24 employees	276,448	13.2	33.8
25 through 99 employees	294,640	14.1	25.6
100 through 499 employees	172,424	8.3	17.1
500 through 999 employees	95,227	4.6	20.3
1,000 or more employees	480,206	23.0	11.6
Not reported	82,627	4.0	unknown.
Total	2,089,800	100.0	21.5

Adapted from U.S. Department of Labor, Bureau of Labor Statistics, *2001 March Current Population Survey*. Online. Available: http://www.bls.census.gov/cps/cpsmain.htm. Accessed: April 8, 2002.

Figure 1.6
Percent of People per Category without Health Insurance by Labor Force Status, 2000

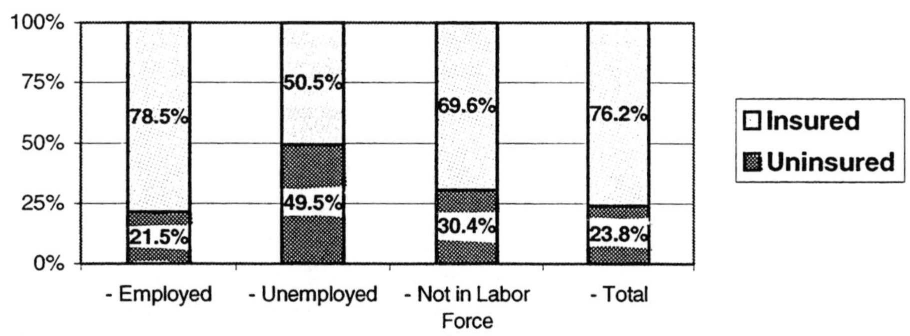

Adapted from: U.S. Department of Labor, Bureau of Labor Statistics, *2001 March Current Population Survey*. Online. Available: http://www.bls.census.gov/cps/cpsmain.htm. Accessed: April 8, 2002.

Note: Data applies to non-retired people aged 18 and older.

Without doubt the likelihood of being uninsured is extremely high among those working in small companies. As shown in Table 1.11 (fourth column), 36 percent of workers of firms with fewer than 10 employees go without health insurance coverage followed by 34 percent among workers of companies with 11 to 25 employees. Smaller percentages are observed for other sectors. Needless to say, firms with less than 10 workers constitute the largest sector in terms of number of economic units.

Citizenship Status

More than three quarters of the uninsured population are U.S. citizens—71.4 percent are native and 4.9 percent are naturalized citizens—and less than a quarter, 23.7 percent, are non U.S. citizens living in the country. One of the results that stands out regarding this issue is the fact that one of every two non-citizens in Texas goes without health coverage (see Table 1.12).

Table 1.12
Uninsured Population By Citizenship Status, Texas, 2000

U.S. Citizen Status	Number	Percentage	Percentage within the same category
U.S. Citizen (Native)	3,213,386	71.4	17.7
U.S. Citizen (Naturalized)	219,393	4.9	26.9
Not a U.S. Citizen	1,067,874	23.7	51.8
Total	4,500,653	100.0	21.4

Adapted from: U.S. Department of Labor, Bureau of Labor Statistics, *2001 March Current Population Survey*. Online. Available: http://www.bls.census.gov/cps/cpsmain.htm. Accessed: April 8, 2002.

Methodology

The data for the demographic profile was prepared by the Research Department of the Texas Health and Human Service Commission and was developed with information that comes from the U.S. Census Bureau's March 2001 Current Population Survey (CPS) for Texas.[5] It should be kept in mind that information is collected from a representative sample of the civilian population and that estimates obtained using surveys are always subject to statistical errors. About 7,700 Texans comprise the sample size for the state.[6] For CPS sampling and non-sampling errors the readers should refer to "Source and Accuracy of the Data for the March 2001."[7] Data from the March 2001 CPS apply to the year 2000.

Some of the advantages of using March CPS data derive from the fact that the survey consists of a large sample of households and that it is designed to produce state-level estimates. Also, the survey is available on a timely and regular basis, plus it provides information for many key socio-demographic subgroups of the population.

In terms of disadvantages associated with the March CPS, it is suspected the survey may overestimate the number of persons that go without insurance during an entire one-year period and that it tends to reflect the health care coverage status of the population as of the month of March only. For example, CPS estimates of the number of persons covered by Medicaid during the previous year are lower than what actual Medicaid program records maintained by the state reflect for the same time period. However, the same CPS estimates come reasonably close in comparison to the actual number of persons that were covered by Medicaid as of the month of March.[8]

Understanding the Differences in Data Sources

There are many different data sources for measuring insured and uninsured rates in the United States. Each data source has specific strengths and weaknesses when using it, along with individual differences among the sources. However, researchers typically rely on one data source with other data sources supplementing this information. It is generally believed that the Current Population Survey (CPS) from the United States Census Bureau provides the most complete and most reliable data. There are three other federal surveys that are major sources of data on the uninsured. These surveys—the Medical Expenditure Panel Survey (MEPS), the National Health Interview Survey (NHIS), and the Survey of Income and Program Participation (SIPP)—can each provide useful estimates of the number of uninsured individuals. Two additional private sector surveys, the National Survey of America's Families (NSAF) and the Community Tracking Study (CTS), also provide uninsured estimates. This report will also rely heavily on the NSAF from the Urban Institute. This note will explain some of the major reasons why estimates of the uninsured from these surveys differ. Depending on the data source researchers use, estimates for the insured and uninsured will differ because of the different methodologies each survey uses.[9]

General Survey Descriptions

Current Population Survey

Conducted by the U.S. Census Bureau, the CPS is a monthly survey designed to collect data on the population's employment status. For questions about health insurance coverage, a March supplement to the CPS asks additional questions covering health insurance topics. The most recent data from the CPS is from March 2001 and provides information about coverage in the prior year (2000). The data is widely employed because they often have the largest household survey sample size of 50,000 households, or about 132,324 individuals. This survey is designed to produce credible state-level estimates. However, as with most surveys, the CPS has been subject to questions regarding over-reporting and under-reporting. Specifically, it is thought that the CPS over-counts the number of individuals who have been uninsured for an entire year, possibly because respondents answer based on current, rather than previous, coverage status. Additionally, the CPS has respondents recall back to a period of 14 months. Most survey methodologists believe that the longer the recall period, the more inaccurate their responses will be.[10]

National Health Interview Survey and Medical Expenditure Panel Survey

Administered by the National Center for Health Statistics (NCHS), since 1956 the NHIS has been a continuous household interview survey of the civilian, non-institutionalized population. The NHIS collects information on public insurance status, type of coverage, measures of health status, health care utilization, and socio-demographic characteristics of members from the sampled households. It provides estimates of the number of persons uninsured at a point-in-time, uninsured for a full-year, and ever uninsured during the year. NHIS also collects data on illnesses, injuries, activity limitations, chronic conditions, health behaviors, and other health topics, which are associated characteristics and risks factors for uninsurance status. Like MEPS and SIPP, the NHIS does not contain a representative sample from each state; however, the sample size is large enough to make state-level estimates of larger states. NHIS surveys 39,832 households or about 103,477 individuals.[11]

The MEPS uses NHIS as a sample frame. MEPS is a two-year panel survey that collects information about health care use and expenditures and is administered by the Agency for Healthcare Research and Quality (AHRQ). MEPS data on an individual's health insurance status are collected several times a year and have the capacity to produce a variety of estimates of health insurance coverage, including point-in-time, monthly, and annual estimates. It is also used as a longitudinal survey, allowing research on health insurance dynamics and changes in coverage. MEPS data can be used to analyze the relationship between insurance status and a variety of individual and household characteristics, including use of and expenditures for health care services. Data on sources of payment for health care are collected and can be used to add greater accuracy and precision to the insurance status estimates. The MEPS sample is smaller than the CPS sample: 9,400 households or about 24,000 individuals. Also, MEPS data cannot be used to make state-level estimates because it does not contain a representative sample from each state.[12]

Survey of Income and Program Participation

SIPP is a 36-month longitudinal panel survey that is also administered by the United States Census Bureau. SIPP collects information on health insurance status, income, labor force activity and federal program participation. It measures the duration of time without health insurance and provides health insurance estimates for various periods, such as point-in-time, monthly, annual, or over the full panel. As part of the core data collected in the SIPP, health insurance data can also be linked to other sections of the survey, such as utilization of health care services, child well being, and disability. The SIPP sample is smaller than the CPS and NHIS samples with about 20,000 households surveyed or about 51,000 individuals. It does not contain a representative sample from each state, and thus cannot be used to make state-level estimates.[13]

National Survey of America's Families

Recently started by the Urban Institute as a part of their Assessing the New Federalism project, the NSAF collects information on the economic, health, and social characteristics of children and non-elderly adults in 13 states. It also provides nationwide estimates by surveying an additional nationally representative sample. The NSAF over-samples the populations below 200 percent of the Federal Poverty Level and provides data on health care access, utilization, health status, and various health insurance estimates. The NSAF also measures if a person was uninsured for a full year, point-in-time, and ever uninsured during the year. However, it is a relatively new survey started in 1997, with data most recently conducted in 1999. It can be used as a source for state-level estimates with 44,000 households or about 100,000 individuals, but only for the 13 states that were surveyed. The 13 states surveyed include Alabama, California, Colorado, Florida, Massachusetts, Michigan, Minnesota, Mississippi, New Jersey, New York, Texas, Washington, and Wisconsin.[14]

Community Tracking Study

Administered by the Center for Studying Health System Change, CTS tracks changes in health systems relating to providers and consumers. One of its components, the household survey, provides information on health insurance status, health care access, utilization, delivery, quality and cost and focuses on 60 selected communities while providing national estimates. Regarding health insurance status, CTS can provide point-in-time and full year uninsured estimates. While the 1996 survey could not determine if individuals had two different types of coverage simultaneously, subsequent surveys will be able to do so. CTS is also a new survey, surveying 33,000 households or about 60,446 individuals. Like most household surveys, the CTS sample does not contain a representative sample from each state and cannot be used to make state-level estimates.[15]

State Comparisons

In comparisons between states, Texas often ranks among the lowest in health related data. According to Table 1.13, Texas' uninsured rate in 2000 was 21.5 percent. For every five individuals in the state, at least one of them did not have some form of insurance. The only other state that had a higher uninsured rate was our neighbor state, New Mexico, with 23.8 percent. Both California and New York, also large states with very large populations, have uninsurance rates lower than Texas, 18.1 percent and 15.2 percent respectively. All these states have large immigrant populations. Texas' higher number of uninsured could be partially accounted for by the unusually large border we share with Mexico. Hispanic rates of uninsurance are extremely high, and Texas has a large Hispanic population due to its proximity to Mexico.

Table 1.13
Percent of People in U.S. without Health Insurance Coverage throughout the Year by State, 2000

State	Without Insurance	State	Without Insurance
Alabama	13.5%	Montana	18.5%
Alaska	19.3%	Nebraska	9.9%
Arizona	16.1%	Nevada	15.6%
Arkansas	13.9%	New Hampshire	6.9%
California	18.1%	New Jersey	12.6%
Colorado	13.3%	New Mexico	23.8%
Connecticut	7.9%	New York	15.2%
Delaware	10.4%	North Carolina	13.0%
District of Columbia	14.4%	North Dakota	11.4%
Florida	17.3%	Ohio	10.9%
Georgia	14.6%	Oklahoma	19.3%
Hawaii	10.1%	Oregon	13.7%
Idaho	15.6%	Pennsylvania	7.6%
Illinois	13.5%	Rhode Island	5.9%
Indiana	12.0%	South Carolina	11.9%
Iowa	8.7%	South Dakota	11.8%
Kansas	11.5%	Tennessee	10.3%
Kentucky	12.9%	Texas	21.5%
Louisiana	19.1%	Utah	13.4%
Maine	11.5%	Vermont	10.6%
Maryland	9.8%	Virginia	12.7%
Massachusetts	9.5%	Washington	13.3%
Michigan	9.9%	West Virginia	14.3%
Minnesota	9.0%	Wisconsin	7.1%
Mississippi	13.1%	Wyoming	14.3%
Missouri	10.6%	United States	14.0%

Adapted from: U.S. Department of Labor, Bureau of Labor Statistics, *2001 March Current Population Survey*. Online. Available: http://www.census.gov/hhes/hlthins/hlthin00/hi00td.html. Accessed: April 8, 2002.

In Table 1.14, Texas falls just below the average of all 50 states, and the District of Columbia, in the percentage of people covered by Medicaid, at 11.8 percent. Again, comparing Texas to California and New York, Texas has a lower percentage of people receiving Medicaid coverage. One-fifth of all Californians receive Medicaid, 21.7 percent while 16.9 percent of New Yorkers received coverage under Medicaid. And, Texas has a higher percent of its population living in poverty.

Table 1.14
U.S. Medicaid Recipients as a Percentage of the Population by State, 1998

State	Medicaid Recipients		State	Medicaid Recipients
Alabama	12.1%		Montana	11.5%
Alaska	12.1%		Nebraska	12.7%
Arizona	10.9%		Nevada	7.3%
Arkansas	16.7%		New Hampshire	7.9%
California	21.7%		New Jersey	10.0%
Colorado	8.7%		New Mexico	19.0%
Connecticut	11.6%		New York	16.9%
Delaware	13.6%		North Carolina	15.5%
District of Columbia	31.9%		North Dakota	9.8%
Florida	12.8%		Ohio	11.5%
Georgia	16.0%		Oklahoma	10.3%
Hawaii	15.5%		Oregon	15.6%
Idaho	10.0%		Pennsylvania	12.7%
Illinois	11.3%		Rhode Island	15.5%
Indiana	10.3%		South Carolina	15.5%
Iowa	11.0%		South Dakota	12.3%
Kansas	9.2%		Tennessee	33.9%
Kentucky	16.4%		Texas	11.8%
Louisiana	16.5%		Utah	10.3%
Maine	13.7%		Vermont	21.0%
Maryland	10.9%		Virginia	9.6%
Massachusetts	14.8%		Washington	24.8%
Michigan	13.9%		West Virginia	18.9%
Minnesota	11.4%		Wisconsin	9.9%
Mississippi	17.7%		Wyoming	9.6%
Missouri	13.5%		United States	15.0%

Adapted from: Health Care Financing Administration, *Medicaid Financial Statistics Tables, HCFA-64 Report.* Online. Available: http://www.hcfa.gov/medicaid/m64.htm. Accessed: May 2, 2002.

Texas pays out about $4,129 to each Medicaid recipient. In Table 1.15, this is slightly above the United States average of $4,040. As Texas is one of the largest states in the Union, Texas has the third highest number of Medicaid recipients, behind California and New York. California has three times the number of Medicaid recipients as Texas and about twice as many as New York. Also, while California has the largest number of recipients, it also has the lowest payout to those recipients, $2,293. New York on the other hand has a large number of Medicaid recipients it also has the highest payouts to recipients, $7,980. Although Texas has a higher percentage of children living in poverty it covers a smaller percentage of them and this population is cheaper to cover per capita.

Table 1.15
Payments per Medicaid Recipient by State, 1998

State	Recipients	Total Payments	Payments Per Recipient
Alabama	527,078	$2,201,307,097	$4,176
Alaska	74,508	$364,110,087	$4,887
Arizona	507,668	$1,740,017,249	$3,427
Arkansas	424,727	$1,313,630,245	$3,093
California	7,082,175	$16,240,099,854	$2,293
Colorado	344,916	$1,523,356,381	$4,417
Connecticut	381,208	$2,932,104,706	$7,692
Delaware	101,436	$409,213,692	$4,034
District of Columbia	166,146	$796,084,288	$4,791
Florida	1,904,591	$6,447,889,401	$3,385
Georgia	1,221,978	$3,584,015,676	$2,933
Hawaii	184,614	$628,742,323	$3,406
Idaho	123,176	$423,261,391	$3,436
Illinois	1,363,856	$6,503,829,004	$4,769
Indiana	607,293	$2,493,114,385	$4,105
Iowa	314,936	$1,262,327,643	$4,008
Kansas	241,933	$1,028,739,139	$4,252
Kentucky	644,482	$2,571,547,988	$3,990
Louisiana	720,615	$3,055,407,383	$4,240
Maine	170,456	$1,090,325,858	$6,397
Maryland	561,085	$2,706,411,626	$4,824
Massachusetts	908,238	$5,509,187,324	$6,066
Michigan	1,362,890	$5,560,326,710	$4,080
Minnesota	538,413	$2,746,987,575	$5,102
Mississippi	485,767	$1,702,265,458	$3,504
Missouri	734,015	$3,142,586,502	$4,281
Montana	100,760	$392,064,609	$3,891
Nebraska	211,188	$731,656,067	$3,464
Nevada	128,144	$489,276,626	$3,818
New Hampshire	93,970	$731,879,670	$7,788
New Jersey	813,251	$5,478,127,337	$6,736
New Mexico	329,418	$945,547,063	$2,870
New York	3,073,241	$24,525,116,698	$7,980
North Carolina	1,167,988	$4,529,992,284	$3,878
North Dakota	62,280	$331,970,747	$5,330
Ohio	1,290,776	$6,443,156,403	$4,992
Oklahoma	342,475	$1,195,881,195	$3,492
Oregon	511,171	$1,544,061,944	$3,021
Pennsylvania	1,523,120	$8,075,706,681	$5,302
Rhode Island	153,130	$917,489,179	$5,992
South Carolina	594,962	$2,152,056,132	$3,617
South Dakota	89,537	$331,629,892	$3,704
Tennessee	1,843,661	$3,434,971,957	$1,863
Texas	2,324,810	$9,600,126,934	$4,129
Utah	215,801	$626,662,383	$2,904
Vermont	123,992	$358,490,340	$2,891
Virginia	653,236	$2,274,509,097	$3,482
Washington	1,413,208	$3,197,051,126	$2,262
West Virginia	342,668	$1,193,977,808	$3,484
Wisconsin	518,595	$2,573,586,437	$4,963
Wyoming	46,121	$194,261,299	$4,212
United States	39,665,703	$160,246,138,893	$4,040

Adapted from: Health Care Financing Administration, *Medicaid Program Statistics, HCFA-2082 Report* (1999). Online. Available: http://www.hcfa.gov/medicaid/mstats.htm. Accessed: May 2, 2002; and Health Care Financing Administration, *Medicaid Financial Statistics Tables, HCFA-64 Report* (1999). Online. Available: http://www.hcfa.gov/medicaid/m64.htm. Accessed: May 2, 2002.

Likewise, New York has the highest total cost of long term care expenditures (Table 1.16), over three times that of Texas. Texas spends about two billion in long term care while New York spends over seven billion dollars. Pennsylvania spends the second largest amount on long term care with over three billion dollars. Due to Texas' large population size, it would correspond that they spend a larger amount on long-term care.

Table 1.16
Long Term Care Expenditures by State, 1997

State	Total		State	Total
Alabama	$581,877,726		Montana	$115,411,333
Alaska	$47,632,334		Nebraska	$259,420,536
Arizona	$16,479,936		Nevada	$90,531,782
Arkansas	$409,913,770		New Hampshire	$206,220,161
California	$2,470,664,034		New Jersey	$1,539,368,116
Colorado	$346,534,908		New Mexico	$154,720,595
Connecticut	$1,046,534,125		New York	$7,354,424,450
Delaware	$108,572,867		North Carolina	$1,142,940,368
District of Columbia	$241,143,862		North Dakota	$153,736,155
Florida	$1,512,980,018		Ohio	$2,209,252,784
Georgia	$742,367,719		Oklahoma	$390,896,390
Hawaii	$148,032,014		Oregon	$244,429,900
Idaho	$135,504,556		Pennsylvania	$3,397,088,197
Illinois	$1,906,315,361		Rhode Island	$228,931,080
Indiana	$976,290,749		South Carolina	$458,398,633
Iowa	$467,334,434		South Dakota	$119,568,187
Kansas	$321,704,739		Tennessee	$873,372,159
Kentucky	$535,819,698		Texas	$1,986,826,184
Louisiana	$811,048,638		Utah	$131,926,059
Maine	$247,639,596		Vermont	$71,998,564
Maryland	$585,928,255		Virginia	$559,492,687
Massachusetts	$1,567,436,789		Washington	$650,566,739
Michigan	$1,331,831,671		West Virginia	$293,370,041
Minnesota	$1,096,876,255		Wisconsin	$962,728,830
Mississippi	$428,600,974		Wyoming	$65,048,321
Missouri	$783,157,471		United States	$42,528,890,750

Adapted from: Health Care Financing Administration, *Medicaid Financial Statistics Tables, HCFA-64 Report* (1999). Online. Available: http://www.hcfa.gov/medicaid/m64.htm. Accessed: May 2, 2002.

According to NSAF's collection of data from the 13 states it focuses on, there are about 162.8 million adults living in the United States and 17 percent of these people are uninsured. That is close to 28 million uninsured adults. Poverty can be an indicator of uninsurance. There are more people that are uninsured at lower Federal Poverty Levels (FPL). There are 41.5 percent of the people below 100 percent FPL that are uninsured, while only 6.2 percent of people above 300 percent FPL are uninsured. Likewise, adults with and without children follow the same pattern, higher percentages of uninsured the lower ones FPL.

People at higher Federal Poverty Levels have a higher percentage of employer-sponsored insurance, but rates for private insurance are generally equalized across incomes. Unsurprisingly, there are a greater number of lower FPL individuals receiving Medicaid.

Table 1.17
Nonelderly Adult Health Insurance Coverage, by Income and Family Type, 1999

	Total (millions)	Employer-Provided	Medicaid	Other Private	Other Public	Uninsured
All Adults	162.8	69.1%	5.1%	5.8%	3.1%	17.0%
Below 100% FPL	20.3	21.6%	26.0%	7.4%	3.6%	41.5%
100-199% FPL	27.4	46.9%	7.1%	7.1%	5.5%	33.5%
200-299% FPL	27.8	71.3%	2.4%	5.4%	4.1%	16.9%
≥300% FPL	87.3	86.3%	0.4%	5.1%	1.9%	6.2%
Adults with Children	63.8	70.2%	7.2%	3.5%	2.5%	16.5%
Below 100% FPL	9.4	17.6%	34.9%	3.0%	2.5%	42.0%
100-199% FPL	13.2	53.6%	7.4%	4.1%	4.0%	31.0%
200-299% FPL	12.6	79.5%	2.0%	3.4%	3.4%	11.8%
300% of FPL above	28.6	91.1%	0.4%	3.5%	1.5%	3.5%
Adults without Children	99.1	68.3%	3.7%	7.2%	3.5%	17.3%
Below 100% FPL	10.9	25.1%	18.3%	11.1%	4.6%	41.0%
100-199% FPL	14.2	40.7%	6.8%	9.9%	6.8%	35.8%
200-299% FPL	15.2	64.4%	2.7%	7.0%	4.7%	21.2%
>300% FPL	58.8	84.0%	0.4%	5.9%	2.2%	7.5%

Adapted from: Urban Institute, *1997 National Survey of American's Families*. Online. Available: http://newfederalism.urban.org/html/series_b/b14/b14.html. Accessed: January 21, 2002.

In **Error! Reference source not found.**, of the adults below 200 percent FPL, they account for 64 percent of the uninsured in the United States. While over half of all Hispanics are uninsured, they only account for less than a third of the low-income uninsured. White, non-Hispanics account for half of the total low-income uninsured and a third of the low-income uninsured as a percentage of all adult uninsured.

Table 1.18
Demographic Characteristics of Low-Income (<200% FPL) Uninsured Adults, 1997

	Number (millions)	**Uninsurance Rate**	**Percent of Low-Income Uninsured**	**Low-Income Uninsured Adults as a Percentage of All Uinsured Adults**
All	17.6	37%	100%	64%
Age				
18-34 (Male)	4.9	47%	28%	18%
18-34 (Female)	4.7	38%	27%	17%
35-54	6.4	35%	36%	23%
55-64	1.5	23%	8%	5%
Race/Ethnicity				
White Non-Hispanic	8.7	31%	50%	31%
Black Non-Hispanic	2.8	34%	16%	10%
Other Non-Hispanic	1	43%	6%	4%
Hispanic	5.1	53%	29%	19%
Family Structure				
Married with Children	5.3	37%	30%	19%
Married without Children	2.6	34%	15%	9%
Single with Children	2.7	33%	15%	10%
Single without Children	7.0	40%	40%	25%
Work Status				
Two or More Full-Time Workers	2.5	37%	14%	9%
One Full-Time Worker	9.0	39%	51%	32%
Part-Time Worker	2.4	42%	13%	8%
No Workers	3.7	30%	21%	13%
Health Status				
Excellent/Very Good	7.7	32%	44%	28%
Good	5.4	41%	31%	19%
Fair/Poor	4.5	41%	26%	16%
Limiting Condition	3.2	30%	18%	11%

Adapted from: Urban Institute, *1997 National Survey of American's Families*. Online. Available: http://newfederalism.urban.org/html/series_b/b14/b14.html. Accessed: January 21, 2002.

Summary

The following are the most remarkable demographic characteristics of the uninsured population in Texas, according to analysis drawn from the 2001 March Current Population Survey on data for the year 2000. Younger adults between 18-34 are more likely to lack health insurance; more than a third of the population that fall into this age group is uninsured. Education is also associated with a lower level of coverage; 70 percent of all uninsured Texan over 18 years of age have not attained a college education or higher. Employed adults account for almost three quarters of the uninsured population, more than half of them working for either small firms (less than 10 employees) or large firms (more than 500 employees). Forty percent of uninsured Texans fall under the 100 percent federal poverty level, confirming that lower levels of income are more likely associated with a lack of health insurance. Minorities run at a higher risk of lacking any type of health insurance, especially Hispanics; 58 percent of the uninsured population in Texas is of Hispanic origin.

While Texans have many things to be proud of, health insurance is not one of them—it has previously been shown that Texas falls short when compared to other states in the country. Texas has a higher percentage of people who are uninsured; both New York and California, similar in size and population, have 3 to 6 percent fewer people who lack health insurance. Again, of those receiving Medicaid, Texas ranks lower than both New York and California, but falls in the middle when compared to all 50 states. While health issues and the problems that are associated with them will always be a problem for the United States, research and critical analysis should be continued in order for us to reach a more stable and perfected form of health care.

Notes

[1] U.S. Department of Labor, Bureau of Labor Statistics, *2001 March Current Population Survey.* Online. Available: http://www.bls.census.gov/cps/cpsmain.htm. Accessed: April 8, 2002.

[2] Texas Department of Human Services, *Reference Guide 2000.* Online. Available: http://www.dhs.state.tx.us/publications/refguide/2000/StateRankings.html. Accessed: April 10, 2002.

[3] U.S. Census Bureau, *United States Census 2000.* Online. Available: http://www.census.gov/main/www/cen2000.html. Accessed: April 8, 2002.

[4] U.S. Department of Labor, Bureau of Labor Statistics, *2001 March Current Population Survey.* Online. Available: http://www.bls.census.gov/cps/cpsmain.htm. Accessed: April 8, 2002.

[5] Ibid.

[6] Texas Health and Human Service Commission, *Demographic Profile of Texans Without Health Insurance Coverage* (2000) Online. Available: http://www.hhsc.state.tx.us/budget/cons_bud/dssi/brt/brtchchap3.pdf. Assessed: January 05, 2002.

[7] U.S. Department of Labor, Bureau of Labor Statistics, *Annual Demographic Survey, March Supplement, Source and Accuracy of the Data for the March 2001.* Online. Available: http://www.bls.census.gov/cps/ads/2001/ssrcacc.htm#accuracy. Accessed: February 10, 2002.

[8] Texas Health and Human Service Commission, *Demographic Profile of Texans Without Health Insurance Coverage* (March 2000). Online. Available: http://www.hhsc.state.tx.us/budget/cons_bud/dssi/brt/brtchchap3.pdf. Assessed: January 05, 2002.

[9] Department of Health and Human Services, Office of the Assistant Secretary for Planning and Evaluation, *Understanding Estimates of the Uninsured: Putting the Differences in Context* (January 2001). Online. Available: http://aspe.hhs.gov/health/reports/hiestimates.htm#7 Accessed: January 28, 2002.

[10] U.S. Department of Labor, Bureau of Labor Statistics, *Current Population Survey.* Online. Available. http://www.bls.census.gov/cps/cpsmain.htm. Accessed: April 24, 2002.

[11] Centers for Disease Control and Prevention, National Center for Health Statistics, *National Health Interview Survey.* Online. Available. http://www.cdc.gov/nchs/nhis.htm. Accessed: April 24, 2002.

[12] U.S. Department of Health and Human Services, Agency for Healthcare Research and Quality, *Medical Expenditure Panel Survey.* Online. Available: http://www.meps.ahrq.gov/. Accessed: April 24, 2002.

[13] U.S. Census Bureau, *Survey of Income and Program Participation*. Online. Available: http://www.bls.census.gov/sipp. Accessed: May 6, 2002.

[14] Urban Institute, *National Survey of America's Families*. Online. Available: http://www.urban.org/ Content/Research/NewFederalism/NSAF/Overview/NSAFOverview.htm. Accessed: April 24, 2002.

[15] Center for Studying Health System Change, *Community Tracking Survey*. Online. Available: http://www.hschange.com/index.cgi?data=01. Accessed: April 24, 2002.

Chapter 2. Expansion Through Waivers

by Leah Kegler

The Development of Medicaid and SCHIP

> The passage of Title XIX marks the beginning of a new era in medical care for low-income families. The potential of this new title can hardly be overestimated, as its ultimate goal is the assurance of complete, continuous, family-centered medical care of high quality to persons who are unable to pay for it themselves. The law aims to much higher than the mere paying of medical bills, and States, in order to achieve its high purpose, will need to assume responsibility for planning and establishing systems of high quality medical care, comprehensive in scope and wide in coverage.[1]

This statement made 35 years ago by The Bureau of Family Services proclaims the untapped power of the Medicaid program. Medicaid is administered through individual state programs; although there are federal guidelines, the programs and their implementation are left largely up to the states. Today in 2002, this quotation still rings true. As the nation enters a period of economic downturn, the potential of full utilization of Medicaid will become essential. This quote refers to the need of family-centered medical care in 1966, and the United States continues to work for a Medicaid system that offers services to low-income families in 2002. If Medicaid is to be truly more than the mere paying of medical bills for the states, federal and state governments must develop creative ways to tap the potential power of this large and complicated state and federal program, which can still potentially help so many Americans obtain the health care they need.

This paper will generally explain the federal and state relationships that occur in the Medicaid Program and the State Children's Health Insurance Program (SCHIP). It will also highlight the implementation of these programs in Texas. One of the recent initiatives in several states has been the expansion of health insurance to low-income adults. This paper will broadly address possible options for expansion to this population and relate these to options available to the state of Texas. Finally, a set of policy prescriptions detailing the cost of expansion will be presented which focus on publicly funded health care options in Texas.

The Federal Aspects of Medicaid

Medicaid is a jointly administered state and federal entitlement program that provides health insurance for eligible low-income children, pregnant women, disabled individuals, and elderly individuals. The program, which was part of President Lyndon Baines Johnson's Great Society agenda, was established by Congress under Title XIX of the Social Security Act of 1965. Every state offers Medicaid benefits, but variations exist between every state's Medicaid programs. Variations in the programs exist on many levels including but not limited to benefits, eligible populations, reimbursement policy, and program structure.

In Federal Fiscal Year (FFY) 2000, the federal and state governments spent over 202 billion dollars on the Medicaid program to serve more than 42 million low-income individuals in the United States.[2] States are allowed to administer and tailor their state Medicaid program within federal guidelines. In participating in Medicaid, each agrees at least to cover a set of mandatory beneficiaries with a package of specified services set by the federal government. Beyond the set federal minimums states have the flexibility to cover other optional groups and cover optional services for both the mandatory and optional populations. And, even within the mandated benefits, states have the authority to limit the extent of coverage in a variety of ways. States are also allowed to cover additional populations and services through the use of Section 1115 waivers of the Social Security Act. As a result of this flexibility, each of the 56 Medicaid programs in the United States (including Washington, D.C., and the five U.S. territories) have a different approach toward their State's Medicaid Program. Table 2.1 lists the federal Mandatory, Optional and Expansion Medicaid Populations. Table 2.2 lists the federal Mandatory and Optional Medicaid Services.

Table 2.1
Federal Medicaid Populations: Mandatory, Optional and Expansion

Federally Mandated Medicaid Eligible Populations	Optional Medicaid Eligible Populations	Populations covered under Expansion through 1115 waivers
Section 1931 Recipients: Low-income families with children who meet that state's AFDC plan requirements as of July 16, 1996*	Children with incomes and/or assets greater than federal mandatory minimum	Childless adults (1115 waiver)
	Children under age 21 who meet income and resource requirements for AFDC, but who are otherwise ineligible	Individuals diagnosed with HIV/AIDS
Supplemental Security Income (SSI) Recipients	Adults in families with children with incomes and/or assets greater than Section 1931 minimums	
Infants born to Medicaid-eligible pregnant women	Recipients of State Supplemental Payments	
	Disabled and elderly individuals with incomes greater than SSI eligibility levels	
Children under age 6 and pregnant women whose family income is less than 133% of the FPL	Disabled and elderly individuals who qualify through home and community-based service	
Children under age 19 whose family income is less than 100% of the FPL	Elderly nursing home residents with incomes and resources below specified limits	
Recipients of Adoption Assistance and Foster Care under Title IV-E of the Social Security Act	TB-infected persons who would be financially eligible for Medicaid at the SSI level	
	Low-income, uninsured women screened and diagnosed with through a Centers for Disease Control Early Detection Program and in need of treatment for breast or cervical cancer	
	Beneficiary groups of Ticket to Work and Work Incentives Improvement of 1999	
	Medically needy: 133 1/3% of the 1996 AFDC level; this benefit covers those who spend-down a specified level of income	

Adapted from: Centers for Medicare and Medicaid Services, *Medicaid Eligibility.* Online. Available at http://hcfa.hhs.gov/medicaid/meligib.htm. Accessed: September 5, 2001; and John Holahan, *Restructuring Medicaid Financing: Implications of the NGA Proposal* (Washington, D.C.: The Kaiser Family Foundation, 2001), p. 3.

* AFDC is the abbreviation used for the welfare program Aid to Families with Dependent Children. The program was replaced with Temporary Aid to Needy Families (TANF) in 1996.

Table 2.2
Federal Medicaid Benefits: Mandatory and Optional

Federally Mandated Medicaid Services	Optional Medicaid Service
Early periodic screening, diagnosis and treatment for those under 21 (EPSDT)	Prescription drugs
Physician services	Podiatrist services
Laboratory and x-ray services	Optometrist services
Federally qualified health center services	Chiropractor services
Family planning services and supplies	Psychologist services
Inpatient and outpatient hospital services	Private duty nursing
Rural health clinic services	Nurse anesthetist services
Nurse midwife services	Medical social worker services
Certified nurse practitioner services	Transportation services
Nursing facility care	Rehabilitation services
Home health care services (for individuals entitled to nursing facility care)	Dental services
	Case management services
	Physical therapy
	Speech, hearing, and language disorder therapy
	Emergency hospital services
	Diagnostic services
	Screening services
	Occupational therapy
	Hospice care services
	Preventative services
	Personal care services
	Respiratory care services
	TB-related services
	Other clinical services
	Medical equipment (prosthetic devices, eyeglasses, dentures)
	Intermediate care facility services for the mentally retarded
	Nursing facility services for under age 21
	Inpatient hospital services for 65+ or seniors in institutions
	Inpatient psychiatric for services under age 21
	Nursing facility services for 65+ or seniors in institution for mental disease
	Christian Science sanitoriums
	Christian Science

Adapted from: The Kaiser Commission on Medicaid and the Uninsured, *Medicaid "Mandatory" and "Optional" Eligibility and Benefits* (Washington, D.C.: June 2001), p. 8; and Families USA, *The Current Medicaid Federal-State Partnership: Already a Good Deal for the States* (Washington, D.C., August 2001), pp. 4-9.

The History of Medicaid in Texas

The federal approach to Medicaid does not tell the entire story of Medicaid in Texas. It has been historically conservative in its approach to social policy including its Medicaid program. Thus, the evolution of the Texas Medicaid program has been molded by the state political philosophy and federal initiatives.

The Administration of Medicaid in Texas

The Texas Health and Human Services Commission (HHSC) is the single state agency administering Medicaid from the perspective of the federal government. However, the Texas Department of Human Services, Texas Department of Health, Texas Department of Mental Health and Mental Retardation, and Texas Department of Protective and Regulatory Services provide key administrative services to specific populations. Other state agencies that receive Medicaid funding include Texas Commission for the Blind, Interagency Council on Childhood Intervention, Texas School for the Blind, Texas School for the Deaf, Texas Rehabilitation Commission, and the Texas Commission on Alcohol and Drug Abuse. The Texas Attorney General's Medicaid Fraud and Control Unit is responsible for fraud investigation and enforcement activities. In addition, the federal government provides oversight through the Centers for Medicare and Medicaid Services (CMS) of the U.S. Department of Health and Human Services.[3]

Early Medicaid Expansion

The Texas Medicaid Program was implemented in 1967. Medicaid has since evolved from programs narrowly targeted at those eligible for federal/state programs providing matches for cash assistance, known at that time as Aid to Families with Dependent Children (AFDC) and Aid to the Aged, Blind and Disabled (AABD), into a large and rather complex program. In 1972, federal law established the Supplemental Security Income (SSI) program. This program formalized cash assistance to the elderly and disabled poor. Health care coverage to this population was mandatory for states with established Medicaid programs.[4]

The Federal Medicaid Mandates

The 1980s were a turbulent era for the Medicaid program. Despite attempts at cutbacks by the Reagan Administration, several federal mandates passed in the 1980s required certain individuals not on AFDC or SSI to be eligible for Medicaid and increased the scope of the services offered by Medicaid. Beginning with the Deficit Reduction Act of 1984, a series of federal mandates and optional expansions were put into place to protect AFDC families and expand state Medicaid programs. The Consolidated Omnibus Budget Reconciliation Act of 1985, the Omnibus Budget Reconciliation Act (OBRA) of 1986 and OBRA 1987 created new optional categories for children and pregnant women for states to add to their Medicaid programs. Finally, through the Medicare Catastrophic Coverage Act of 1988 (MCCA), the Family Support Act of 1988, OBRA 1989, OBRA 1990, and OBRA 1993 many of the newly created optional categories were mandated. States were required to cover children under age six in families with incomes of less than

133 percent of the federal poverty level (FPL) and children born after September 30, 1983, up to 100 percent of poverty.[5] This meant that as of October 1, 2001, states were mandated to cover all children under 100 percent of the FPL.[6] And, all children covered by Medicaid were eligible for any service provided to children in the Medicaid program, in any state. (Other mandates were also added to the Medicaid Program addressing the needs of disabled, SSI eligibles, elderly, and nursing home populations.)

In short, these expansions covered uninsured low-income pregnant women and their newborn infants, children in low-income families not receiving cash assistance, and low-income disabled poor and elderly with the need for more comprehensive health care coverage. These mandates also opened up a wide range of services to children on Medicaid. As a result, the number of individuals eligible and costs for the Medicaid program expanded greatly.

Some states, including fiscally conservative states such as Texas, also took advantage of the early optional expansions, which allowed the states to cover pregnant women and children over 133 percent of the federal poverty level. Texas covers pregnant women and infants under age one up to 185 percent of the FPL, an option made available through OBRA 1987. Other states utilized Section 1902(r)(2) of the Social Security Act, which allows states to cover children and pregnant women with incomes above the mandated and optional levels through income disregards.

Overall, this series of Medicaid mandates caused individual state Medicaid programs to become more uniform across the nation by linking the Medicaid program for children and pregnant women to the federal poverty guidelines rather than AFDC eligibility levels, which differed across the states. Budget constraints in richer states forced states to shrink their Medicaid program, while those in poor states expanded their program, because of the mandates and the incentive to draw down more Medicaid dollars through the higher federal match entitled to poorer states for the reimbursement of Medicaid services. Further, wealthier states had more optional benefits to cut than those poorer states like Texas that traditionally offered less rich Medicaid benefits.

Disproportionate Share Hospital Funds

Simultaneous with the creation of the Medicaid mandates, the Disproportionate Share Hospital (DSH) funds program was created through the Omnibus Budget Reconciliation Act of 1981 to reimburse hospitals that serve a disproportionate number of Medicaid and uninsured patients. Through the federal-state matching program, DSH became increasingly popular with states searching for ways to fund the federal mandates. In fact, between 1989 and 1992 the DSH program grew from $600 million to $17 billion. This tremendous growth was due to three primary reasons: increased state participation in the program, the swelling of the Medicaid rolls as a result of the declining economy and federal mandates, and general health care inflation.[7]

By 1992, the DSH program accounted for 15 percent of total Medicaid spending. Congress was concerned about this unrestrained growth and in 1991 established an aggregate national limit on DSH of 12 percent of total Medicaid spending and established DSH capitations for each state.[8] With the third largest DSH program in the country,

Texas has taken full advantage of this program, drawing down 100 percent of available federal matching funds. Despite the forced decline in federal DSH funds over the last few years, the cap on federal DSH funds for Texas for FFY 2001 and FFY 2002 is $765 million.[9]

Attempting a Section 1115 Waiver in Texas

As a direct result of the federal mandates, caseload expenditures in Texas increased from $6.6 billion in the 1990-91 biennium to $14.9 billion in the 1994-95 biennium. Sensing a financial crisis, Lieutenant Governor Bob Bullock issued an interim charge to Chairwoman Judith Zaffirini and the Senate Health and Human Services Committee to review the possible options and make recommendations to accomplish the goal of significant savings in state fiscal years 1996 and 1997.[10]

As a result of this charge, the Texas State Medicaid Office and the Texas Health and Human Services Commission worked together to study the ballooning Medicaid budget and produced a set of findings entitled *Prescription for Change*, which was published in November of 1994. This document broadly described the difficulties facing Texas Medicaid and options to address these issues.

From this series of options, the state decided to submit a research and demonstration waiver proposal to the Secretary of DHHS. This type of proposal is known as a Section 1115 waiver, as it asks the secretary to waive federal rules pertaining to Medicaid for a particular state. Texas submitted a Section 1115 waiver that proposed the following reforms:[11]

- Expand Medicaid coverage and reduce the rate of uninsurance by combining state and local dollars.
- Improve access to primary care providers through managed care.
- Through managed care, control costs by focusing on prevention and reducing inappropriate utilization of costly services.
- Maximize limited resources to meet Texan's health care needs through coordination of state and local efforts.
- Control rising health care and insurance costs.

Specifically, this waiver would have required certain local public entities (hospital districts in large urban areas, medical schools, and state teaching hospitals) to "give" the state the public funds they spend on indigent health care in order for the state to obtain a federal Medicaid match for these funds. In return, these local public entities would receive, following the matching process, at least as much money as they originally made available to the state. County Indigent Health Care Programs also would have had the option to put up the public funds they spend on indigent health care. This program also encouraged individual counties and hospital districts that provide matching resources to create a nonprofit entity called an intergovernmental initiative (IGI) to design and administer a managed care program in their service area. The State would provide managed care in areas of the state that did not create an IGI.[12]

This waiver would have not only changed the funding structure of Medicaid in Texas, but it would have also expanded eligibility in the program to the following groups:[13]

- Parents of children with income up to 45 percent of the FPL;
- Children age 6 and older with family incomes below 133 percent of the FPL;
- Single Adults without children with income up to 45 percent of the FPL; and
- Childless couples with family income up to 45 percent of the FPL.

The proposal would have helped to insure a substantial number of Texans and brought together hospital districts, public hospitals and counties to fund the expansion. It also had the potential to take some of the pressure off the Texas health care safety net, which continues to struggle to meet the needs of many different populations in Texas.

For a variety of reasons, political and structural, this waiver was not approved by DHHS. Questions posed by the federal government related to the waiver proposal were never addressed by the state.[14] Although a second less robust waiver was submitted in October 1996, this waiver, which focused on expanded health care to children through managed care, was later abandoned because of the Balanced Budget Act (BBA) of 1997 and the creation of the State Children's Health Insurance Program (SCHIP), which will be discussed in further detail in subsequent sections of this paper. Texas was left to continue with its Medicaid structure, highly dependent on a patchwork local safety net system for many low-income individuals in the state.

Welfare Reform

In 1996, major welfare reform legislation was passed at the federal level. The AFDC program was eliminated, and a new program called Temporary Assistance to Needy Families (TANF) was created. At this point, Medicaid and welfare became delinked. This means that those eligible for Medicaid no longer have to be eligible or receiving cash assistance to receive Medicaid services although those who are receiving TANF in Texas are automatically eligible for Medicaid (federal law provides that all people on SSI are automatically eligible for Medicaid). In Texas, the changes to the welfare system decreased the number of individuals/families who qualified for cash assistance. As an unintended result, the number of individuals in the Medicaid program decreased, because eligible recipients were not fully aware that they could still receive Medicaid benefits even if they were not participating in the TANF program.

Another reason for the decrease in the number of Medicaid enrollees can possibly be attributed to the changes that welfare reform had upon immigrant populations. The Personal Responsibility and Work Opportunity Reconciliation Act (PRWORA), the federal welfare reform act of 1996, gave states the option to decide whether or not to continue providing Medicaid to most legal immigrants. However, most immigrants entering the United States after August 22, 1996, would be subject to a five-year "bar" period, during which no federal Medicaid funds could be used for their care. Every state but Wyoming decided to continue treating so-called "qualified aliens" who were in the

U.S. prior to August 22, 1996, the same as U.S. citizens for purposes of Medicaid eligibility.

As originally drafted, PRWORA would have revoked SSI coverage of legal immigrants who were in the U.S. before the bill was signed; however, the BBA of 1997 restored SSI benefits for legal immigrants who arrived in the United States prior to August 22, 1996. Those arriving after this date are still banned from the SSI program, and because Texas limits Medicaid coverage of elderly and disabled largely to SSI beneficiaries, post-1996 entrants qualifying for Medicaid will be fewer in number. In July of 1996, about 101,000 out of two million Texas Medicaid enrollees were recorded as legal immigrants, and sixty percent of these were SSI beneficiaries. (Later analysis by the Texas Department of Human Services revealed that many of these enrollees had in fact become U.S. citizens, so the actual number of legal immigrants was somewhat lower.) These policy changes especially affect Texas with its large Hispanic population. The primary immigration-related impact on Texas Medicaid enrollment resulted not from actual changes in eligibility, but from fear and uncertainty among mixed-immigration status families about the impact that a family member's use might have on another family member's ability to get a green card or eventually naturalize. Federal guidance issued by the Immigration and Naturalization Service (INS) in May 1999 clarified that Medicaid use by an immigrant or his family member, would not, except in rare cases affect immigration status, but some immigration lawyers and immigrants remain reluctant to access Medicaid, including US citizen children of non-citizen parents.[15]

The Introduction of the State Children's Health Insurance Program

The BBA of 1997 created the State Children's Health Insurance Program (SCHIP) for low-income children who need health insurance but do not qualify for Medicaid. The SCHIP program allotted to the states nearly $50 billion over 10 years to create health insurance programs for uninsured low-income children with family incomes that are just above the requirements for the states' Medicaid programs. Texas has created with their SCHIP allotment a program that covers children up to 200 percent of the FPL not covered by the state's children's Medicaid program.

Medicaid Eligibility in Texas

Medicaid eligibility for children relates to the income and assets of the child's family. In Texas, Medicaid covers infants less than one year old, if they are living in families who earn less than 185 percent of the FPL. Children age one until their sixth birthday are eligible for Medicaid in Texas if their family income is at or below 133 percent of the FPL. Children from age six through 18 are eligible for coverage, if they are living in families with incomes that are 100 percent of the FPL or less. Finally, if families make 200 percent of the FPL or less and do not qualify for Medicaid because of their income or assets, they are eligible for the SCHIP program in Texas.[16] Table 2.3 illustrates the relationship between the Texas Children's Medicaid Program and SCHIP.

Table 2.3
Children's Public Health Insurance Status According to Income and Age

Age	0-100% FPL	100-133% FPL	134-150% FPL	151-185% FPL	186-200% FPL
<1	Medicaid	Medicaid	Medicaid	Medicaid	SCHIP
1-5	Medicaid	Medicaid	SCHIP	SCHIP	SCHIP
6-18	Medicaid	SCHIP	SCHIP	SCHIP	SCHIP

Adapted from: Anne Dunkelberg, and Cathy Schechter, *Every Child Equal: What Texas Parents Want from Children's Medicaid* (Center for Public Policy Priorities, Austin, Tex., September 2000), p. 14.

To qualify for Medicaid in Texas, adults must have a "countable" income of less than 34 percent of the federal poverty level.[17] Pregnant women who earn less than 185 percent of the FPL qualify for Medicaid with coverage lapsing two months after the birth. Low-income elderly and disabled Texans are also eligible for Medicaid; they must be at or below the income level to qualify for SSI or the low-income nursing home benefit. (To qualify for SSI, an individual must have an income of less than 74 percent of the FPL. To qualify for the nursing home benefit, the individual's income cannot exceed 223 percent of the FPL. There are also Medicaid programs that provide partial coverage available to qualified elderly and disabled Medicare beneficiaries.) The low-income nursing home benefit is available for individuals with incomes up to three times the SSI eligibility level. Texas also offers a frail elderly program that is available to those with incomes up to three times the SSI level and who qualify for admission to a nursing home, which offers home-care.

In Texas to qualify for Medicaid, one must also have limited assets to be eligible for Medicaid. Individuals and families who qualify for Medicaid are allowed to have up to $2000 in countable resources; there is no assets test for SCHIP. Table 2.4 lists the Federal Medicaid Population Guidelines in Relation to Texas.

Table 2.4
Federal Medicaid Population Guidelines in Relation to Texas

Federally Mandated Medicaid Eligible Populations	Optional Medicaid Eligible Populations served in Texas	Optional Medicaid Eligible Populations NOT served in Texas and Populations covered by 1115 waivers in other states
Section 1931 recipients	TANF recipients[1]	Childless adults (1115 waiver)
		Parents of children over 34% of the Federal Poverty Level not receiving TANF
SSI recipients	Pregnant women with family incomes less than 185% of the FPL[2]	Elderly not receiving SSI but below 100% of the Federal Poverty Level
Children under 1 year old with family incomes at or below 185% of the FPL; children 1 to 6 years old with family incomes at or below 133% of the FPL; and all other children under 19 years old with family incomes less than 100% of the FPL	Medically needy: Adults with children under age 19 with 133 1/3% of the 1996 AFDC income eligibility level; this means in Texas, this benefit covers those who spend-down to 24% of the FPL	Breast and cervical cancer patients through the Breast and Cervical Cancer Treatment Act of 2000
		Beneficiary groups of Ticket to Work and Work Incentives Improvement of 1999
		Medically Needy for the Aged and the Disabled

Adapted from: Texas Health and Human Services Commission, *Texas Medicaid in Perspective, Third Edition* (Austin, Tex., February 1999), pp. 49-50; and Families USA, *Expanding Medicaid State Options: Could Your State Do More?* (Washington, D.C., 1999), pp. 4-5.

[1] In Texas, individuals receiving TANF are automatically eligible for Medicaid. Federal law requires six months of Transitional Medicaid for those leaving 1931 eligibility due to increased earnings. Texas currently provides 12 months under terms of its AFDC waiver, which expires in 2002.

[2] Covering pregnant women up to 133 percent of the FPL is mandatory.

Services Covered by Texas Medicaid

As mentioned, federal law requires that states cover specific services within their Medicaid programs. Texas, like other states, has chosen to cover some services deemed as optional. (See Table 2.5, first column). States are allowed to implement optional services as long as they are adequate in amount, duration, and scope (all optional services are required to be provided to individuals under age 21 if the service is medically necessary). States are not allowed to limit the amount, duration, or scope of a covered service "solely on the basis of an individual's diagnosis, types of illness, or condition."[18] For example a state would not be allowed to exclude AIDS patients from the Medicaid prescription drug benefit. States are also required to offer the same Medicaid services throughout the state. There are also optional Medicaid services that are not offered in

Texas. (See Table 2.5, second column). No co-payment, in the form of a premium or a deductible, is currently required to receive Medicaid benefits in Texas.

Table 2.5
Federal Medicaid Service Guidelines in Relation to Texas

Optional Medicaid Service offered in Texas	Optional Medicaid Services NOT offered in Texas for adults
Limited birthing center	Christian Science nurses
Case management for certain groups	Clinic services (except for maternity and family planning)
Certified registered nurse anesthetists	Routine dental care
Chiropractic (limited)	Dentures
Christian Science sanitarium	Diagnostics, screening, preventive, and rehabilitative services
Day activity and health Service	Durable medical equipment such as wheelchairs, walkers and crutches, except when provided by a Medicaid home health agency
Emergency medical	Institutions for mental disease, persons over 65
Licensed professional counselor	Occupational, hearing, or speech therapy
Licensed Master of Social Work/Advanced Clinical Practitioner	Diagnostic services: Assessment of persons with mental retardation
Hearing instruments and other related audiology	
Hospice care	
Intermediate Care Facilities for people with mental retardation/developmental disabilities	
Maternity care clinic (limited)	
Medically necessary surgery and dentistry	
Optometry and eyeglasses	
Personal care services in the home	
Physical therapy	
Podiatry	
Prescription drugs	

Adapted from: Texas Health and Human Services Commission, *Texas Medicaid in Perspective, Third Edition* (Austin, Tex., February 1999), pp. 70-71.

The Cost of Medicaid

The states and the federal government jointly fund the Medicaid program. In FFY 2001, Texas received a 60.6 percent federal match for each state dollar spent providing Medicaid services. States are allowed to use funding from a variety of sources, including local government funding, provider taxes and fees, and state general revenue. In SFY 2000, the Texas Medicaid program cost approximately $11.3 billion.[19]

The Number of Texans Covered by Medicaid

The size of the Texas Medicaid population may be expressed in two ways, the monthly average count and the unduplicated count. In 2000, the average monthly count was approximately 1,767,800 Texans.[20] Of the individuals who are covered at some point during the year (the unduplicated count), 60 percent were under 20, 30 percent were non-elderly/non-disabled adults, and 10 percent 65 years old or over. Twenty-three percent were SSI recipients (this number reflects all Medicaid recipients for the year).[21]

Almost one of every eight Texans is enrolled in Medicaid at some point during the year. Although Medicaid rolls declined significantly from 1996 to 1999, they stabilized in 1999 and began to increase in 2000, an average of approximately 1.77 million people were enrolled in 2000, down from the high of 2.1 million in 1996. The reduction is attributed to confusion concerning federal and state welfare reforms.[22] However, it is important to note that it is estimated that approximately 50 percent of the Medicaid eligible population in Texas is not enrolled in the program.[23]

Texas has a significantly less generous Medicaid program than many other states. The enrollment process, although recently simplified for children, is rather burdensome, and the benefit package is less rich than that offered by other states. Much of the Texas labor market is composed of low-paying small business jobs that often do not offer private insurance options; only 53 percent of Texans have private insurance while the national average is 58 percent. This coupled with the state only covering 10 percent of its population through Medicaid leads to a high rate of uninsured. In fact in 1999, Texas had the highest rate of uninsurance among all of the states.[24] Methods exist to curtail this problem, and Texas has the proven ability to address this type of problem. The success of the State Children's Health Insurance Program is a prime example.

The State Children's Health Insurance Program in Texas

The State Children's Health Insurance Program (SCHIP) was created by Congress as part of the Balanced Budget Act (BBA) of 1997. SCHIP insures children in low-income working families whose incomes are too high for Medicaid but too low to be able to afford private health insurance. As of July 1, 2000, 50 states, the District of Columbia, and five U.S. Territories have implemented SCHIP.[25] According to the most recent data available, 4.6 million children have been enrolled in SCHIP nationally.[26, 27]

A Brief History of SCHIP in Texas

In Texas the SCHIP program has been given the name TexCare Partnership to represent the partnership between the federal and state governments and the private sector. As mentioned, the BBA established the SCHIP program in 1997; however, it took the state of Texas three years to fully implement the TexCare Partnership program.

The Texas SCHIP program was developed in two phases. Phase I began on July 1, 1998, and expanded Medicaid to children ages 15 to 18 in families with incomes below 100 percent of FPL. Texas used SCHIP funds to implement this expansion, which was federally mandated. Then in 1999, the Texas Legislature passed Senate Bill 445, which created Phase II of the Texas Children's Health Insurance Program. The bill assigned the statutory authority to oversee SCHIP in Texas to the Texas Health and Human Services Commission. Birch & Davis was selected to be the SCHIP program administrator. The state also contracted with several other private sector entities, which include: Sherry Mathews Advertising and Public Relations (the media services contractor) and approximately 50 community based organizations (CBO) contractors.

Enrollment in Texas began on April 3, 2000, and SCHIP coverage began May 1, 2000. Within the first seven months, the state of Texas enrolled an estimated 44.74 percent of its eligible population; the next best state, Arizona, enrolled 23.75 percent of its population during the first seven months of its program.[28] In the fall of 2001, the Texas SCHIP reached its goal of enrolling 428,000 children and has since continued to enroll thousands more children.[29] As of February 18, 2002, the state had enrolled an estimated 530,300 children in the SCHIP program.[30]

The Need to Expand Medicaid and SCHIP in Texas

The recent federal and state initiatives to reduce the number of uninsured children have had impressive results. Another group, low-income adults, has received much less attention despite the fact that there are 27 million uninsured adults versus 9 million uninsured children in the United States. Furthermore, the majority of this population resides in households with at least one full-time worker.[31]

In Texas, 47 percent of nonelderly adults (ages 19-64) with family income below 200 percent of the federal poverty level (FPL) are uninsured; nationally 35 percent of this population is uninsured. Another 8 percent of this population in Texas is covered through public or state-sponsored insurance compared to 15 percent nationally.[32] Low-income nonelderly adults include both those individuals with and without minor children. It is possible to expand health insurance to low-income parents in Texas by amending the state Medicaid plan through Section 1931 of the Social Security Act, but it is not possible to offer Medicaid coverage to childless adults unless the state pursues a Section 1115 waiver.

At least 50 percent of uninsured low-income nonelderly adults in Texas work.[33] More specifically it is estimated that 42 percent of workers earning less than $20,000 per year cannot access affordable health insurance through their employer.[34] Overall, Texans have a more difficult time accessing health care coverage than the rest of the nation. One major circumstance behind this reality is the Texas economy. Many of the jobs available to low-income Texans are the least likely to have health care benefits. These jobs include low-paying service jobs, agriculture, part-time or temporary work, small businesses, and non-union employment in large industries that tend to be unionized in other states.[35]

The Benefits of Expanding Medicaid

Access to high-quality health care is essential to the livelihood of states and the entire nation. Especially in economically unstable times, health care is an essential portion of the national economy. Rising unemployment among low-income adults could lead to the erosion of coverage and encourage reductions within the health industry, which could add to the economic downturn. Therefore, providing health insurance to low-income individuals and families is essential to both the recipients of the care and the unstable economy.[36] It follows, then, that in a state like Texas where health insurance coverage is historically low that the state should address the problem before it declines further. In recent years, much attention has been placed on the health care needs of children and significant progress has been made. Many feel it is now time to address the needs of low-income adults with and without children.

Providing health care for low-income adults may improve the health of their children. Parents with health care coverage are more likely to support and access health care for their children's needs when they are also insured because they are more likely to understand the benefits that health care provides their children. Research has shown that the uninsured are more likely to be in poor health, lack a usual source of care, rely on emergency rooms, and have unmet health care needs.[37]

Parents

Understanding benefits and accessing health care is a difficult venture that is further exaggerated for low-income families who are struggling to make ends meet. These families may not have time to understand the delivery system where they access health care, especially when parents and children are covered under multiple policies. Parents are more likely to be effective advocates for their children's health care needs when they are covered by the same insurance as their children because they are familiar with the particular system.[38] On the other end of the spectrum, parents who are not familiar with the health benefit system are likely to be the least effective in accessing high quality health care for their children.

Of all low-income parents with children having public insurance in the United States, 35.5 percent are uninsured and 55.4 percent have public coverage as their children do. This means that over one-third of children on Medicaid and SCHIP have uninsured parents who may not be able to advocate for their insurance needs as well as those parents who are covered under of the same system. According to 1999 data from the Urban Institute, 57 percent of parents of low-income children in Texas receiving public insurance are uninsured and only 39.5 percent of this population receives public insurance similar to that of their children.[39]

Childless Adults

Low-income adults without children under the age of 19 are the group least able to access health care in the United States. Generally, Medicaid does not cover childless adults at any income unless they are pregnant, disabled, or elderly. A few states have used 1115 waivers to expand to some of this population, but most states are left to care for this population themselves. For example, Texas law requires that counties provide care for their indigent populations, which includes childless adults, at or below 21 percent of the

FPL. Indigent care is provided through a variety of mechanisms including hospital districts, public hospitals, and County Indigent Health Care Programs (CIHCP).[40]

Childless adults are vulnerable in difficult economic times, just as parents are, but categorical restrictions keep them out of the Medicaid program. Further, childless adults are not eligible to receive benefits through the "medically needy" category.[41] When a childless adult is unable to pay for their health care needs, the state is often forced to take on an expensive charge. Nationally, 33.8 percent of low-income childless adults were uninsured in 1999 and historically; parents are more likely to be covered by insurance than this population.[42] Thus, it is important when considering options to reduce the number of uninsured individuals and provide quality health care to the people of Texas to address this significant piece of the uninsured population.

Ways to Expand

Two types of Medicaid expansions are currently being used by states to insure low-income parents and childless adults. Specifically, Texas could amend its state plan using Section 1931, or apply for a Medicaid and/or SCHIP Section 1115 waiver. Texas could pursue either of these options to decrease the number of uninsured adults in the state. As previously noted, studies have also shown that offering public coverage to parents can also potentially decrease the number of uninsured children in the state.[43]

Section 1931

Section 1931 of the Social Security Act is available to states that want to amend their State Medicaid Plan to insure low-income parents through the use of increased income and resources disregards. These mechanisms allow the state to adopt methods of determining countable income and resources that are less restrictive than those required prior to the implementation of welfare reform in 1996. For example using Section 1931 flexibility, some states have disregarded all resources, disregarded a car of any value, disregarded the cash value of a life insurance policy, disregarded the actual cost of child care, disregarded more income than required by federal law, or eliminated the time limits on the state's earned income disregard policy.[44] There is no limit to the size of disregards that can be offered to the parents through the states. States usually limit themselves based on their state budgets. This provision is similar to Section 1902(r)(2) of the Social Security Act, which was used extensively in the early 1990s to insure pregnant women and children with incomes above the optional and mandated levels.[45] Section 1931 is a relatively easy way for Texas to decrease the number of uninsured parents in the state.

Section 1115 Waiver

Section 1115 of the Social Security Act provides flexibility to states to alter the operation of their Medicaid and SCHIP programs through research and demonstration projects. This statute confers authority to the Secretary of Health and Human Services to waive specific provisions of some "grant-in-aid" programs including Medicaid and SCHIP. In the past, the waivers have been used to test new ideas on ways to better serve those enrolled in the Medicaid program, while making a more efficient use of state and federal dollars. In July 2000, the Clinton Administration released guidance describing how Section 1115 waivers can be applied to SCHIP.

Section 1115 waivers can be used to expand eligibility and/or the population covered by the program. New adult populations that can be covered through this authority include pregnant women over 185 percent of the FPL, parents of any income level, children who age out of Medicaid or SCHIP eligibility while being treated for a specific condition, and childless adults.

The use of research and demonstration waivers has the potential to help insure a specific population, but the waivers are often difficult to obtain, as they require that the proposal be budget neutral. This means that the state applying for the waiver must prove that the demonstration will not increase projected federal expenditures for the program over the expenditures that would be made without a waiver. Detailed descriptions of Section 1931 and Section 1115 waivers follow in the next two sections of this report.

Expanding through Section 1931

Section 1931, through the use of less restrictive income and assets tests, allows states to offer health insurance benefits in the form of Medicaid to low-income parents regardless of whether they are currently receiving welfare benefits. This type of expansion was implemented through the welfare reform act of 1996, The Personal Responsibility and Work Opportunity Reconciliation Act (PRWORA). It was added to the Medicaid Program to ensure that those eligible prior to the passage of PRWORA would continue to be eligible for Medicaid. Besides allowing those who would have been eligible prior to the new legislation to continue to be eligible for Medicaid, this program gave greater flexibility to states in their administration of Medicaid benefits. States only need to alter their state plan to increase the Medicaid eligibility for low-income parents.

This federal legislation mandated that the receipt of TANF benefits no longer entitled individuals to Medicaid benefits, and conversely, ineligibility for TANF does not necessarily make individuals ineligible for Medicaid benefits. Section 1931 provides states with viable options that they can utilize to create state standards to determine who is eligible to receive the Medicaid benefit. These options are especially powerful because unlike a Section 1115 waiver, Section 1931 does not put a federal budget constraint on the expansion. Under Section 1931, states are given the flexibility to cover more low-income parents and receive the federal Medicaid match by using the following measures: income disregards, asset disregards, and increasing income and asset limits.[46]

Not only are there these broad reasons to expand through Section 1931, other reasons exist as to why Texas would benefit from this type of expansion. This list was developed in part by researchers with funding through The Commonwealth Fund:[47]

- **Scope of benefits:** There are not set rules on what medical needs must be covered under the Medicaid benefit for adults. Each state is able to determine the amount, scope, and length of time the patient receives benefits, particularly for adults receiving benefits, although any changes in these limits made through Section 1931 will be applied to all adults who receive Medicaid, not just low-income parents (adults who receive Medicaid through SSI are excluded from this authority to reduce the amount, scope, and length of the benefit). Texas could use this flexibility to insure low-income parents at the most basic level, and then expand to more services, if they see the need for more services.

- **Ability to control the cost of expansion:** Limiting the scope of benefits is just one way to control expansion costs. Other options exist for Texas in this arena. Specifically, if expansion becomes too fiscally demanding on the state, it is allowed to scale back or eliminate optional expansion of coverage, such as the coverage to low-income parents. If this were to happen, coverage to low-income parents already enrolled would continue under the original legislation.

- **Cost-sharing:** Cost-sharing is defined as the out-of-pocket payments that Medicaid beneficiaries make in relation to the receipt of covered services. States are allowed to add a cost-sharing option into the Medicaid coverage for the adults insured under Section 1931. There are three main forms that cost-sharing takes: deductibles (specified dollar expenditures), copayments (fixed amounts), and coinsurance (percentage of the cost for service). The element of cost-sharing may help patients to consider whether visiting the doctor is medically necessary.

Along with these explicit benefits, 1931 gives states the freedom to simplify their application processes. Correspondingly, states are not able to make Medicaid eligibility standards stricter than they were in July of 1996.[48] Income disregards are also given to families for any child care and child support income based on the July 1996 AFDC level.

Many states have taken advantage of 1931 by aligning their Medicaid program with their TANF eligibility requirements, ensuring automatic Medicaid coverage to those eligible for TANF. Since TANF is available to both single parent and two-parent families, Section 1931 is a method that can be used to insure low-income adults in families with eligible children.

States have the ability to determine the level at which the benefit is available to parents. The states are then given the regular Medicaid match for the adults while their children receive the Medicaid/SCHIP match. Section 1931's ability to cover adults can be directly linked to SCHIP benefits, if the state chooses. This allows the entire family to be insured under one plan.[49]

Section 1931 was designed to meet the needs of states by being flexible. It authorizes states to use phase-in expansion, which allows states to monitor and evaluate the program's success and make the necessary program changes. Section 1931 also has the capability to create enrollment limits by allowing states to treat recipients and those currently applying differently. Finally, states are required to offer the core services, but the scope of the services are up to the state, as is the copayment option.[50]

Ultimately, Section 1931 of the SSA can be used to improve health care access in states in different ways depending on the needs of the individual states. Table 2.6 lists the states that have adopted more generous eligibility standards through 1931 and the income level and whether or not they have an assets test.

Table 2.6
State Medicaid Expansions to Parents through Section 1931

State	Income Test (Percent of FPL)	Assets Test (Yes or No)
California	107 %	Yes
Connecticut	157 %	Yes
Washington, D.C.	200 %	No
Maine	157 %	Yes
New Jersey	133 %[1]	Yes
Ohio	100 %	No
Rhode Island	100 %[2]	No

Adapted from: The Center on Budget and Policy Priorities, *Expanding Family Coverage: States' Medicaid Eligibility Policies for Working Families in the Year 2000* (Washington, D.C., 2002), p. 18.

[1] Granted a SCHIP Waiver to receive enhanced match to cover parents between 133-200 % FPL in January 2001.

[2] Granted a SCHIP Waiver to receive enhanced match to cover parents between 100-192 % of the FPL.

Section 1931 in Texas

Texas has not taken advantage of many of the opportunities that are offered through Section 1931. By disregarding income and assets more parents would be eligible for Medicaid. The state would receive the federal match for these populations but would also have to pay the state share of the cost enrollment for these parents.

Although there is some cost to the state involved in this type of expansion, benefits do exist for states like Texas that take advantage of Section 1931 who have a substantial population of uninsured low-income adults. The Center for Budget and Policy Priorities advocates state expansion through 1931 for the following reasons: [51]

- **Federal Medicaid match:** Section 1931 allows states to receive the federal matching funds to expand coverage without the hassle of a waiver;
- **Coverage promotes work and may reduce the need for welfare:** Not only will health insurance ease the transition off welfare, it will also promote job retention by helping workers avoid illness that could potential force them to miss work;
- **It gives low-income working parents the same access to health care as parents who are not employed:** This encourages more expedient entry into the workforce rather than dependence on welfare.

As this description of Section 1931 points out, there are ways to decrease the rate of the uninsured, utilize federal funds, promote welfare reform, and help those most in need of health insurance in Texas. Section 1931 enables states to expand coverage to parents through an amendment to their state Medicaid plan, which is both easier and faster than obtaining a waiver. States need only to apply for Section 1115 waivers if they want to change the rules of their current federally and state funded public health insurance programs or if they want to expand coverage to new populations not currently covered by these programs, namely childless adults. Thus, if states just wish to add additional optional benefits they do not need a Section 1115 waiver. However, states may want to consider a waiver to cover other populations such as SCHIP parents, childless adults, HIV patients, and those in need of family planning services. A combination of Medicaid and SCHIP Section 1115 waivers may help a state to reach multiple groups more efficiently.[52]

Expanding through Section 1115 Waivers

A major source of state diversity in Medicaid policy is Section 1115 waivers. Section 1115 of the Social Security Act gives the Secretary of the Department of Health and Human Services the authority to authorize research, pilot, or demonstration projects that are likely to assist in the objectives of certain federally subsidized "welfare programs." These waivers provide states with greater flexibility by enabling them to receive federal funding for trying out new and innovative methods to fulfill the objectives of these two programs. The federal government has traditionally promoted 1115 waivers as a way to encourage states to expand benefits or to provide services more efficiently to a larger population while at the same time reducing, or at least maintaining, current Medicaid and SCHIP expenditures.

The authority under Section 1115 furnishes each presidential administration's Secretary of Health and Human Services with the discretion to steer the objectives of many social programs. This ability to alter federal law is especially monumental in the case of Medicaid, a costly and often controversial federal and state administered social program.

Through the Public Welfare Amendment of 1962, Public Law 87-543, Section 1115 was added to the Social Security Act. The original intent of this law was to allow states to waive any provision of cash assistance programs, currently known as Temporary Aid to Needy Families (TANF), for demonstrations that are "likely to assist in promoting the objectives" of the program. Authority to create Medicaid demonstrations was established with the enactment of the program in 1965, while the authority to create SCHIP waivers was granted in 2000.[53]

Before explaining the considerable potential of Section 1115 waivers, it is important to note its limitations. They are specifically limited to use in demonstrations that investigate issues of interest to the Centers for Medicare and Medicaid Services (CMS, the agency formerly known as the Health Care Financing Administration, or HCFA), test a program, or otherwise fulfill a research purpose.[54] These research programs typically have a five-year life to demonstrate outcomes, but the waiver can be renewed. In fact, Arizona has run its Medicaid program through an 1115 waiver since 1983. A final requirement of the waivers is budget neutrality, meaning they cannot cost the federal government more than what they would have spent on Medicaid and/or SCHIP if the program had not been implemented.

As mentioned, two types of Section 1115 waivers can be used to research expansion options; the type is based upon the program that the waiver alters: Medicaid and SCHIP.

Medicaid underwent several modifications in the 1980s on the national level; then, in the early to mid-1990s individual states took an active role in modifying their Medicaid program through the authority of Section 1115 waivers. This process was facilitated by guidance released by the Clinton Administration that defined and explained the waiver application process. Many of the changes sought and granted through this authority culminated in national policy changes enacted in the BBA of 1997. In July 2000, HCFA released waiver guidance that would allow states to apply for Section 1115 waivers through SCHIP. Use of this authority was limited to states that had met certain requirements in their Medicaid program and SCHIP.

How can States use Medicaid Section 1115 waivers?

Since the first major Medicaid research and demonstration waiver was awarded to Arizona in 1983, three broad concepts have emerged that states have used to pursue improvements to their Medicaid programs.[55] States have sought to:

- **Waive Federal Program Requirements:** Federal Medicaid law has continually developed throughout the past 36 years from the original potentially broad-reaching legislation to a program with a plethora of rules and regulations. Some of these pertain to benefits, cost-sharing, use of managed care, provider participation and compensation and all have been the basis of Section 1115 waivers.
- **Increase access to federal coverage for the categorically ineligible:** Increasing access to the otherwise ineligible has been a motivating factor that has encouraged many states to pursue a Section 1115 waiver. Without a waiver, federal funding for Medicaid is limited to specific groups outlined in Medicaid statute. (See Table 2.1) Non-disabled adults, 19-64, without dependent children under age 19 are a frequently targeted population for increased eligibility.
- **Redirect Federal Funds:** Redirecting federal funds from one expenditure of the Medicaid program to a newly recognized expenditure is the third provision that states often seek through a Section 1115 waiver.[56] Budget neutrality is required of all Section 1115 waivers. In the past, several states redirected funds from Medicaid's Disproportionate Share Hospital (DSH) Program, which typically allocate additional Medicaid funds to hospitals that serve a larger portion of Medicaid and uninsured patients, to achieve budget neutrality.

Thus, by using Section 1115 waivers, each state is able to create more viable Medicaid programs and, in many cases, to reduce the number of uninsured individuals in the state.

There are certain rules under Medicaid law that are mandatory and may only be waived by an 1115 waiver. In short, these include statewide application and equal services and benefits for all beneficiaries that are adequate in duration and scope. Therefore, while it is somewhat ambiguous as to what CMS might allow under an 1115 waiver, states use waivers to alter one or more of these rules. Examples of requirements that have been waived in the past include:

- Allowing provision of services to specific populations or regions within a state as opposed to serving all eligible populations,
- Offering different benefits to one group and not another group,
- Making enrollment in a managed care plans mandatory, and
- Expanding coverage to groups like childless adults or parents.[57, 58]

Table 2.7 lists the states with Medicaid expansions to adults under the authority of Section 1115.

Table 2.7
State Medicaid Expansions to Adults under Section 1115

State	Income Test (Percent of FPL)
Arizona[1]	107
Delaware	107
Hawaii	100
Massachusetts	133
Minnesota[2]	275
Missouri	107
New York	150
Oregon	100
Tennessee[3]	400
Vermont	192

Adapted from: The Center on Budget and Policy Priorities, *Expanding Family Coverage: States' Medicaid Eligibility Policies for Working Families in the Year 2000* (Washington, D.C.: 2002), p. 18.

[1]Arizona received a waiver in January 2001 to cover all eligible populations up to 107 percent of the FPL. In December 2001, the state was awarded the first Health Insurance Flexibility and Accountability Demonstration Initiative Waiver through the Bush Administration to expand coverage up to 200 percent of the FPL using the state's remaining funds from their SCHIP allotment.

[2] Minnesota expanded coverage up to 275 percent through a state funded program. They received a Medicaid waiver in 2000 to expand eligibility to parents earning the regular Medicaid Match in June 2001; they received a SCHIP waiver that allows the state to receive an enhanced match for parents who earn between 100 and 200 percent of the FPL.

[3] Enrollment in Tennessee is currently closed to adults unless they qualify for coverage under the state's Section 1931 eligibility category, they are uninsurable, or meet other specified conditions. Parents with higher incomes that were enrolled in the program prior to the cap are still being served.

How can States use SCHIP Section 1115 waivers?

SCHIP provides states with a capped entitlement for 10 years. Each year the state accesses a piece of their allotment. States are required to spend state dollars to actually receive the enhanced SCHIP dollars. The funding began in 1998, but many states were unable to utilize their entire allotment that year because of the challenge of creating and enrolling eligible individuals in a new program. Under the SCHIP financing rules, states have three years to spend their allotments. If states fail to use these funds, they are redistributed to states that can potentially use them in their SCHIP program. States have one year to use these redistributed funds, and then, the funds are returned to the U.S. Treasury.[59] States have built up reserves in their SCHIP allotments because of the length of time it takes to create and enroll people in newly funded programs. The excess funds from a states allotment are a potential source of budget neutral funds necessary in the creation of a Section 1115 waiver. A three-year dip in the SCHIP allotment starting in FFY 2002, occurring because of budget restraints, however, may lead to a shortfall in SCHIP by FFY 2004, making it difficult for some states to pursue SCHIP waivers.[60] States with rapidly rising expenditures and growing enrollment should consider this issue, as an 1115 waiver through SCHIP may cost the state more than their existing program.

The SCHIP demonstration projects under Section 1115 waivers allow states to implement a tailored state program not ordinarily allowed under Title XXI of the Social Security Act. One reason that states choose to apply for an 1115 SCHIP waiver as opposed to an 1115 Medicaid waiver is because of the enhanced federal match that they receive under the SCHIP program. States can expand SCHIP to cover parents so that it can receive a higher federal match.[61]

In the State Medicaid Directors letter dated July 31, 2000, the U.S. Department of Health and Human Services (DHHS) stated that any state applying for an 1115 waiver under SCHIP must first meet certain requirements. These requirements include the following:

- The state's SCHIP program must have been in operation for at least one year;
- States are required to conduct evaluations of the SCHIP program and must have submitted the required reports pertaining to these evaluations;
- Each state must have submitted its enrollment reports;
- The state must prove that it has met the primary objective of the SCHIP program, which is to insure children up to age 19 in families with incomes up to 200 percent of the federal poverty level; and
- If granted a waiver, states cannot have a waiting list nor can they close registration and enrollment of eligible children during the life of their demonstration projects.[62]

In states that apply to cover populations other than low-income children, the state must also meet at least three of the following five guidelines in their SCHIP program.[63] The states listed in Table 2.8 have met these requirements and have received and implemented SCHIP 1115 waivers.

1. Use a joint mail-in application and common application process for SCHIP and Medicaid;
2. Eliminate assets tests;
3. Have 12-month continuous eligibility;
4. Have presumptive eligibility; and/or
5. Have simplified procedures for redetermination of coverage; so it can be done through the mail, and have a seamless system in which participants can shift between SCHIP and Medicaid without a new application or lapse in coverage.[64]

Table 2.8
Covering Adults with Children through SCHIP Funds

State	Method	Income Eligibility (Percent of the FPL)
Arizona	HIFA Waiver[1]	100-200% of the FPL
Minnesota	SCHIP Waiver[2]	100-200% of the FPL
Rhode Island	SCHIP Waiver[3]	100-192% of the FPL
Wisconsin	SCHIP Waiver	100-185% of the FPL

Adapted from: The Center on Budget and Policy Priorities, *Expanding Family Coverage: States' Medicaid Eligibility Policies for Working Families in the Year 2000* (Washington, D.C.: 2002), p. 18.

[1] In December 2001, the state was awarded the first Health Insurance Flexibility and Accountability (HIFA) Demonstration Initiative Waiver granted by the Bush Administration. HIFA waivers, which can tap a state's unused federal SCHIP allotments, will be discussed in a subsequent section of this report. Arizona used a HIFA waiver to expand coverage to parents up to 200 percent of the FPL using the state's remaining funds from their SCHIP allotment. Arizona already had a Medicaid 1115 waiver that expanded coverage to parents under 107 percent of the FPL.

[2] In June 2001, Minnesota received a SCHIP waiver that allows the state to receive an enhanced match for parents who earn between 100 and 200 percent of the FPL. At that time, Minnesota had already expanded coverage up to 275% through a state funded program. They also received approval for a Medicaid waiver in 2000 to expand eligibility to parents up to 100 percent of the FPL with the regular Medicaid match.

[3] Rhode Island originally expanded coverage through Section 1931 but was granted a SCHIP Waiver in January 2001 to allow the state to receive enhanced match to cover parents between 100-192 of the FPL.

SCHIP Waiver in Texas

The Texas Legislature passed a Medicaid simplification bill in the 2001 legislative session. The bill, SB 43, underwent much negotiation and in the end, the simplification measures were not as broad as many had expected. For instance, the bill signed into law kept the assets test for the children's Medicaid program. In November 2001, the Texas Department of Human Services (DHS) published its proposed rules in the Texas Register. The bill required DHS to address four major areas:

1. Application Simplification;
2. Continuous Eligibility and Eligibility Transition with SCHIP;
3. Health Care Orientation (HCO);
4. Participation in Texas Healthy Steps (THSteps).[65]

Currently, Texas is in the process of updating and implementing the published rules. The rules became effective near the end of January 2002. The policies explain how the separate Medicaid and SCHIP applications will be merged into one and how enrollment procedures will be affected. This allowed the state, beginning in January 2002, to utilize a joint application and a common application process for SCHIP and Medicaid. The state is also working on implementing phased-in continuous eligibility for children under age 19, with six months continuous eligibility by February 2002 with the possibility of 12 months continuous eligibility as early as September 2002. [66] Thus, Texas has not yet met the 12-month continuous eligibility requirement.

Texas did not adopt any children's presumptive eligibility requirements as part of their simplification package. Texas is working to set-up a simplified redetermination process, but the state has encountered obstacles on this front. As part of SB 43, parents who enroll their children in Medicaid are required to go through a Health Care Orientation (HCO). HCOs did not exist prior to the Medicaid simplification bill. The proposed rule created a set of administrative guidelines for the HCOs. The rule leaves open the possibility of required face-to-face Medicaid renewal. Thus, when implemented, Texas will not be creating simplified procedures for redetermination that can be completed through the mail.

At this point, the state's chances at a SCHIP 1115 waiver are uncertain. Texas has only truly met only one of the simplification requirements out of a possible five that enable a state to apply for a Section 1115 SCHIP waiver under the 2000 guidance. Until Texas meets at least three of these requirements or DHHS changes the policy, SCHIP waivers are not an option.

Obtaining a Section 1115 Waiver

Despite the bleak prospects for a SCHIP waiver in Texas without further steps to simplify the Texas Medicaid program, Texas can and should be aware of the potential of both Medicaid and SCHIP Section 1115 waivers. These waivers have specific requirements including budget neutrality and an application process that must be fulfilled to be approved for a waiver by the Secretary of DHHS; the budget neutrality requirements and application procedures are outlined below. Several states have successfully fulfilled these requirements and are also discussed. Finally, a brief discussion of the current Bush Administration's concept of Section 1115 waivers describes the federal political feasibility of a waiver in Texas.

Budget Neutrality

One of the key concepts entrenched in the concept of all Section 1115 waivers is budget neutrality. This concept much like the rest of Medicaid and SCHIP has a cumulative history. Changes by several administrations have encouraged the development of the current policy regarding budget neutrality.

The Carter Administration establishes the concept of budget neutrality in Section 1115 waivers. Budget neutrality refers to the concept that total federal expenditures under the Section 1115 waiver can not be any greater than expenditures would have been in the absence of the demonstration for comparable services for the same beneficiaries.[67] Through codification of the Paperwork Reduction Act of 1980, the Reagan Administration established the authority of the Office of Management and Budget (OMB) to approve the budget neutrality of Section 1115 waivers.[68] The explicit definition of budget neutrality was not publicly described until 1994 when the Clinton Administration published a description of policies and procedures in the *Federal Register.*[69]

The Clinton Administration established general definitions for budget neutrality, duration of the waiver, evaluation, timeliness and administrative complexity, and state notice procedures, but specifically stated,

> This notice is intended to inform the public and the States regarding procedures the Department ordinarily will follow in exercising the Secretary's discretionary authority with respect to State demonstration proposals under section 1115. This notice does not create any right or benefit, substantive or procedural, enforceable at law or equity, by any person or entity, against the United States, its agencies or instrumentalities, the States, or any other person.[70]

This statement explains the procedures published in 1994 that were being used in authorizing Section 1115 waivers at that point in time, but that administration along with future administrations are not legally bound to following these guidelines. Using this approach to promote and explain the usage of Section 1115 waivers gives the acting administration a critical and amorphous tool to continue to shape Medicaid policy. The new Bush Administration has already begun to mold the Medicaid program to meet its goals through the Health Insurance Flexibility and Accountability (HIFA) demonstration initiative, which will be discussed subsequently in this report.

The Application Process

The federal government has developed a five-step process through which the waivers are reviewed, awarded, and evaluated. Initially, states are encouraged to develop a concept paper and submit it to the DHHS for discussion. Next, states submit a proposal, which is evaluated by the Secretary's Office, the Assistant Secretary on Management and Budget, and the Office of Management and Budget. States are given feedback and expected to respond to questions developed through these agencies. Finally, if all of the issues and questions raised are taken care of in satisfactory manner, the Centers for Medicare and Medicaid Services (CMS) within DHHS develop an operating plan for the waiver.[71]

The third stage of the waiver process is known as the pre-implementation phase; it follows approval of the waiver and is when the state prepares to implement the waiver. Meanwhile, CMS must also determine that the state is prepared to operate the waiver. When this is determined and the state also feels that it is ready, the waiver is implemented and new and/or modified services are available to defined beneficiaries. Finally, the state must evaluate its project.[72] Typically, demonstrations are awarded for five years and three-year extensions are available. In the previous administration, evaluation was not as stringently monitored; strong emphasis was placed on the proposal and implementation process. The following steps depict the steps in the Section 1115 waiver process.

1. State prepares a concept paper;
2. Formal proposal submitted;
3. If approved, develops an operating plan;
4. Implementation; and
5. Evaluation.[73]

As mentioned, the reasons that so much emphasis is placed upon the contents of the proposal is the requirement that states must enact a waiver that is budget neutral. This concept has developed over time and was not part of the original law authorizing Section 1115 waivers but is now the most essential requirement pertinent throughout the entire process.

Research and Demonstration Waivers in the Bush Administration

President Bush's budget for FFY 2001 estimated $128 billion in federal Medicaid spending; over 20 percent of which, $27 billion, was allocated to individual states to fund Medicaid Section 1115 research and demonstration waivers alone.[74] To put this Section 1115 spending into perspective, it was five times the federal allotment for SCHIP in FY 2001. Further, if the proportion of funds expended on 1115 waivers remained constant, their cost over the next ten years would be an estimated $400 billion. Currently, Section 1115 waivers provide health insurance to nearly two million uninsured Americans, allow states to change their Medicaid delivery system, and target benefits to specific populations.[75] Seventeen states have Section 1115 waivers that operate comprehensive health care demonstrations.

President Bush and the Secretary of Health and Human Services, Tommy Thompson, are both former governors, and much has been said and written about how responsive they will be to the needs of states. Their work on Medicaid policy will be a prime indicator how their discourse will interact with their policies. In early August, President Bush announced an initiative "to empower states to propose reforms tailor to the needs of their citizens."[76] The plan would allow states to trim certain optional benefits and use the savings to expand to other uninsured populations using Section 1115 waivers. This program nearly mirrors a proposal brought forth by the National Governors Association (NGA) earlier this year. Unlike the NGA proposal, this plan does not offer an enhanced match to states that offer Medicaid to new optional and expansion populations.

Health Insurance Flexibility and Accountability

The Center for Medicare and Medicaid Services (CMS) introduced the Health Insurance Flexibility and Accountability (HIFA) demonstration initiative in August 2001. HIFA is a new approach to Section 1115 research and demonstration waivers for Medicaid and SCHIP created by the Bush Administration. The overriding goal of HIFA is to encourage states to develop new approaches to increase the number of individuals with health insurance under 200 percent of the FPL using their current level of Medicaid and SCHIP resources, although the HIFA demonstration does not limit the upper eligibility level.

The National Governors Association Plan's Theoretical Foundations

The basic ideas behind the initiative were proposed by state governors attending the National Governors Associations February 2001 meeting. Three strong Medicaid recommendations were publicized in an effort to illustrate the growing consensus of the governors of the United States. These recommendations laid the theoretical foundation for the HIFA initiative. The first of these highlighted the need to restructure Medicaid to rid the program of the "all or nothing" approach to benefits, which was the residue of legislation in place prior to Medicaid. Secondly, governors wanted the ability to create appropriate cost-sharing arrangements that would encourage responsible utilization of the limited services available. Finally, the governors hoped to encourage prompt review of Medicaid waivers and state plan amendments. It should be noted that the original NGA proposal also included an enhanced match similar to SCHIP for the expansion populations, but this recommendation has not been enacted, as it would take legislative action. The HIFA initiative is a product of administrative policy, not legislation.

Overall, NGA has supported the Bush Administration's program as an important step toward the creation of a Medicaid program that meets the needs of health care in the 21st century, but they have also maintained that flexibility is not enough.[77] The federal government needs to provide states with an enhanced match according to Matt Salo, the Director of Health Legislation at the NGA, especially since most state budgets are falling short due to the current economic downturn. "In a time of serious state fiscal situations, without the enhanced match, few states will be able to come up with the money to propose significant expansions."[78]

Creating a HIFA waiver

Through the HIFA initiative, states are given the ability to create programs that utilize savings from providing more limited benefits and imposing cost-sharing on certain groups of existing Medicaid beneficiaries and expansion populations. As previously noted, no new money accompanies this initiative and states applying for a HIFA waiver must still meet the requirement of budget neutrality; further, there is no written requirement that states must spend savings from the initiative on health care in the state. The initiative has been met with staunch criticism from advocacy communities, who are concerned that this program will encourage states to cut benefits to certain groups of disabled, elderly, pregnant women, and children that are defined under Medicaid statute as optional populations.

Another concern that has arisen since the announcement of the HIFA program is the condition of state budgets. Even prior to the events of September 11, 2001, the American economy was experiencing a downturn while Medicaid spending was on the rise. These factors, in addition to current increases in unemployment, are sure to cause growth in Medicaid spending and place financial pressure on the states that were already facing budget shortfalls in the recent sluggish economy.

The paramount goal of the HIFA initiative is to expand health insurance to adults under 200 percent of the FPL, but when the initiative was announced, few had any idea that state economies were going to reach their current tenuous conditions. Many states may not see Medicaid and SCHIP expansions as the answer to their budget problems, although states may be motivated by the flexibility that allows them to tap the unused portions of their SCHIP allotments for the federal portion of the HIFA waiver's funding. This means that states may be able to provide health care coverage to parents and childless adults while also receiving the enhanced SCHIP match. Thus, despite the economic downturn, HIFA tries to provide states with the ability to develop expanded coverage to Medicaid populations while managing the utilization of health care services.

In the initial announcement the Bush Administration stated that HIFA will work with the individual states to:

- Encourage innovation to improve how Medicaid and SCHIP funds are used to increase health insurance coverage for low-income individuals.
- Give states the programmatic flexibility required to support approaches that increase private health insurance coverage options.
- Simplify the waiver application process by providing clear guidance and data templates.
- Increase accountability in the state and federal partnership by ensuring that Medicaid and SCHIP funds are being used effectively to increase health insurance coverage, including substantially more private health insurance coverage options.
- Give priority review to state proposals that meet the general guidelines of the HIFA demonstration project.[79]

These broad goals are delineated below within the context of the initial guidance published describing the HIFA demonstration initiative.

Program Innovation

The first goals described by the administration aim to encourage states to be innovative by using existing Medicaid and SCHIP funds in new ways to address the needs of low-income uninsured individuals. One of the chief potential sources of HIFA funding is states' unused SCHIP allotments. SCHIP provides states with a capped entitlement for 10 years. Each year the state is allowed access part of their allotment. Similar to the funding of the Medicaid program, states are required to spend state dollars to receive the enhanced SCHIP match from the federal government. Funding began in FFY 1998, but many states were unable to utilize their entire allotment that year because of the challenge of creating, administering and enrolling eligible children into the new programs.

SCHIP financing rules were then developed to allow states to have up to three years to spend their state allotments. If states fail to use these funds, they are to be redistributed in the fourth year to other states that can use them in their SCHIP program. States have one year to use these redistributed funds, and then, the funds are returned to the U.S. Treasury.[80] Over the past four years, states have built up reserves in their SCHIP allotments because of the lengthy process of creating and enrolling people in newly funded programs.

The Bush Administration has identified these excess funds from states' allotments as a potential source of budget neutral funds necessary in the creation of a SCHIP Section 1115 waiver and more specifically a HIFA waiver. When calculating the excess allotment amounts states must note that there is a three-year dip in the SCHIP allotment starting in FY 2002. This is a result of budget restraints written into the BBA of 1997. Thus, this may lead to a shortfall in SCHIP funding for the states by FFY 2004 making it difficult for states with robust programs to pursue SCHIP waivers.[81] States with rapidly rising expenditures and growing enrollment should consider this issue, as a Section 1115 waiver through SCHIP may cost the state more than their existing program.

With this in mind, the Office of the Actuary at CMS estimated that at the beginning of FFY 2002, states have $11 billion in prior years unspent SCHIP allotment. This money plus FY 2002 allotment of $3.1 billion means that states will have $10.5 billion dollars for program expansion following the use of a projected $3.6 billion in FY 2002. Only one state, Rhode Island, is expected to utilize all of its available SCHIP funding in FY 2002.[82] Therefore, it is reasonable for states to at least recognize the existing excess in state allotments.

Defining the Populations

The Medicaid program offers benefits to different categories of individuals; in Section 1902(a)(2) of the Social Security Act, the federal government requires states to cover certain groups known as the mandatory population. Certain benefits offered through the Medicaid program are also mandatory. States are allowed to draw down federal funding for specified optional populations; these groups are described in 42 Code of Federal Regulations (CFR) Part 435, Subpart C.[83] These populations are added to a state's Medicaid programs through an amendment to their Medicaid state plan. According to CMS guidelines, expansions made to state programs through Section 1902(r)(2) and Section 1931 of the Social Security Act will be considered optional populations. Finally, expansion populations may be covered through the cost-saving achieved through a HIFA waiver; however, the administration has made it clear that states applying for a HIFA waiver must demonstrate that the states has a high level of uninsured under 200 percent of the FPL.[84] Table 2.9 lists some of the Medicaid populations that fall into these categories.

Table 2.9
Medicaid Populations in HIFA Categories

Category	Eligibles
Mandatory Populations	• Infants up to age one under 185 percent of the FPL • Children and pregnant women up to 133 percent of the FPL • Children between the ages of 6 and 18 under 100 percent of the FPL • Section 1931 recipients: low-income families with children who meet that State's AFDC plan requirements as of July 16, 1996 • SSI Recipients • Recipients of Adoption Assistance and Foster Care under Title IV-E of the Social Security Act
Optional Populations	• Children covered under Medicaid above the mandatory levels stated above • Children covered under the SCHIP program • Parents covered under Medicaid Section 1931 (excluding those defined as mandatory) • Parents covered under SCHIP • Recipients of State Supplemental Payments • Certain disabled and elderly individuals with incomes greater than SSI eligibility levels as defined by the state • disabled and elderly individuals who qualify through Home and Community-based service • Low-income, uninsured women screened and diagnosed with through a Center for Disease Control Early Detection Program and in need of treatment for breast or cervical cancer • Beneficiary groups of Ticket to Work and Work Incentives Improvement of 1999 • Medically needy as defined by individual states
Expansion Populations	• Childless non-disabled adults • Pregnant women above age 19 covered by SCHIP • Parents outside family coverage in SCHIP

Adapted from: Jennifer M. Ryan, "Health Insurance Family Style: Public Approaches to Reaching the Uninsured." Issue Brief No. 767 (Washington, D.C.: National Health Policy Forum, September 24, 2001), p. 7; and Centers for Medicare and Medicaid Services, *Medicaid Eligibility*. Online. Available: http://hcfa.hhs.gov/medicaid/meligib.htm. Accessed: September 5, 2001; and John Holahan, "Restructuring Medicaid Financing: Implications of the NGA Proposal" (Washington, D.C.: The Henry J. Kaiser Family Foundation, 2001), p. 3.

Defining the Benefits

The HIFA language explicitly gives states the authority to modify the benefit packages offered to the optional Medicaid and SCHIP recipients. The HIFA guidance describes the minimum benefits that must be offered to optional Medicaid and SCHIP children; these requirements coincide with the packages listed for SCHIP under Title XXI. The benefits listed for other optional populations are less rigid stating that they should include basic service including inpatient and outpatient hospital services, physician surgical and medical services, laboratory and x-ray services, well-baby and well-child care including age appropriate immunizations.[85] Thirty-three optional services are available to states through state plan amendments.[86]

Through HIFA, states are given more flexibility in the design of the benefit packages for expansion populations. CMS describes this package as a basic primary care package that must include "services customarily furnished by or through a general practitioner, family physician, internal medicine physician, obstetrician/gynecologist, or pediatrician."[87] However, the flexibility granted for expansion population benefit packages is limited; the Secretary of the Department of Health and Human Services must approve the package, which must be comprehensive enough to illustrate consistency with the goals of the HIFA demonstration initiative.[88] This initiative's principle purpose is to decrease the number of uninsured citizen in the United States. HIFA waivers are consistent with other Section 1115 waivers in that the cost of adding the expansion populations to the state Medicaid program must not exceed the cost of the program without the waiver; this, of course, is known as budget neutrality.

Cost-Sharing

Cost-sharing for all mandatory populations applied through the HIFA waiver initiative must continue to be the nominal amounts described in federal regulation. Similar to SCHIP guidance issued in June 2001, cost-sharing imposed on optional children receiving either the Medicaid or SCHIP benefits is not allowed to exceed five percent of the family's income per child. A caveat to this limitation remains, states are allowed to define the level of cost-sharing imposed upon the other optional and expansion populations. Therefore, the state has potentially the unfettered ability to impose higher levels of cost-sharing upon the parents of the children whose cost-sharing is limited to five percent.

Low-income families could potentially thus spend a large percentage of their income on cost-sharing for adults receiving health care benefits. This policy may have the unintended consequence of discouraging entire families from enrolling in programs if they realize the potentially detrimental effects of high levels of cost-sharing. This could also have the negative effect of keeping parents and children out of the same health care program. Research has shown that children are more likely to have higher take-up rates of public health care benefits, if the program's benefits are also available to their parents.[89] Defining cost-sharing will be a potentially difficult obstacle for states that choose to attempt to obtain HIFA waivers. Cost-sharing can create savings through revenue and the responsibility that it places on health care recipients to monitor their utilization, but it may also discourage those truly in need from accessing health care.

Private Insurance

President Bush has been a strong supporter of private insurance options; two of three ways that he promised to support health care during his presidency are directly related to private insurance. Early in his presidency, refundable tax-credits were proposed to reach nearly six million of the uninsured.[90] Nothing has been enacted on this front but the issue was a point of contention during the economic stimulus talks of late 2001 and has returned in the president's budget for FFY 2003. The other way that the Bush Administration has advocated for private health insurance is through the HIFA initiative. The second goal listed in the HIFA guidance assures states that the administration will work with states to create flexible programs that utilize private insurance options.

The HIFA guidance maintains that the administration strongly encourages states to create proposals that work to further integrate, or minimally coordinate, Medicaid and SCHIP with private health care options available in the states.[91] By permitting more flexibility within the optional and mandatory population's benefits and cost-sharing, the Secretary of DHHS will also support premium assistance programs that are based upon private health plans. No specific cost effectiveness test for premium assistance programs will be enforced, as has been the case in the past. Instead the programs will be tested as part of the comprehensive waiver program that aims to decrease the number of uninsured in the state below 200 percent of the FPL. An overall test of budget neutrality will be used to determine whether the cost of both the premium assistance program and other reforms proposed by the state are less than the direct cost of the Medicaid program without the waiver in place.

Allowing states to cover low-income individuals through employer-sponsored insurance through employer buy-in programs is a lynchpin of the HIFA initiative. According to the report *State of the States* the partnering of states and the private sector through an employer buy-in is "a win-win technique for the states."[92] The report contends that the state and private employer can share the cost of insuring a low-income employee through the employer-based system. This concept is politically popular with both the states, who are working to decrease the number of low-income individuals in their states, and the employers, who want to provide benefits but are unable to fully finance increasingly costly health insurance benefits.[93] Further, buy-ins help to provide single insurance plans for an entire family and encourage continuity of coverage for those who may cycle on and off a more traditional Medicaid program.

Simplifying the Waiver Application

An important change added to help simplify the waiver process is the availability of an online application template. States are encouraged to use the standardized online application available through the CMS website. The use of a standardized form is different than past procedure related to Section 1115 waivers. Historically, states were required to create their own application when applying a waiver, with DHHS taking the stance that a standardized Section 1115 application would hinder states' flexibility. On the other hand, a template, like the one used for the HIFA initiative, helps to demystify the Section 1115 application process and provide states with a framework to help them conceptualize what they must do to obtain a waiver.

Accountability

The HIFA initiative guidance also specifically states its desire to increase the accountability of the federal and state partnership by ensuring that Medicaid and SCHIP are being used effectively to promote the goal of reducing the number of uninsured individuals. In the past, the federal and state governments have not always collaborated in the design and implementation of the Medicaid and SCHIP programs. States have found loopholes in federal statutes to draw down billions, while the federal government has forced unfunded mandates upon the states. Acknowledging that the federal and state governments play an essential role in the success of a Medicaid and/or SCHIP expansion is both an important policy and rhetorical statement. The states need assurance that the federal government, for the length of the waiver, will support the decisions that they make especially during fiscally difficult times. Further, the federal government must feel comfortable "bending" the rules of Medicaid for the individual state. Accountability is key to successfully implementing state-level reforms in programs based upon the principles of federalism.

Priority Review

DHHS has promised that states that apply for a Section 1115 waiver through the HIFA initiative will experience expedited review of their waiver proposal. States that use the HIFA template will be granted priority review. In the case of the Arizona HIFA waiver, the only one submitted and approved thus far, the review process has moved swiftly. Arizona submitted their HIFA waiver September 18, 2001, and received approval less than three month later on December 12, 2001. Past waiver applications have typically taken at least six months and often longer to be approved by the Secretary of DHHS.

HIFA's Opponents

Many groups are skeptical of this initiative calling it a zero-sum gain for states and for the administration. Tim Westmoreland, Counsel for Representative Henry Waxman (D-CA) and former Director of Medicaid and State Operations at HCFA and a state health advocate, argues that through HIFA, "The only way to increase coverage is to cut benefits or raise cost-sharing for current beneficiaries and if states don't do that there isn't any more (money) there for expansions."[94]

Health care advocates have publicly criticized the program because it permits states to decrease benefits and add cost-sharing elements to Medicaid coverage received by optional groups of low-income individuals in order to save money to insure new individuals referred to as the expansion population. Opponents of the plan argue that lessening the benefits will cause hardship and reduce quality of health care for a needy population. Those in favor of the initiative believe that HIFA will give states a concrete means to insure more individuals using creative strategies.[95]

Prospects for a Section 1115 waiver in Texas

The uninsured in Texas could benefit if it chose to pursue an 1115 HIFA demonstration waiver, as it would allow Texas to cover childless adults, a group that can only be covered through Medicaid with the aid of a Section 1115 waiver. In the mid-1990s, Texas tried unsuccessfully to obtain an 1115 waiver but never received final approval of either proposal submitted. An 1115 waiver may be the only way that Texas will be able to insure certain individuals, but if Texas is to pursue such a waiver, increases in cost-sharing and reduction of benefits would have to be carefully analyzed. As many advocates have pointed out, the zero-sum nature of the HIFA initiative has the potential to help more than harm, especially since Texas is a step behind the health care expansions that have occurred in other states. Texas has not covered many of its very low-income through its Medicaid program; thus, the state must be aware of the potential implications of high cost-sharing and the basic of benefit packages on populations that will not be able to pay cost-sharing or afford services not offered through the basic package.

On the other hand, since Texas has not insured many of the optional populations designated in federal statute, it may be able to create a HIFA waiver that uses this to its advantage. The next section describes how Texas can bring in a new optional population (parents) through a Section 1931 state plan amendment and then use the increased federal cost to the state's advantage when projecting budget neutrality for a subsequent HIFA waiver. One benefit to this approach would be that no populations currently receiving Medicaid packages would experience benefit reductions.

Texas and the Bush Administration

Understanding the Bush HIFA initiative is important as it provides clues as to how the administration plans to approach Section 1115 waivers. Thus far, the Bush Administration has taken an extremely active and accountable role in the waiver process. Hundreds of other programmatic waivers have been processed and approved since President Bush took office in January 2001. Texas should utilize this information when constructing an 1115 waiver, by having an open dialogue with CMS throughout the waiver process. The state is also in an amiable position being the home state of the President; as the former Governor of Texas, George W. Bush knows the State's position in relation to the uninsured. As a result, Texas may be more likely to propose programs that push the envelope with its waiver proposal and receive direct feedback on these proposals because of the Administration's ties to the State. A more open dialogue with the federal government may prove helpful when deciding whether or not to pursue a HIFA waiver or even the traditional Section 1115 waiver.

Estimating the Cost of Expansion

Before any attempts to expand coverage to low-income parents and childless adults, the state must be able to estimate clearly the cost of such an initiative, especially in the current tenuous budget climate. Several components must come together to produce an accurate cost estimate for each year of the expansion. The essential equation for such a calculation is:

Cost in Year X = State match rate x Number of eligible people x Participation Rate x Phase-in Factor for Year X x Cost per participant in base year x Inflation factor[96]

State Match Rate

The Texas Federal Medical Assistance Percentage (FMAP) for FY 2003 is 59.99 percent, and the enhanced SCHIP match is 71.99 percent. This means that Texas receives 59.99 cents back from the federal government for every dollar that it spends on its Medicaid program and 71.99 cents for every dollar that it spends on SCHIP. Medicaid is an entitlement program; this means that there is no limit to the amount that the federal government will match the Texas dollars. In contrast, SCHIP is a capped entitlement; Texas is limited in the number of dollars that it can draw down by its designated SCHIP allotment. State officials are tight-lipped concerning the amount of excess SCHIP allotment; therefore, most of the proposed models here will utilize Medicaid financing.

Number of Eligible People

Computing an estimate of the number of people eligible for expansion can be calculated through survey data. Using the Census Bureau's Current Population Survey (CPS), it is possible to estimate the number of individuals in the range of an expansion based on their income and also estimate how many of those individuals are uninsured. Two the advantages of using March CPS data are that the survey consists of a large sample of households and that is designed to produce state-level estimates. A second advantage is that the survey is available on a timely and regular basis, providing information for many key socio-demographic subgroups of the population.[97]

When estimating the number of the uninsured, CPS data is often averaged over three years to improve the stability of the data.[98, 99] Table 2.10 provides an estimate of the total number of Uninsured Parents by income. Table 2.11 provides similar estimates for childless adults.

Table 2.10
Total Number of Uninsured Parents by Income in Texas

Percent of the Federal Poverty Level	Number of Uninsured Parents
Under 50%	74,299
50 - 99%	211,814
100 - 149%	185,862
150 - 199%	152,252
200 - 249%	120,925
250% or higher	135,381
Total	880,532

Adapted from: U.S. Department of Labor, Bureau of Labor Statistics, *1999 March Current Population Survey*. Online. Available: http://www.bls.census.gov/cps/cpsmain.htm. Accessed: April 8, 2002; U.S. Department of Labor, Bureau of Labor Statistics, *2000 March Current Population Survey*. Online. Available: http://www.bls.census.gov/cps/cpsmain.htm. Accessed: April 8, 2002; and U.S. Department of Labor, Bureau of Labor Statistics, *2001 March Current Population Survey*. Online. Available: http://www.bls.census.gov/cps/cpsmain.htm. Accessed: April 8, 2002.

Table 2.11
Total Number of Adults Under 65 with no Children under Age 18 by Income in Texas

Percent of the Federal Poverty Level	Number of Childless Adults
Under 50%	243,428
50 - 99%	224,736
100 - 149%	322,016
150 - 199%	268,065
200 - 249%	262,369
250% or Higher	853,707
Total	2,174,320

Adapted from: U.S. Department of Labor, Bureau of Labor Statistics, *1999 March Current Population Survey*. Online. Available: http://www.bls.census.gov/cps/cpsmain.htm. Accessed: April 8, 2002; U.S. Department of Labor, Bureau of Labor Statistics, *2000 March Current Population Survey*. Online. Available: http://www.bls.census.gov/cps/cpsmain.htm. Accessed: April 8, 2002; and U.S. Department of Labor, Bureau of Labor Statistics, *2001 March Current Population Survey*. Online. Available: http://www.bls.census.gov/cps/cpsmain.htm. Accessed: April 8, 2002.

The uninsured population estimate of those who qualify should be further refined through application of the policy rules such as income disregards, assets tests, immigrant status, and number of years living the U.S. In a high immigration state like Texas, it is necessary to subtract recent immigrants from the eligibility count to properly estimate the cost of a waiver, since the federal government does not provide federal match for legal immigrants living in the U.S. less than five years.[100] Since CPS provides information on the year of entry, an estimate of the percentage of the total immigrant population that entered the United States less than five years ago can be made. This percentage can then be used to determine those who should be excluded from the waiver because of federal Medicaid law. In this model, it was assumed that 50 percent of the foreign-born are undocumented aliens; the use of this assumption compensates for the insufficient information collected by the CPS pertaining to the legal status of the foreign-born population. The assumption is consistent with estimates used by the Urban Institute.[101]

The CPS is not a faultless estimator; generally, researchers agree that it tends to overestimate the number of the uninsured. It is important to note the disadvantages of the CPS data, as they also tend to reflect the health care coverage status of the population in the month of March, the month when the telephone and personal surveys are administered. Some researchers argue that the March CPS does not accurately represent the insurance status of the population over an entire year, as many assume it does. In fact, CPS data estimate that the number of persons covered by Medicaid during the previous year are lower than what actual Medicaid program records maintained by the state over the same time period, but the same CPS estimates come reasonably close in comparison to the actual number of persons that were covered by Medicaid as of the month of March.

Population growth can also be factored into the eligibility estimates but were not included in the model presented, which attempts to achieve budget neutrality over five years. Table 2.12 and Table 2.13 estimate the number of documented immigrants and citizen uninsured parents and childless adults, respectively, eligible for Medicaid. These are the numbers used in the model to represent those eligible for the Medicaid waiver.[102]

Table 2.12
Documented and U.S. Citizen Uninsured Parents Eligible for Medicaid Expansion by Income

Percent of the Federal Poverty Level	Number of Uninsured Parents
Under 50%	58,029
50 - 99%	176,256
100 - 149%	150,070
150 - 199%	125,243
200 - 249%	99,129
250% or Higher	99,448
Total	708,175

Adapted from: U.S. Department of Labor, Bureau of Labor Statistics, *1999 March Current Population Survey*. Online. Available: http://www.bls.census.gov/cps/cpsmain.htm. Accessed: April 8, 2002; U.S. Department of Labor, Bureau of Labor Statistics, *2000 March Current Population Survey*. Online. Available: http://www.bls.census.gov/cps/cpsmain.htm. Accessed: April 8, 2002; and U.S. Department of Labor, Bureau of Labor Statistics, *2001 March Current Population Survey*. Online. Available: http://www.bls.census.gov/cps/cpsmain.htm. Accessed: April 8, 2002.

Table 2.13
Documented and U.S. Citizen Uninsured Adults with no Children Under Age 18 Eligible for Medicaid Expansion by Income

Percent of the Federal Poverty Level	Number of Uninsured Childless Adults
Under 50%	199,176
50 - 99%	129,025
100 - 149%	224,432
150 - 199%	195,003
200 - 249%	203,497
250% or Higher	757,277
Total	1,708,410

Adapted from: U.S. Department of Labor, Bureau of Labor Statistics, *1999 March Current Population Survey*. Online. Available: http://www.bls.census.gov/cps/cpsmain.htm. Accessed: April 8, 2002; U.S. Department of Labor, Bureau of Labor Statistics, *2000 March Current Population Survey*. Online. Available: http://www.bls.census.gov/cps/cpsmain.htm. Accessed: April 8, 2002; and U.S. Department of Labor, Bureau of Labor Statistics, *2001 March Current Population Survey*. Online. Available: http://www.bls.census.gov/cps/cpsmain.htm. Accessed: April 8, 2002.

Participation Rate

The participation rate aims to identify those who are uninsured that will participate in the program. Research by the Urban Institute has shown that between 50 to 70 percent of eligible parents that are uninsured would participate in a free Medicaid expansion.[103] Cost-sharing requirements are often used to deter recipients from enrolling and utilizing unneeded services. States, who utilize cost-sharing requirements, must strike a balance by setting rates that do not deter recipients from preventative services but function to help eliminate improper use of certain health care services (i.e., emergency room visits for non-emergency events). Furthermore, cost-sharing can be used to instill a sense of responsibility in recipients and help to eliminate the "welfare stigma" associated with public assistance programs.

When contemplating cost-sharing requirements, the state should recognize the administrative burden of implementing any cost-sharing. Some states have created cost-sharing program based upon a monthly premium system. Premiums are used to offset the cost of the program, and actual cost-sharing is used to deter utilization. Either way, the state must create an administratively feasible system to collect and account for payments received through cost-sharing mechanisms.

As Table 2.14 shows, research indicates that the greater the co-payment the less likely a parent is likely to take-up the Medicaid program. The models put forth in this paper use three participation rates estimates based on this research, as participation rates are calculated based upon cost-sharing levels. First, the assumption is made that if there is no cost-sharing there would be a 67 percent take-up rate. Second, it is assumed that if a 2 percent of family income cost-sharing requirement is imposed, a 45 percent take-up rate would result. Finally, a 5 percent of family income cost-sharing rate is estimated to lead to a 17 percent participation rate.[104]

Table 2.14
Participation Rate Estimation based on Cost-Sharing

Cost of Recipient Premiums as a Percent of Family Income	Estimated Participation Rate
0% of income	67%
1%	57%
2%	45%
3%	34%
4%	25%
5%	17%
6%	12%
7%	8%
8%	5%
9%	3%
10%	2%

Adapted from: Leighton Ku and Teresa Coughlin, "Sliding Scale Premiums: Four States' Experiences," *Inquiry*, vol. 36, no. 4, pp. 471-80 (Rochester, MN: Blue Cross and Blue Shield Association, 2000), p. 476.

Participation rates are also affected by several aspects pertaining to the administration of the program including: assets test, public acceptance of the program: the degree of the "welfare stigma," the length of application, difficulty of the application process, outreach, and other barriers to enrollment.

Of this set of variables that have potential impact upon the participation rate, it is necessary to specifically address the assets test in Texas. The State of Texas requires that most Medicaid households not have countable assets greater than $2,000. In the model utilized within this paper, an assets test is not applied to the expansion adults. The expansion populations that could potentially receive benefits through any of the expansion models discussed below would not receive full adult Medicaid benefit coverage, and with this in mind, the assets test was eliminated.[105, 106]

Another consideration to make when increasing the number of adults covered through Medicaid and SCHIP is the effect on children's enrollment when an adult expansion occurs. An increasing number of researchers have uncovered a trend that suggests extending coverage to parents may have the effect of increasing the number of eligible children enrolled in Medicaid and SCHIP. The Urban Institute, the Commonwealth Fund, and the Center on Budget and Policy Priorities have all found indications that extending coverage to parents may lead to the enrollment of eligible children.[107] If this were to prove true, the state would need to adjust children's Medicaid and SCHIP cost projections upward (this assumption was not included in our model).

Phase-In Factors

The cost of the expansion program is phased in rather than budgeted for a fully functioning program from its initiation. Expansion programs, as was the case with

SCHIP, take time, effort, and outreach to enroll those eligible in the program. Since the offices administering Medicaid and SCHIP may already have information pertaining to families with previously enrolled children in many expansion families, the enrollment process should be expedited.

For the sake of simplicity, a three-year phase-in was applied to the model. This estimate acknowledges that any expansion program will not be an overnight success. To reach the predicted participation rate in three years, some outreach and enrollment procedures will have to be strategically planned and implemented. The Texas CHIP Program, which utilized an extensive outreach and enrollment programs, was serving most of its target population within a year and a half of implementation.

Cost per Participant

The cost of providing Medicaid to non-pregnant, non-elderly, non-disabled adults in Texas cost approximately $253 per member per month, which totals $3,036 per person for State Fiscal Year (SFY) 2002.[108] This is the average acute care, which includes everything Medicaid covers including prescription drugs, transportation, and other services. Prescription drug costs account for approximately 20 percent of this cost, and a little over 6.5 percent of the costs are in a poorly defined category we call "cost reimbursed."[109] Approximately two dollars is also added to the monthly rate for the cost of medical transportation. The Director of Actuarial Analysis at the Texas Health and Human Services Commission stated, "There are a number of cost-related issues that would have to be considered depending on who you want to cover under Medicaid. However, the $253 is a good starting point."[110]

Inflation Factors

To find the most accurate cost estimate, an inflation factor should be applied to the proposed expansion. States are allowed to choose between two options to account for inflation. The first of these is the Medical Consumer Price Index (MCPI). The MCPI for between January 2001 and January 2002 was 5 percent and rising. The second option used to estimate inflation, which was used in the model presented, allows states to look at the historical trends for the last five years in the Medicaid program.[111] According to this standard, the Director of Actuarial Analysis at the Texas Health and Human Services Commission believes that the most accurate overall trend to use is about 6 percent per year when estimating for a future year.[112] Six percent is a more conservative estimate and was, therefore, used in this model

Model for Expansion

The assumptions discussed in this paper are the basis for a model for expansion, which aims to reduce the number of uninsured in Texas (see Figure 2.1). The model takes a three-part approach. Figure 2.1 provides a visual representation of this process. The first step in the model to expand Medicaid to adults in Texas proposes that the state contemplate a Section 1931 expansion. This type of expansion only requires a state plan amendment and entitles full Medicaid benefits to all parents of children under age 19 up to a specific income. The hypothetical plan would offer the current Texas benefit plan of the Medicaid program and not impose any new forms of cost-sharing. Although it should be noted that the state will not actually pursue a Section 1931 expansion unless the rest of the expansion plan is enacted; therefore, this expansion concept is often referred to as a hypothetical 1931. The hypothetical expansion would not require a waiver but would effectively serve as the "without the waiver" expenditure projection in a test for the budget neutrality when a Section 1115 waiver is proposed in the next steps in the model.[113]

Figure 2.1
List of Assumptions Applied to the Three-part Approach to Expansion

Matching Rate
- Texas Federal Match Rate $.5999 for 2002
- State pays $.401 for every Medicaid dollar spent
- Used Same Rate for all five years of the waiver

Number of Eligibles
- Used March CPS averaged over three years
- Eliminated those not eligible for federal match

Participation Rate
- 0%, 2%, and 5% of family income cost-sharing and utilized participation rates of 67%, 45%, and 17%, respectively
- Based on research published by Inquiry journal
- Assets test not applied

Phase-in Factor
- Used three year phase-in over five years: 50%, 75%, and 87.5% of population expected to participate

Cost per Participant
- The cost of providing Medicaid to non-pregnant, non-elderly, non-disabled adults through Medicaid Managed Care will cost approximately $253 per member per month
- $3,036 per person for State Fiscal Year 2002
- Average acute care estimate, which includes every thing adult Medicaid offers including drugs and transportation

Inflation Factors
- 6 %, which looks at the historical inflation trends in Medicaid the past five years

The second step in the expansion process has the state propose a HIFA Section 1115 waiver. This would allow Texas to create a reduced package and impose higher levels of cost-sharing on recipients. For example, Texas could request a waiver to limit the extent of coverage for specific benefits. CMS describes the minimum requirements for a HIFA package as a basic primary care package that must include "services customarily furnished by or through a general practitioner, family physician, internal medicine physician, obstetrician/gynecologist, or pediatrician."[114] The federal Medicaid program offers states the choice of implementing 33 optional benefits to all populations served by Medicaid and of these benefits; Texas offers 21 optional services to adult participants.[115] Table 2.15 lists optional benefits offered by Texas that are offered by less than two-thirds of the states. Texas could use this information to analyze the needs of certain optional populations and apply to waive the requirement that optional populations must receive the same benefits as mandatory populations.

Table 2.15
Optional Benefits offered in Texas Available in Less than Two-Thirds of the States

Optional Benefit	Number of States Offering the Benefit
Chiropractic Services	27
Psychological Services	27
Nurse Anesthetists	23
Medical Social Worker Services	7
Emergency Room Hospital Services	31
Preventive Services	28
Personal Care Services	31
Respiratory Care Services	15
Christian Science Sanitariums	13

Families USA, "The Current Medicaid Federal-State Partnership: Already a Good Deal for the States," (Washington, D.C., August 2001), p. 2.

The other area in which the HIFA waivers pledge flexibility is in cost-sharing. Texas could create savings through the cost-sharing revenue and add this to the budget neutral component the waiver. According to the HIFA guidance, it is possible for states to impose a higher level of cost-sharing on optional and expansion populations.

The final step in this approach utilizes the savings from the reduced benefit package and cost-sharing to offer Medicaid benefits to childless adults under a set income. The package offered to these individuals would parallel the reduced benefit package with cost-sharing offered to the newly covered Section 1931 expansion population. It would also be possible to cap the number of people covered under this expansion, unlike the Section 1931 expansion, to control state costs.

Finally, it is important to note that if the proposed waiver were not approved, the state would not have to go ahead with the hypothetical Section 1931 expansion through a state plan amendment. This approach discussed in this paper has never been approved by CMS, but it builds upon precedent in past waiver proposals and the new HIFA guidance. This approach would give a large number of low-income Texans health insurance. Although, it does not provide the traditional rich Medicaid benefit package, it does not take coverage for any services away from any current Medicaid eligibility groups; rather, it extends coverage to those without health insurance.

Figure 2.2
Proposed Approach to Expansion

Hypothetical Section 1931 Expansion to Parents

↓

Propose a HIFA waiver Reducing Benefits and Applying Cost-Sharing to this Newly Covered Population

↓

Propose a HIFA waiver to Expand a Reduced Benefits Package and Cost-Sharing to Uninsured Childless Adults

Adapted from: Charles Milligan, "Section 1115 Waivers and Budget Neutrality: Using Medicaid Funds to Expand Coverage" (Washington, D.C.: State Coverage Initiatives of the Robert Wood Johnson Foundation, 2001), p. 4.

Possible Medicaid Benefit Packages Using Model

By utilizing the approach described above, Texas would be able to offer uninsured parents and childless adults access to health care coverage. Depending upon the amount of money the state chooses to budget for an expansion, the populations that it explicitly chooses to cover and the cost-sharing that it plans to impose, Texas has a range of options using the aforementioned Medicaid expansion model. Table 2.16 lists several of these options. The first column describes the ratio of the percent of the FPL covered by the Section 1931 expansion (parents) to the percent of the FPL covered by the Section 1115 waiver (childless adults); it also indicates the amount of cost-sharing imposed as a percentage of family income, which affects both the percent of uninsured who choose to participate in the expansion and the amount of state revenue needed depending upon how cost-sharing is applied.

The second column in Table 2.16 represents the percentage of the full Medicaid benefit package that Texas can offer parents and childless adults who qualify based on each particular scenario. This percentage is found by dividing the cost of the Section 1931 expansion (parents) by the cost of the Section 1931 expansion (parents) plus the Section 1115 waiver expansion (childless adults). The equation follows in Figure 2.3:

Figure 2.3
Percentage of Benefits Package in relation to Mandated TANF Adults

Cost of offering full Section 1931 benefits / (Cost of offering full Section 1931 Benefits + Cost of offering full benefits to Childless Adults)	=	Percentage of the full benefit package per member that can be offered under the Section 1115 constraint of budget neutrality

The third column multiplies the per member per month cost of the mandated TANF Managed Care benefit package by the percentage in column two. This provides the estimated per member per month cost of the benefit package. The fourth column estimates the cost of the expansion to the state over five years using the FFY 2003 state match rate of .401 cents on each dollar. The fifth lists the amount of general revenue needed in the next biennium to begin funding the expansion. Finally, the sixth column provides an estimate of how many Texans would be covered under each of the scenarios described in the table.

Table 2.16
Selected Models of a HIFA Medicaid Waiver in Texas

FPL of Parents/ FPL of Childless Adults: Cost-sharing Imposed	Percent of Benefits Package in relation to Mandated TANF Adult	Per Member per Month Premium	Amount of State Revenue Needed over Five Years	Amount of State Revenue Needed for the Next Biennium	Number of Uninsured Texans Covered
100/50: 0%	54.05%	$136.75	$958,482,000	$360,197,000	290,419
150/50: 0%	65.87%	$166.64	$1,572,433,000	$590,920,000	390,966
200/50: 0%	71.90%	$181.90	$2,084,811,000	$783,472,000	474,879
200/100: 0%	60.83%	$153.89	$2,084,811,000	$783,472,000	561,325
100/50: 2%	54.05%	$136.75	$643,756,000	$241,924,000	195,058
150/50: 2%	65.87%	$166.64	$1,056,112,000	$369,887,000	262,589
200/50: 2%	71.90%	$181.90	$1,400,246,000	$526,212,000	318,948
200/100: 2%	60.83%	$153.89	$1,400,246,000	$526,212,000	377,010
100/50: 5%	54.05%	$136.75	$243,197,000	$91,393,000	73,688
150/50: 5 %	65.87%	$166.64	$398,976,000	$149,935,000	99,200
200/50: 5%	71.90%	$181.90	$528,982,000	$198,792,000	120,492
200/100: 5%	60.83%	$153.89	$528,982,000	$198,792,000	142,426

Note: Calculations for each column explained above.

Analysis of the Benefit Packages

None of the benefit packages found in Table 2.16 are as rich as the mandatory package offered through Medicaid, but some of the packages allow the Medicaid program to offer more benefits than others. The decision about how to best apply this model should not rely solely on the size of the benefit package. When cost-sharing is imposed on the expansion population, the cost to the state decreases. This occurs for two reasons. First, the percentage of the uninsured choosing to take-up the program increases if as less cost-sharing is imposed. (Participation rates decrease as cost-sharing increases.) Second, the cost of the expansion is reduced by premiums paid in by those enrolled in the program.

If Texas chooses to cover more parents through a Section 1931 expansion, it will be able to offer a better benefit package to parents and childless adults. Conversely, covering more childless adults reduces the funds available to purchase each benefit package. For example, covering parents up to 200 percent of the FPL and childless adults up to 50 percent of the FPL with no cost-sharing allows the state to offer a benefit package that is nearly 72 percent of the mandatory package, but by increasing the number of childless adults covered in the expansion up to 100 percent of the FPL the package reduces to 61 percent. Either of these packages would cost the state same amount of general revenue, but the latter would cover more individuals with less comprehensive services than the former. Thus, if the state were to adopt a model similar to those described above, it would have to decide upon the amount benefits it would be willing to offer and to which expansion populations.

It is important to note that in the Medicaid model described above two financing mechanisms are not utilized. First, no DSH reductions are being proposed. In this waiver, no DSH funds will be used to create a budget neutral waiver. Second, the waiver model does not attempt to redistribute the SCHIP allocation. The next section of this paper highlights how a SCHIP waiver could possibly be implemented.

Achievement of budget neutrality in the Medicaid waiver described above depends only on benefit reductions and cost-sharing. Again, it should also be noted that those receiving reduced benefit packages though this model are currently uninsured; no benefits are taken from those currently receiving Medicaid in Texas.

Possible SCHIP Benefit Packages Models through HIFA

Another possible option is for the Texas to apply for a HIFA waiver using the excess funds from its SCHIP allocation. This option is complicated by the fact that the amount of excess SCHIP funds that the state has access to has not been released. In a conversation with a state SCHIP official, it was disclosed that there are some excess allotment funds, but the Texas Health and Human Services Commission believes that, using "a rather conservative estimate," it will be using all of the current federal annual allotment and carry-forward funds by SFY 2007. At that point, the projected annual federal allotment might not be adequate.[116] If Texas starts to use federal funds for other purposes, such as insuring parents and childless adults, this money would run out sooner. Thus, it is difficult to estimate how much federal allotment Texas will have at specific points in time and whether it would be feasible to use the federal allotment to expand health care coverage to parents and childless adults.

SCHIP Waiver Guidelines

The possibility of devising a SCHIP HIFA waiver is further complicated by guidelines set for a state pursuing a SCHIP waiver during the Clinton Administration.[117] As mentioned previously in this paper, Texas has not technically met the guidelines set in July 2000 in order to be deemed eligible to apply for a SCHIP waiver. Again, these requirements include:

1. Use a joint mail-in application and common application process for SCHIP and Medicaid;
2. Eliminate assets tests;
3. Have 12-month continuous eligibility;
4. Have presumptive eligibility; and/or
5. Have simplified procedures for redetermination of coverage; so it can be done through the mail, and have a seamless system in which participants can shift between SCHIP and Medicaid without a new application or lapse in coverage.

Texas has only truly met one of the simplification requirements, the joint mail-in application and common application process, out of a possible five that enable a state to apply for a Section 1115 SCHIP waiver. Until Texas meets at least three of these requirements, SCHIP waivers are not an option.

On the other hand, an argument could be made that since current state law states that 12-month continuous eligibility will be phased in as early as September 2002 and no later than June 2003 that Texas has met the 12-month continuous eligibility guideline. Texas continues to work on setting-up a simplified redetermination process, but the state has faced many obstacles on this front. As part of Senate Bill 43, the Medicaid simplification bill, in the 77th Legislature, parents who enroll their children in Medicaid are required to go through a process known as a Health Care Orientation (HCO). HCOs did not exist prior to the Medicaid simplification bill. The promulgated rule for the HCOs leaves open the possibility of required face-to-face Medicaid renewal. Again, depending upon how the rule is interpreted, Texas may, as the guideline states, "be creating a simplified procedures for redetermination so it can be done through the mail." Thus, how the current administration reads these guidelines will determine whether Texas can be deemed eligible for a SCHIP waiver by officially meeting one of the guidelines and creatively meeting two others. With these technicalities in mind, a model for a SCHIP Section 1115 HIFA waiver is described in the following paragraphs.

Amount of SCHIP Allotment being Utilized

SCHIP waivers are different than Medicaid waivers because budget neutrality is contained by the capped SCHIP allotment. Following the creation of SCHIP by the federal government, Texas was slow in creating and implementing their SCHIP program.

In FFY 1998, the state spent only 0.2 percent of its allotment. Allotment expenditures the next two years were 6.9 percent and 8.2 percent, respectively. Then, expenditures soared with the State utilizing an estimated 60 percent of the federal allotment in FFY 2001.[118] In FFY 2002 states' federal SCHIP allocations begin a three-year dip, and Texas is slated to have SCHIP expenditures that are 135.9 percent of the FFY 2002 allotment.[119] Therefore, Texas will have to tap into its unused allotments from previous years to cover children on the program. This will further reduce the amount of money available to cover parents though SCHIP funding.

Description of Possible Models

With all this in mind, the following is an explanation of several possible models that Texas could utilize to apply for a SCHIP Section 1115 waiver through the HIFA initiative. At this point in time, the amount of unused federal funds available for the next several years is not clear. Thus, this paper simply outlines options and what they would cost not whether or not they are fiscally feasible.

Table 2.17 lists several possible parameters of a HIFA SCHIP waiver in Texas. The first column designates the income cap placed on the parents to be covered through the expansion. It is followed in the second column by the cap for childless adults to be covered by the waiver. These groups correspond to those in the Medicaid HIFA model described above. The Texas could choose any income level cap for either group as long as the state had the funds through match and federal allotment to pay for the expansion.

The third column lists potential levels of cost-sharing to impose upon each group. Again these were used in this example because they correspond with the information presented in the illustration of a possible Medicaid waiver. Texas could choose other values, apply different cost-sharing to different group, or apply cost-sharing on a sliding-scale based upon income. The fourth column presents the amount of State revenue needed over five years to implement a waiver without any reduction to the full Medicaid benefit package given to TANF adults. This number assumes that there is enough federal SCHIP allotment to cover the expansion, but this issue has not been fully investigated in this research. The fifth column provides an estimate of the number of uninsured Texans that will receive coverage based on each set of variables.

Table 2.17
Possible Models of a HIFA SCHIP Waiver in Texas

FPL of Parents	FPL of Childless Adults	Cost-Sharing Imposed	Amount of State Revenue Needed over Five Years without Benefit Reduction*	Number of Uninsured Texans Covered
100%	50%	0%	$1,238,676,000	290,419
150%	50%	0%	$1,667,524,000	390,966
200%	50%	0%	$2,025,422,000	474,879
200%	100%	0%	$2,394,129,000	561,325
100%	50%	2%	$831,947,000	195,058
150%	50%	2%	$1,119,979,000	262,589
200%	50%	2%	$1,360,358,000	318,948
200%	100%	2%	$1,607,997,000	377,010
100%	50%	5%	$314,291,000	73,688
150%	50%	5%	$423,103,000	99,200
200%	50%	5%	$513,913,000	120,492
200%	100%	5%	$607,465,000	142,426

Note: Calculations for each column explained above.

* Revenue numbers are rounded to the nearest thousand dollars.

The state cost of a HIFA SCHIP waiver is further delineated in Table 2.18. The first column describes the FPL of the parents and the FPL of childless adults included in the waiver. The percentage of cost-sharing imposed on recipients is also listed. Again, the application of cost-sharing does not have to be the same on all individuals, but it is in these scenarios. The second column simply lists the cost Texas using the parameters listed in the first column. This data coincides with that listed in the fourth column of Table 2.17.

A benefit package reduction is applied to the traditional TANF adult package by the percent in the third column. The percentage represents the reduction in the cost of the benefit package. Unlike the Medicaid model described, Texas has more control over the amount of the benefit package reduction, since it can simply add childless adults without devising a method to prove its budget neutrality, if there was federal SCHIP allotment available to cover the expansion. Next, the fourth column presents the state cost of offering the reduced benefit package to the specified population. Finally, the fifth column restates the number of uninsured Texans covered by each scenario.

Covering uninsured adults through a reduced benefit package utilizing SCHIP funds has tremendous potential; although before such an expansion can be undertaken, more information is needed. State employees and legislators must work together to project how many children will be covered in the future and what cost. Once this is soundly estimated, discussion may begin on the best way to expand health insurance to adults. The final section will address what issues stakeholders will have to wrestle with if they were to choose to implement a HIFA waiver through SCHIP or the Medicaid program.

Table 2.18
Cost of Possible Models of a HIFA SCHIP Waiver in Texas

FPL of Parents: FPL of Childless Adults: Cost-Sharing	State Cost without Benefit Reduction*	Benefit Reduction	State Cost with Benefit Reduction*	Number of Uninsured Texans Covered
100:50:0%	$1,238,676,000	60%	$743,206,000	290,419
150:50:0%	$1,667,524,000	60%	$1,000,514,000	390,966
200:50:0%	$2,025,423,000	60%	$1,215,253,000	474,879
200:100:0%	$2,394,129,000	60%	$1,436,477,000	561,325
100:50:0%	$1,238,676,000	70%	$867,073,000	290,419
150:50:0%	$1,667,524,000	70%	$1,167,267,000	390,966
200:50:0%	$2,025,422,000	70%	$1,417,795,000	474,879
200:100:0%	$2,394,129,000	70%	$1,675,890,000	561,325
100:50:0%	$1,238,676,000	80%	$990,941,000	290,419
150:50:0%	$1,667,524,000	80%	$1,334,019,000	390,966
200:50:0%	$2,025,422,000	80%	$1,620,337,000	474,879
200:100:0%	$2,394,129,000	80%	$1,915,303,000	561,325
100:50:2%	$831,947,000	60%	$499,168,000	195,058
150:50:2%	$1,119,979,000	60%	$671,987,000	262,589
200:50:2%	$1,360,358,000	60%	$816,214,000	318,948
200:100:2%	$1,607,997,000	60%	$964,798,000	377,010
100:50:2%	$831,947,000	70%	$582,363,000	195,058
150:50:2%	$1,119,979,000	70%	$783,985,000	262,589
200:50:2%	$1,360,358,000	70%	$952,251,000	318,948
200:100:2%	$1,607,997,000	70%	$1,125,598,000	377,010
100:50:2%	$831,947,000	80%	$665,557,000	195,058
150:50:2%	$1,119,979,000	80%	$895,983,000	262,589
200:50:2%	$1,360,358,000	80%	$1,088,286,000	318,948
200:100:2%	$1,607,997,000	80%	$1,286,397,000	377,010
100:50:5%	$314,291,000	60%	$188,574,000	73,688
150:50:5%	$423,103,000	60%	$253,862,000	99,200
200:50:5%	$513,913,000	60%	$308,348,000	120,492
200:100:5%	$607,465,000	60%	$364,479,000	142,426
100:50:5%	$314,291,000	70%	$220,004,000	73,688
150:50:5%	$423,103,000	70%	$296,172,000	99,200
200:50:5%	$513,913,000	70%	$359,739,000	120,492
200:100:5%	$607,465,000	70%	$425,226,000	142,426
100:50:5%	$314,291,000	80%	$251,433,000	73,688
150:50:5%	$423,103,000	80%	$338,482,000	99,200
200:50:5%	$513,913,000	80%	$411,130,000	120,492
200:100:5%	$607,465,000	80%	$485,972,000	142,426

Note: Calculations for each column explained above.

* Costs are rounded to the nearest thousand dollars.

The Dilemmas of Implementing a HIFA Waiver

When creating a HIFA waiver, decisions related to whether the number of people covered through public means is more valuable than the wealth of the benefit package will be arduous. Similarly, debates on the cost expansion will surely be impassioned, especially in this era with Texas facing a severe budget crisis. Legislators, county officials, hospital administrators, providers, health care advocates, and health care consumers should also be brought into this important policy discussion. This section highlights some of the difficult questions that stakeholders in Texas will face, if they choose to craft a HIFA waiver that covers the state's uninsured population.

Possible Dilemmas

Availability of State Funds

The premise of the HIFA initiative presented in this research is to expand coverage to low-income Texans, but the state's fiscal situation may inhibit many stakeholders from fully realizing the benefits of an expansion. Stakeholders will need to engage in discussion focusing on the inadequacies in the health care financing in Texas and the state's tax structure. Once the state addresses these concerns, the key decision for any health care expansion can be addressed: how much will the state of Texas be willing to spend to extend health insurance to low-income uninsured parents and childless adults?

Reduced Benefits Package

After critical funding decisions have been made, Texas stakeholders must begin to consider the merits of a reduced benefit package. Essentially, they must debate and work toward the answer of one question: What does it mean to have health insurance in Texas? The answer to this question will affect the answer to other essential questions.

- How will the Texas HIFA waiver in Texas affect access to care for its target populations and their children?
- Is minimal health care coverage for those with no health insurance better than no coverage?

Cost-sharing

Notably, the benefit package offered can be enriched through cost-sharing mechanisms. In private plans, cost-sharing is used to both reduce the cost of coverage and to produce cost consciousness among health care consumers, but as was noted in the discussion of participation rates, minimal cost-sharing among low-income populations can prevent low-income individuals from enrolling in programs offering public health insurance.[120] Thus, the following questions regarding cost-sharing arise:

- Can parents and childless adult earning less than the federal poverty level afford to share in the cost of their health care needs?

- At what income level should low-income adults be asked to contribute to their health care costs and at what level?
- How would the enactment of premiums and enrollment fees affect those who choose to participate?

All of these questions should be addressed in any discussion of the merits of cost-sharing. Some stakeholders may believe that cost-sharing is attractive for many reasons. For instance, one might argue that recipients are encouraged to participate in a program that appears more like private coverage. This point is often made in relation to Texas CHIP, which charges families a sliding scale premium to cover their children. Others might argue that cost-sharing encourages adverse selection.

In fact, the most critical question regarding cost-sharing asks whether or not healthy low-income individuals will be discouraged from enrolling in a program charging premiums? Since sick people are more willing to pay premiums than healthy people, stakeholder will need to determine whether or not premiums will result in a disproportionate number of sick people enrolling in the waiver program because, if that were to be the case, the cost of coverage per participant may elevate above the agreed-upon budget-neutral level. This would, in turn, cost the state, not the federal government.[121]

Finally, in the cost-sharing discussion, Texas must assess if cost-sharing arrangements will shift costs to providers. For instance, if recipients are not able to pay deductibles and cost-sharing will the burden be passed along to hospitals and providers who provide their care? If this is the case, hospital administrators and providers must understand the potential for this scenario and decided whether assured Medicaid reimbursement for their services to this previously uninsured population is worth the risk.

Conclusion

Throughout this report, it has become clear that trade-offs between the number of Texans covered through a HIFA expansion and the size of the benefit package will need to be addressed. Is it more important for Texas to cover more low-income uninsured adults through an expansion with a bare-bones benefit package, or is it more important to address the needs of the most vulnerable members of this population with a more comprehensive benefit package? This difficult decision must be addressed if Texas is to take advantage of the flexibility offered to states under the auspices of the HIFA initiative.

A strong commitment to financing health care policy innovation in Texas is the fundamental component of reducing the number of uninsured individuals in Texas. It is only after such a commitment is made that Texas can pursue the exciting and flexible health care policy options discussed throughout this report. Then, maybe the new era of medical care for low-income families that the Bureau of Family Services spoke of over 35 years ago can actually begin.

Notes

[1] U.S. Department of Health, Education and Welfare, Welfare Administration, Bureau of Family Services, "Medical Assistance Programs Under Title XIX of the Social Security Act," *Handbook of Public Assistance Administration, Supplement D* (Washington, D.C., 1966), Sec. D-5140.

[2] Katharine Levit, and Cynthia Smith, Cathy Cowan. Helen Lazenby, and Anne Martin, "Inflation Spurs Health Spending in 2000," *Health Affairs,* vol. 21, no. 1, p. 176; and Brian Bruen, and John Holahan, *Medicaid Enrollment and Spending Trends* (Washington, D.C.: The Kaiser Commission on the Uninsured, February 2001), p.1.

[3] Texas Health and Human Services Commission (HHSC), *Texas Medicaid in Perspective, Third Edition* (Austin, Tex., February 1999), pp. 14-15.

[4] Ibid., pp. 19-21.

[5] The General Accounting Office, *Major Federal Expansion of Medicaid Eligibility and Services (1984-1993*), HEHS95-122 (Washington, D.C., 1995), pp. 56-62.

[6] Ibid.

[7] Jean Hearne, "Medicaid Disproportionate Share Payments" (Washington, D.C.: Congressional Research Service, 2001), p.4.

[8] Ibid.

[9] HHSC, *Texas Medicaid in Perspective*, p. 66.

[10] Letter from Bob Bullock, Lieutenant Governor, State of Texas, to The Honorable Judith Zaffirini, State Senator, March 15, 1994.

[11] Texas Health and Human Services Commission, "Texas Medicaid 1115 Summary," (Austin, Tex., 1995), pp. 8-11.

[12] Ibid, p. 11.

[13] Ibid, p. 24.

[14] DeAnn Friedholm, Executive Director, Children's Defense Fund of Texas, Class Presentation, Lyndon B. School of Public Affairs, Austin, Texas, November 6, 2001.

[15] Interview by Michelle Harper and Leah Kegler with Anne Dunkelberg, Senior Policy Analyst, Center for Public Policy Priorities, Austin, Texas, March 5, 2001.

[16] The Center for Public Policy Priorities, *Every Child Equal* (Austin, Tex: The Texas CHIP Coalition, September 2000), p. 14.

[17] The income eligibility level is based on a three-person family with only one wage earner. It is also assumed that the family's only source of income is from earnings. The income level takes into account Texas's treatment of earnings, but not other income deductions such as child care expenses. Source: Families USA, *Uninsured Parents and Medicaid Information, State-by-State* (Washington, D.C.: Families USA Health Action Annual Conference, January, 2001), p.1.

[18] The Henry J. Kaiser Family Foundation, *Medicaid: A Primer* (Washington, D.C., 1999), p. 4.

[19] Texas Department of Human Services, *Title XIX Expenditure History List*, (Austin, Tex.,, November 2000).

[20] Texas A & M University System Health Science Center, *Health Insurance Stati*stics, 2000. Online. Available: http://srph.brc.tamus.edu/srphis. Accessed: February 13, 2001.

[21] Texas Health and Human Services Commission, *Texas Medicaid in Perspective*, Third Edition (Austin, Tex, February, 1999), pp. 51-52.

[22] Ibid., pp. 51-52.

[23] Families USA, *Deep in the Heart of Texas: Uninsured in the Lone Star State* (Washington, D.C., 2000).

[24] Kaiser Family Foundation, *State Health Facts Online.* Online. Available: http://www.statehealthfacts.kff.org. Accessed: November 16, 2001.

[25] Health Care Financing Administration, "The State Children's Health Insurance Program: Preliminary Highlights of Implementation and Expansion" (Washington, D.C., July 2000), p. 1.

[26] Center for Medicare and Medicaid Services, "The State Children's Health Insurance Program Annual Enrollment Report," February 6, 2002. Online. Available: http://www.hcfa.gov/init/schip01.pdf. Accessed: March 20, 2002.

[27] Lyndon B. Johnson School of Public Affairs, *Expanding Health Care Coverage for the Uninsured in Texas,* Policy Research Report Series, no. 141 (Austin, Tex., 2001), p. 77.

[28] TexCare Partnership, *CHIP Start Up Comparisons.* Online. Available: http://www.Texcarepartnership.com/CHIP-Comparison-Stats-Page.htm. Accessed: March 7, 2001.

[29] Presentation by Jason Cook, Health and Human Services Commission, at the CHIP Coalition Meeting, Austin, Texas, September 20, 2000.

[30] TexCare Partnership, *Cumulative, Application, Eligibility Determination, and Enrollment Activity for 2-18-02.* Online. Available: http://www.hhsc.state.Tex.us/chip/WeeklySumRpt.pdf. Accessed: February 21, 2002.

[31] John Holahan, and Niall Brennan, *Who are the Adult Uninsured?* (Washington, D.C.: The Urban Institute, 2000), p. 1.

[32] Stephen Zuckerman, Jennifer Haley, and John Holahan, *Health Insurance, Access, and Health Status of Nonelderly Adults* (Washington, D.C.: Urban Institute, 2001), p. 4.

[33] Holahan and Brennan, *Who are the Adult Uninsured?,* p.5.

[34] Ibid.

[35] Presentation by DeAnn Friedholm to "State Budget Crisis: Working Together to Finance a Fair Budget Conference," ProTex, Austin, Texas, November 9, 2001.

[36] Diane Rowland, *Health Insurance for Unemployed Workers* (Washington, D.C.: The Kaiser Commission of the Uninsured, 2001), pp. 13-14.

[37] Jeanne Lawbrew, *Health Insurance: A Family Affair* (Washington, D.C.: The Commonwealth Fund, 2001), p. 1.

[38] Amy Davidoff, Genevieve Kenney, Lisa Dubay, and Alshadye Yemane, *Patterns of Child-Parent Insurance Coverage: Implications for Coverage Expansions* (Washington, D.C.: The Urban Institute, 2001), p. 1.

[39] Ibid, p. 5.

[40] Evan Christman, Research Assistant and PRP Student, Lyndon B. Johnson School of Public Affairs, Class Presentation, Lyndon B. Johnson School of Public Affairs, Austin, Texas, September 11, 2001.

[41] To receive Medicaid through the "medically needy" classification, there must be a child under age 19 in the legal household. Spend downs eligibility is determined on a monthly basis. Each month, to be eligible for Medicaid in that month, a person's medical expenses must equal his/her spend down. When person is approved for the Medicaid spend down, the person will receive a notice giving the spend-down amount. This amount is determined through a formula that subtracts the person's excess income and/or excess assets from the maximum allowed. Once medical expenses equal spend-down, then Medicaid coverage is available to that person for the remainder of the month. For example, if a person's medical expenses equal his spend-down on the 14th day of the month, from the 14th day of the month forward, he will have Medicaid coverage for the remainder of the month.

[42] Zuckerman, Haley, and Holahan, *Health Insurance, Access, and Health Status of Nonelderly Adults*, p. 3.

[43] Leighton Ku and Matthew Broaddus, *The Importance of Family-Based Insurance Expansions: New Research Findings about State Health Reforms* (Washington, D.C.: Center on Budget and Policy Priorities, September 2000), p. 1.

[44] Centers for Medicare and Medicaid Services, *Enrolling and Retaining Low-Income Families in Health Care Coverage* (Washington, D.C., 2001), p. 27.

[45] Lisa Dubay, and Genevieve Kenney, *Covering Parents through Medicaid and SCHIP: Potential Benefits to Low-Income Parents and Children* (Washington, D.C.: The Urban Institute, 2001), p. 7.

[46] Michael Birnbaum, *Expanding Coverage to Parents through Medicaid Section 1931* (Washington, D.C.: The Robert Wood Johnson Foundation, 2000), p. 1.

[47] Jocelyn Guyer and Cindy Mann, *A New Opportunity to Provide Health Care Coverage for New York's Low-Income Families* (Washington, D.C.: The Commonwealth Fund, 1999), p. 11.

[48] Marilyn Ellwood, *The Medicaid Eligibility Maze: Coverage Expands, But Enrollment Problems Persist* (Washington, D.C.: The Urban Institute, 2000), p. 1.

[49] Birnbaum, *Expanding Coverage to Parents through Medicaid Section 1931*, p. 4.

[50] Andy Schneider and Rachel Garfield, *Medicaid Benefits* (Washington, D.C.: The Kaiser Commission on Medicaid and the Uninsured, 2000), p. 18.

[51] Jocelyn Guyer and Cindy Mann, *Taking the Next Step: States Can Now Expand Health Coverage to Low-Income Parents Through Medicaid* (Washington, D.C.: Center on Budget Policy Priorities, 1998), p.3-4.

[52] The Title XXI SCHIP program was created to insure children, therefore, the focus of the program is the expansion of health insurance to kids and therefore states must apply for waivers if they want to extend coverage to parents. In addition, under no circumstances will states be granted the authority to cover childless adults under a Title XXI waiver.

[53] Mark Merlis, *Medicaid: Program and Demonstration Waivers* (Washington, D.C.: Congressional Research Service, 1994), p. 7.

[54] Gabriela Alcalde, *Section 1115 Demonstration Waivers Under the State Children's Health Insurance Program* (Washington, D.C.: The National Conference of State Legislatures, 2001), p. 4.

[55] Jeanne Lambrew, *Section 1115 Waivers in Medicaid and the State Children's Health Insurance Program* (Washington, D.C.: The Henry J. Kaiser Family Foundation, 2001), p. 3.

[56] Ibid, p. 4.

[57] Following the passage of the Balanced Budget Act of 1997, states are able to allow enrollment in managed care programs mandatory without a Section 1115 waiver.

[58] National Association of State Medicaid Directors, *Medicaid 1115 Waivers*. Online. Available: http://medicaid.aphsa.org/waivers/1115waivers.htm. Accessed: January 8, 2001.

[59] The Kaiser Commission on Medicaid and the Uninsured, *Issues Related to Unspent S-CHIP Money* (Washington, D.C.: The Henry J. Kaiser Family Foundation, 2001), p. 2.

[60] Ibid, p. 5.

[61] Letter from Timothy M. Westmoreland, Health Care Financing Administration, Department of Health and Human Services, to State Health Officials, July 31, 2000.

[62] Ibid.

[63] These guidelines were published under the Clinton Administration. The current Bush Administration is not required to make states applying for a SCHIP waiver to these standards.

[64] Letter from Timothy M. Westmoreland, Health Care Financing Administration, to State Health Officials, July 31, 2000.

[65] Texas Health and Human Service Commission, *Children's Medicaid Simplification-Senate Bill 43 Proposed Implementation Outline.*, Online. Available: http://www.hhsc.state.Tex.us/chip/SB43/SB43_Simplification_Intro.html. Accessed: January 27, 2002.

[66] Anne Dunkelberg, *Children's Medicaid Eligibility Simplification Bill, SB 43, Sent to the Governor* (Austin, Tex: Center for Public Policy Priorities, 2002), p. 1.

[67] Jeanne Lambrew, *Section 1115 Waivers in Medicaid and the State Children's Health Insurance Program* (Washington, D.C.: The Henry J. Kaiser Family Foundation, 2001), p. 3.

[68] Mark Merlis, *Medicaid: Program and Demonstration Waivers* (Washington, D.C.: Congressional Research Service, 1994), p. 7.

[69] Office of the Secretary of Health and Human Services, "Medicaid Program: Demonstration Proposals Pursuant to Section 1115(a) of the Social Security Act: Policies and Procedures," *Federal Register* (Washington, D.C., September 27, 1994), 59(186), p. 49249.

[70] Ibid.

[71] Lyndon B. Johnson School of Public Affairs, *Expanding Health Care Coverage for the Uninsured in Texas,* Policy Research Report Series, no. 141 (Austin, Tex., 2001), p. 126.

[72] Ibid.

[73] Ibid.

[74] Analytical Perspectives, *Budget of the United States Government, Fiscal Year 2001* (Washington, D.C.: U.S. Government Printing Office), Table 14-4.

[75] Jeanne Lambrew, Section *1115 Waivers in Medicaid and the State Children's Health Insurance Program* (Washington, D.C.: The Henry J. Kaiser Family Foundation, 2001), p. 6.

[76] George W. Bush, "Radio Address of the President to the Nation: August 4, 2001." Online. Available: http://www.whitehouse.gov/news/releases/2001/08/20010804.html. Accessed August 6, 2001.

[77] Matt Salo, Briefing on President Bush's Medicaid Flexibility Initiative "Medicaid Flexibility for the Uninsured?" (Alliance for Health Reform, Washington, D.C., August 28, 2001).

[78] State Coverage Initiatives, *State of the States* (Washington, D.C.: Academy for Health Care Services Research and Health Policy, 2002), p. 13.

[79] Centers for Medicare and Medicaid Services, *Health Insurance and Flexibility and Accountability Demonstration Initiative* (Washington, D.C.: Department of Health and Human Service, July 25, 2001), p. 1.

[80] The Kaiser Commission on Medicaid and the Uninsured, *Issues Related to Unspent S-CHIP Money* (Washington, D.C.: The Henry J. Kaiser Family Foundation, 2001), p. 2.

[81] Ibid, p. 5.

[82] State Coverage Initiatives, *State of the States* (Washington, D.C.: Academy for Health Care Services Research and Health Policy, 2002), p. 13.

[83] Centers for Medicare and Medicaid Services, *Health Insurance and Flexibility and Accountability Demonstration Initiative,* p. 2.

[84] Jennifer M. Ryan, "Health Insurance Family Style: Public Approaches to Reaching the Uninsured." *Issue Brief No. 767* (Washington, D.C.: National Health Policy Forum, September 24, 2001), p. 7.

[85] Center for Medicare and Medicaid Services, *Health Insurance and Flexibility and Accountability Demonstration Initiative*, p. 3.

[86] Legislative Budget Board, "Spotlight: Health Insurance Flexibility and Accountability (HIFA) Demonstration Initiative," *Federal Fund Watch,* volume 7, no. 4, October 2001, p. 1.

[87] Ibid.

[88] Center for Medicare and Medicaid Services, *Health Insurance and Flexibility and Accountability Demonstration Initiative*, p. 3.

[89] Leighton Ku and Matthew Broaddus, *The Importance of Family-Based Insurance Expansions: New Research Findings about State Health Reforms* (Washington, D.C.: Center on Budget and Policy Priorities, September 2000), p. 1.

[90] Jennifer M. Ryan, "Health Insurance Family Style: Public Approaches to Reaching the Uninsured." *Issue Brief No. 767* (Washington, D.C.: National Health Policy Forum, September 24, 2001), p. 9.

[91] Center for Medicare and Medicaid Services, *Health Insurance and Flexibility and Accountability Demonstration Initiative*, p. 4.

[92] State Coverage Initiatives, *State of the States* (Washington, D.C.: Academy for Health Care Services Research and Health Policy, 2002), p. 14.

[93] Ibid.

[94] Tim Westmoreland. *Briefing on President Bush's Medicaid Flexibility Initiative, Medicaid Flexibility for the Uninsured?* (Washington, D.C.: Alliance for Health Reform, August 28, 2001).

[95] Thomas Scully, *Briefing on President Bush's Medicaid Flexibility Initiative, Medicaid Flexibility for the Uninsured?* (Washington, D.C.: Alliance for Health Reform, August 28, 2001).

[96] Leighton Ku and Matt Broaddus, *How to Review Cost Estimates for Family Coverage Expansions* (Washington, D.C.: The Center on Budget and Policy Priorities, 2001), p.1.

[97] The Assistant Secretary for Planning and Evaluation (ASPE), *Understanding Estimates of the Uninsured: Putting the Differences in Context*. Online. Available: http://aspe.hhs.gov/health/reports/hiestimates.htm. Accessed: November 14, 2001.

[98] Ibid, p.2.

[99] It is important to note that basing estimates only on the uninsured assumes that those with private coverage are not eligible for the expansion. According to Section 1931, states are not allowed to deny eligibility to those with private coverage, but in a Section 1115 waiver, states are allowed to protect against the problem of crowd-out in the conditions of the waiver.

[100] By only subtracting legal immigrants who have been in the United States for less than five years, these estimates assume that Texas will take the federal Medicaid option to reinstate Medicaid benefits to immigrants who have been in the United States over five years in the next legislative session. In the 77th legislature, Governor Perry vetoed Senate Bill 1156, which assured benefits to this population.

[101] Lisa Dubay and Genevieve Kenney, " Covering Parents through Medicaid and S-CHIP: Potential Benefits to Low-Income Parents and Children" (Washington, D.C.: The Henry J. Kaiser Family Foundation, January 2002), p. 12.

[102] Simply having legal immigration status does not mean immigrants have access to Medicaid similar to that of a U.S. citizen. For instance, there is no way for these individuals to obtain SSI because of the 1996 federal welfare reform legislation.

[103] Leighton Ku and Teresa Coughlin, "Sliding Scale Premiums: Four States' Experiences," *Inquiry*, vol. 36, no. 4, pp. 471-80.

[104] No reduction for the state in the cost of services is accounted for based upon the level of cost-sharing implemented. This is because actual amount of money collect by the state depends upon the cost-sharing mechanism in place.

[105] The assumption was made that enforcing an assets test would drastically reduces the overall benefit of providing reduced benefit package insurance to the low-income uninsured adults targeted by this model

[106] A similar approach is used in the Arkansas Medicaid expansion programs, which provides expansion children with a reduced benefit package. Contrary to the Mandatory/Optional Children's Medicaid program in Arkansas, an assets test is **not** required in Arkansas for its Medicaid expansion program. The Kaiser Commission on Medicaid and the Uninsured, "Medicaid Eligibility for Children and Families." Online. Available at: http://www.kff.org/content/archive/2106/eligibility5.html. Accessed: March 3, 2002.

[107] Lisa Dubay and Genevieve Kenney, *The Effects of Family Coverage on Children's Health Insurance Status* (Washington, D.C.: The Urban Institute, 2001), p. 1; Jeanne M. Lambrew, *Health Insurance: A Family Affair* (Washington, D.C.: The Commonwealth Fund, May 2001), p. 3; Leighton Ku and Matthew Broaddus, *The Importance of Family-Based Insurance Expansions: New Research Findings about State Health Reforms* (Washington, D.C.: Center on Budget and Policy Priorities, September 2000), p. 1.

[108] This rate is a general estimate based on a variety of data sources representing the total acute costs for a TANF adult. This type of estimate is used in general knowing a portion would be in managed care. The Director of Actuarial Analysis at HHSC believes that managed care alone would not differ greatly from the general estimate unless focusing on specific geographic areas.

[109] Cost reimbursed covers a variety of services such as Texas Healthy Steps, CCP, family planning, Federally Qualified Health Centers, and case management. Not all of these services would be used by adults, however, thus the small percentage.

[110] David Palmer, Director of Actuarial Analysis, Texas Health and Human Services Commission, "RE: Medicaid Question," Email to Leah Kegler, December 17, 2001.

[111] Bureau of Labor Statistics, "Consumer Price Index Summary." Online. Available at: http://stats.bls.gov/news.release/cpi.nr0.htm. Accessed March 3, 2002.

[112] Ibid.

[113] Charles Milligan, *Section 1115 Waivers and Budget Neutrality: Using Medicaid Funds to Expand Coverage* (Washington, D.C.: State Coverage Initiatives of the Robert Wood Johnson Foundation, 2001), p. 4.

[114] Legislative Budget Board, "Spotlight: Health Insurance Flexibility and Accountability (HIFA) Demonstration Initiative," *Federal Fund Watch,* Austin, Tex., vol. 7, no. 4, October 2001, p. 1.

[115] Families USA, "The Current Medicaid Federal-State Partnership: Already a Good Deal for the States," (Washington, D.C., August 2001), p. 2.

[116] Interview by Leah Kegler and Lisa Ewart with Trey Berndt, Special Assistant for Medicaid/CHIP Operations, Texas Health and Human Services Commission, Austin, Texas, February 15, 2002.

[117] The Bush Administration has not indicated whether or not it will continue to follow these guidelines when granting SCHIP waivers.

[118] Jocelyn Guyer, *Trends in CHIP Expenditures: State-by-State Data* (Washington, D.C.: The Kaiser Commission on Medicaid and the Uninsured, October 2001), p. 7.

[119] Ibid, p. 11.

[120] Cindy Mann, *The New Medicaid and CHIP Waiver Initiatives* (Washington, D.C.: The Kaiser Commission on the Uninsured, 2002), p. 29.

[121] Ibid., p. 28.

Chapter 3. Health Care Access for Immigrants in Texas

by Jennifer Eldridge

Of the 4.6 million uninsured Texans, over half are Hispanic.[1] A large proportion of these individuals are immigrants from Mexico. This population faces many unique barriers to accessing health care, including immigration status issues as well as cultural and language considerations. Therefore, no evaluation of efforts to expand health care access in Texas can be complete without a thorough examination of this seriously underserved population.

There are 6.7 million Hispanics in Texas, or 33 percent of the state's population.[2] Of these Hispanic individuals, 89.6 percent, or 5.7 million, are of Mexican origin.[3] There are an estimated 1.8 million immigrants living in Texas.[4] Because of the state's close proximity to Mexico, Hispanics make up the largest segment (77 percent) of the immigrant population in Texas.[5] There are an estimated 1.4 million immigrants of Hispanic origin living in Texas.[6] It is very difficult to know how many of the immigrants living in Texas are undocumented, however demographers estimate the number at approximately 500,000 people.[7] Again, because the state shares a border with Mexico, it can be safely assumed that the vast majority of the undocumented immigrants in Texas are Hispanic.

Sixty-one percent, or 3.8 million people, of Hispanics living in Texas are considered poor or near-poor, meaning that they fall below 200 percent of the Federal Poverty Level (FPL).[8] To better illustrate this, see the 2001 U.S. Department of Health and Human Services (HHS) poverty guidelines in Table 3.1.

Table 3.1
2001 U.S. Department of Health and Human Services Poverty Guidelines

Size of Family Unit	100% FPL	200% FPL
1	$8,590	$17,180
2	$11,610	$23,220
3	$14,630	$29,260
4	$17,650	$35,260
5	$20,670	$41,340
6	$23,690	$47,380
7	$26,710	$53,420
8	$29,730	$59,460
For each additional person, add	$3,020	$6,040

Adapted from: U.S. Department of Health and Human Services, *The 2001 HHS Federal Poverty Guidelines.* Online. Available: http://aspe.hhs.gov/poverty/01poverty.htm. Accessed: November 18, 2001.

The Current State of Coverage for Hispanics in Texas

Table 3.2 compares insurance coverage for children and non-elderly Hispanics and non-Hispanic whites, both in Texas and nationwide.

Table 3.2
Insurance Coverage for Hispanics and Non-Hispanic Whites by Age

Type of Insurance		Non-elderly 0-64 years		Children 0-17 years	
		U.S.	Texas	U.S.	Texas
Employer-sponsored	Hispanics	46.2%	38.2%	41.7%	32.1%
	Non-Hispanic whites	74.0%	70.5%	73.8%	68.1%
Other Private	Hispanics	2.8%	1.1%	2.3%	1.1%
	Non-Hispanic whites	6.0%	7.0%	4.9%	6.9%
Medicaid/Other Public	Hispanics	19.4%	20.0%	33.2%	34.8%
	Non-Hispanic whites	8.1%	6.3%	12.4%	10.5%
Uninsured	Hispanics	31.6%	40.8%	22.8%	32.1%
	Non-Hispanic whites	11.9%	16.2%	8.8%	14.5%

Adapted from: Urban Institute, *Snapshots of America's Families I: Texas State Data* (Washington, D.C., May 2000), table 4.

Private Insurance

Employer-sponsored insurance (ESI) is the main source of coverage for children and non-elderly adults in the U.S.[9] The rate of ESI in Texas is much lower than the national average. This is due in part to the fact that only 50 percent of private employers in Texas offer insurance to their employees.[10] Hispanics are less likely to have ESI for several reasons. Whether or not a company offers insurance is directly correlated to how many employees it has, and Hispanics often work for small companies, i.e., those with fewer than 25 employees.[11] Furthermore, Hispanics tend to work in fields with high uninsured rates, such as the personal service industry, with a 57.3 percent uninsured rate, and agriculture, with a 47.6 percent uninsured rate.[12]

Public Insurance

Texas's Medicaid program is designed to provide coverage mostly for low-income children and low-income, elderly, or disabled adults. In Texas, infants under one year old are eligible if their family incomes are 185 percent or less FPL. Children from one to five are eligible for Medicaid if their family incomes are 133 percent or less of FPL. Children age six to 18 are eligible if their family incomes are 100 percent or less of FPL. Most adult Texans are ineligible for Medicaid. Pregnant women with incomes at or less than 185 percent of FPL may receive Medicaid benefits to cover the costs related to pregnancy and birth. Non-pregnant adults, on the other hand, are only eligible for Medicaid if they earn less than 34 percent of FPL and are parents of a child who is on Medicaid. Low-income elderly or disabled individuals may receive benefits if they qualify for SSI or the low-income nursing home benefit.

In Texas, 63.9 percent of the children on Medicaid are Hispanic.[13] Fifty-six percent of the uninsured children who are eligible for Medicaid in Texas are Hispanic.[14] The federal welfare reform legislation enacted in 1996 had a severely chilling effect on enrollment for eligible immigrants, as well as having the effect of reducing Medicaid eligibility for both legal and undocumented immigrants. The effects of this legislation on the immigrant population will be discussed in detail in a later section.

Children's Medicaid Simplification

There are an estimated 658,000 uninsured children in Texas who are eligible for Medicaid but are not enrolled.[15] Historically, the need for simplification of children's Medicaid has been a major barrier to enrollment in Texas. Many of these issues were addressed by the Children's Medicaid Simplification Act (SB 43), which was signed into law by the Texas Legislature in May 2001. SB 43 establishes the following reforms:

- eliminates face-to-face interview for application and re-certification;
- adopts documentation and verification standards no more stringent than those for SCHIP; and
- allows for phased-in implementation of 12-month continuous eligibility.

In November 2001, the Texas Department of Human Services (TDHS) published its proposed rules in the Texas Register. The bill required TDHS to address four major areas: application simplification, continuous eligibility and eligibility transition with SCHIP, Health Care Orientation (HCO), and participation in Texas Healthy Steps (THSteps).[16]

Texas is in the process of updating and adopting the published rules. The rules became effective near the end of January 2002. The policies explain how the separate Medicaid and SCHIP applications will be merged into one and how enrollment procedures will be affected. This will allow the state, beginning in January 2002, to utilize a joint application and a common application process for SCHIP and Medicaid. The state also plans to implement phased-in continuous eligibility for children under age 19, with six months continuous eligibility by February 2002 with the possibility of 12 months continuous eligibility as early as September 2002.[17]

Texas did not adopt any children's presumptive eligibility requirements as part of its simplification package. Texas is working to set up a simplified redetermination process, but there have been many obstacles on this front. As part of SB 43, parents who enroll their children in Medicaid are required to go through a Health Care Orientation (HCO), which did not exist prior to SB 43. The proposed rule created a set of administrative guidelines for the HCOs, leaving open the possibility of required face-to-face Medicaid renewal. Thus, it is possible that SB 43 will be implemented in such a way that does not truly simplify children's Medicaid as much as the bill's authors had intended.

The State Children's Health Insurance Program

The State Children's Health Insurance Program (SCHIP) essentially picks up where Medicaid leaves off, offering insurance coverage to children whose families earn too much for Medicaid eligibility but still cannot afford private coverage.

In Texas, SCHIP is referred to as the TexCare Partnership. Since the program began in April 2000, more than 480,000 children have been enrolled across the state.[18] Children in families earning between 100-200 percent of FPL are eligible for SCHIP. [19] Parents are responsible for paying a small enrollment premium of up to $18 per month, as well as office visit co-pay fees of between $2-5 per visit.[20] However, essential services such as well-child exams, immunizations, and preventive care are exempt from cost-sharing.[21]

At 1.3 million, Texas is second only to California in the number of uninsured children.[22] Fifty-six percent, or 800,000, of these uninsured children are Hispanic.[23] Children who are legal immigrants are eligible for SCHIP, regardless of their parents' immigration status. It is estimated that 62 percent of the uninsured children who are eligible for SCHIP in Texas are Hispanic.[24] This suggests that more outreach is needed to inform the Hispanic population regarding SCHIP eligibility.

Uninsured

In terms of barriers to obtaining health care coverage, Hispanics have two major strikes against them: a high rate of poverty, and a large subpopulation of immigrant non-citizens. At 51 percent, or over 2.4 million people, Hispanics make up more than half of Texas' uninsured population.[25] Conversely, 39 percent of the Hispanics living in Texas are uninsured.[26]

Poverty is one major barriers to health care coverage. Fifty-one percent of Hispanics in Texas who earn less than 100 percent of FPL, or approximately 859,000 people, are uninsured.[27] To further break down the uninsured Hispanic population by income level, 36 percent earn less than 100 percent of FPL, 39 percent earn between 100 and 200 percent of FPL, and 25 percent earn more than 200 percent of FPL.[28]

Texas has the fourth largest immigrant population in the U.S.[29] Hispanics make up the vast majority (85.6 percent) of the uninsured immigrant population in Texas.[30, 31, 32] Because uninsurance may lead to poor access to health care, immigrants in Texas are particularly vulnerable. Nationally, 20 percent of children of immigrants are uninsured, versus 10 percent of children with native parents.[33] In Texas, 40 percent of the children of immigrants are uninsured compared to 17 percent of children of natives.[34] Nationwide, 9 percent of children of immigrants are in fair or poor health, as compared to 4 percent of children of natives.[35] In Texas, 14 percent of children of immigrants are in fair or poor health versus 4 percent of children with native parents.[36]

The Impact of Welfare Reform

The 1996 Personal Responsibility and Work Opportunity Reconciliation Act (PRWORA) delinked Medicaid from welfare (Temporary Assistance to Needy Families, or TANF) benefits. Beneficiaries no longer have to be eligible for one in order to receive services from the other. As an unintended result, many people no longer eligible for welfare also dropped out of Medicaid, not realizing they were still eligible.

Following PRWORA, Texas experienced a 7.6 percent decrease in Medicaid enrollees—the second-highest in the nation.[37] This decrease is attributed in large part to the effect that welfare reform had on the immigrant population. PRWORA established the distinction between "qualified" and "not qualified" immigrants when determining eligibility for specific entitlement programs (see Table 3.3). This resulted in confusion among mixed-immigration status families, and people who were lawfully entitled to benefits did not enroll for fear of getting in trouble with the Immigration and Naturalization Service (INS).

Table 3.3
Qualified Immigrant Categories Under PRWORA

Qualified	Not Qualified
Legal permanent residents ("green card" holders)	Parolees for less than a year
Refugees	Temporary residents
Asylees	Aliens granted temporary protected status
Persons granted withholding of removal	Family Unity beneficiaries
Parolees for a year or more	Aliens granted deferred enforced departure status
Cuban and Haitian entrants	Aliens granted deferred action status
Amerasians	Spouse or child with adjustment of status pending
Domestic violence victims and their parents or children	Asylum or withholding of removal applicants
Native Americans who are legal permanent residents	In status aliens
	Undocumented immigrants

Adapted from: National Immigration Law Center, "Immigrant Eligibility for Public Benefits: U.S. and Texas" (Los Angeles, Calif., 2000), pp. 1-9.

PRWORA gave states the option to continue Medicaid coverage for qualified immigrant adults who entered the U.S. before the law was enacted in August 1996, which Texas did. States are required by federal law to provide SCHIP coverage to qualified immigrant children who entered before August 1996. Qualified immigrant adults entering the U.S. after August 1996 are barred from Medicaid coverage for five years from date of entry, although emergency Medicaid is still available during that time. States may opt to use their own funds to cover immigrant children during the five-year bar period; Texas covers these children with SCHIP funds. All qualified immigrant children may receive state-funded care following the five-year bar.

States have the option to cover post-1996 qualified adult immigrants after the five-year bar; however, as the first group of immigrants is now exceeding the five-year bar point, Texas has not yet exercised this option. During the 77th Texas Legislature, Governor Rick Perry vetoed SB 1156, which would have exercised Texas's option to cover post-1996 qualified immigrant adults following the five-year bar period.

PRWORA presents no restrictions on qualified immigrants' access to some other federal programs, including the Maternal Child Health Block Grant (Title V), the Family Planning Grant (Title X), and the Social Services Block Grant (Title XX). [38]

One of the negative impacts of the federal eligibility restrictions is cost-shifting from the federal government to the states, and in turn to counties and localities. States like Texas that do not provide coverage for certain immigrants place the costs of providing care onto locally funded clinics and public hospitals.[39]

In addition to affecting non-citizens' access to health care, PRWORA also affected the many citizen children of immigrant parents. In Texas, 29 percent of citizen children living in families earning less than 200 percent of FPL have at least one immigrant parent.[40] Although children born in the U.S. to immigrant parents are considered full citizens with the same rights to public benefits as children of U.S. citizens, many immigrant parents are afraid of enrolling their citizen children in Medicaid or SCHIP for fear of risking their own immigration status. Outreach efforts are being undertaken in immigrant communities to educate pregnant women on the benefits of enrolling their children in these public programs. By documenting the change in health insurance coverage for immigrant children between 1995 and 1999, Table 3.4 illustrates the adverse effects of PRWORA on rates of coverage nationwide.

Table 3.4
Public Insurance Coverage of Children in U.S. Families with Incomes below 200 Percent FPL

	1995	1999	Change in percentage points, 1995-1999
Immigrant Children			
Medicaid or SCHIP	35.8%	28.1%	-7.7%
Other public insurance	1.1%	0.6%	-0.5%
Uninsured	44.0%	45.6%	1.6%
Citizen Children with Immigrant Parents			
Medicaid or SCHIP	46.5%	43.1%	-3.5%
Other public insurance	1.2%	1.2%	0.0%
Uninsured	28.5%	31.3%	2.8%

Adapted from: Leighton Ku and Shannon Blaney, Center on Budget and Policy Priorities, "Health Coverage for Legal Immigrant Children: New Census Data Highlight Importance of Restoring Medicaid and SCHIP Coverage." Online. Available: http://www.cbpp.org/10-4-00health.htm. Accessed: January 3, 2002.

PRWORA marks the first time that Congress has authorized states to discriminate against legal immigrants in determining eligibility of public benefit programs.[41] This policy stands in stark contrast against our relatively inclusive immigration policy. Clearly, problems are inevitable in a situation where immigrants are being admitted to the U.S. without adequate public programs needed to support them.

Undocumented Immigrants

By the very nature of being "undocumented," it is easy to understand why it is difficult to identify this subpopulation of immigrants. Demographers estimate that there are 500,000 undocumented immigrants living in Texas.[42, 43, 44] One proxy method that is used to estimate the number of undocumented children in the state is to go by the number of children in public schools using substitute identification instead of Social Security numbers.[45] Using this method, one can estimate that there are approximately 330,000 undocumented children in Texas. The Texas Department of Insurance estimates that 19 percent of the uninsured in the state are undocumented immigrants.[46]

Under PRWORA, undocumented and other "not qualified" immigrants are barred from federal public benefits with the following exceptions:

- emergency Medicaid, immunizations, and diagnosis/treatment of communicable disease;
- non-cash assistance to protect life and safety, such as soup kitchens, shelters, and crisis intervention services; and
- short-term emergency disaster relief.[47]

Because most undocumented immigrants are poor and ineligible for any kind of insurance coverage, they largely depend on county-funded programs (such as public hospitals), community health centers (CHCs), and charitable organizations for their health care needs. All of these will be described in more detail later.

Prenatal Care for Undocumented Women

One of the biggest issues with regard to health care for undocumented immigrants is the need for publicly funded prenatal care. Since the children born in the U.S. to undocumented women will be U.S. citizens, it is in the state's best interest to work towards a healthy birth outcome. The Maternal and Child Health Block Grant (Title V) provides health care funds for pregnant women, mothers, infants, and children who do not have access to adequate health care. Because the patient is only required to be a Texas resident and not necessarily a citizen, Title V funds represent a primary source of funding for prenatal care for undocumented women in Texas.

At the federal level, Title V funds are administered by the Maternal and Child Health Bureau (MCHB), one of four bureaus of the Health Resources and Services Administration (HRSA), which falls under the Department of Health and Human Services. The stated mission of MCHB is "to provide national leadership and to work in partnership with states, communities, public-private partners and families to strengthen the maternal and child health infrastructure, assure the availability and use of medical homes and build the knowledge and human resources in order to assure continued improvement in the health, safety and well-being of the MCH population."[48]

In Texas, the Title V program is administered by the Associateship for Community Health and Resources Development under the Texas Department of Health. Contract agencies bill the program for Title V reimbursable services on a capitated fee-for-service basis.[49] To be eligible for Title V services in Texas, the patient must meet the following requirements:

- a child age 0 to 21, a female age 12 to 45, or a male age 21 or over seeking a vasectomy with a family income of less than 185 percent FPL;
- a Texas resident (not necessarily a citizen);

- otherwise uninsured for the service provided; and
- not eligible for Medicaid and has been screened for Medicaid eligibility using the Texas Eligibility Screening System software or another instrument meeting minimum specifications for Medicaid and has been found not to be potentially eligible for Medicaid.[50]

Although Title V funds may be used towards prenatal care for undocumented women, this program has been flat-funded for several years and access has declined correspondingly.[51]

Access for Undocumented Children

This population also lacks access to much needed acute care services, preventive, and primary care for undocumented children. For example, the Center for Public Policy Priorities reports receiving complaints on a weekly basis from school nurses who do not have an outlet for treating undocumented children.[52] These children are often reliant on CHCs for their health care needs, however there is a shortage of such facilities, and children in need of care often must be driven many miles across several counties in order to reach the nearest CHC.[53]

The Texas Health Access Project's March 2001 "Random Access" report cites several anecdotes that illustrate the problem of access for undocumented children, for example:

> Marta S., 40, a mother of four children ages 7, 9, 11, and 13, is undocumented, as are her children and husband. She applied for CHIP, and her children were referred, due to immigration status, to Texas Health Kids Corporation (THKC). The monthly THKC premium for each child was $66.00 per month, compared to the $15 annual family fee available for legal resident or citizen children through CHIP, or free care through Medicaid. The family's income is roughly $180 per week, so their children would qualify for Medicaid if they were U.S. citizens. The family's source of income fluctuates based on availability of employment for undocumented immigrants (i.e., employers who do not require the I-9 form of the INS, or self-employment, e.g., yard work, etc.) The family is registered for medical services at Gateway [Community Health Center in Laredo].[54]

Federal law excludes undocumented children from Medicaid and SCHIP enrollment. However, states may use SCHIP funds to provide "health services initiatives" that do not screen for immigration status, including programs aimed at migrant farmworker communities, low-income immigrant communities, newborn screening, lead testing, health education, and school health programs.[55] These initiatives are subject to a 10 percent cap of the state's SCHIP block grant spending, although a federal waiver may be requested to exceed this cap.[56] In addition to funding health care programs for undocumented children, these funds may also be used to serve legal immigrant children during the five-year freeze-out period.

Why Provide Health Care for the Undocumented?

There are many compelling reasons to serve the undocumented immigrants of Texas:

- It makes sense to provide the citizen children of immigrant (legal or undocumented) parents the best opportunity for a healthy birth outcome, which means providing prenatal care to pregnant women, regardless of immigration status.
- Communicable disease poses a public health threat to everyone—regardless of immigration status—and so diagnosis and treatment benefits the general public.
- County-funded programs bear the burden of caring for undocumented immigrants in hospital emergency rooms. Providing primary and preventive care to these people would be less costly than waiting until acute conditions are presented in hospital emergency rooms.
- All employed people, regardless of immigration status, are contributing to county-funded programs through sales and property taxes. Even people working in the "cash economy" are contributing to these programs through the sales tax.[57]

Migrant Farmworkers

A migrant farmworker is defined as one who must be absent from his or her permanent place of residence in order to seek employment in agricultural work. Migrant farmworkers are one of the poorest and most underserved populations in the U.S. and in Texas. Most are not offered health insurance, and those who are undocumented immigrants are not eligible for public assistance. Historically, farmworker migration was though to have occurred in three "streams": Western, Midwestern, and Eastern, with those based in Texas traveling up the Midwestern stream.[58] However, it now seems evident that the patterns of movement are more complex.

Migrant farmworkers largely depend on the national network of migrant health centers (MHCs) to meet their health care needs; this network was developed in response to the Migrant Health Act of 1962.[59] Texas does not have any standalone MHCs *per se*, however there are 12 operating out of community health centers (CHCs) in El Paso, Laredo, and the Lower Rio Grande Valley.[60]

Special Health Issues for Migrant Farmworkers

Migrant farmworkers suffer an especially high incidence of common conditions and ailments due to poor nutrition, substandard and overcrowded housing, and poor sanitation.[61] Because of poor education and limited access to care, many conditions go untreated for a long time and become more serious. In addition, farm work is considered the second most dangerous occupation in the U.S. behind mining.[62]

Diabetes, cardiovascular disease, asthma, and tuberculosis are seen in especially high numbers in the migrant farmworker community.[63] A lack of sufficient prenatal care among migrant farmworkers leads to a high incidence of premature births, preeclampsia, other complications.[64] Farm work poses its own set of specific health risks, including repetitive motion injuries and pesticide exposure.[65]

Reciprocity and Portability Programs

A basic problem faced by migrant farmworkers and their families is access to care while working outside of Texas (or, "in stream"). Although most migrant farmworkers in Texas are immigrants, many of their children are U.S. citizens.[66] Approximately 35,000 children of migrant farmworkers spend part of the year in stream, and even if they have Medicaid or SCHIP coverage in Texas, they often cannot access care outside of the state.[67] Without a Medicaid or SCHIP reciprocity or portability program, most states will only provide emergency services to non-residents.[68] The nature of the job makes it necessary for migrant farmworkers to move from state to state often—sometimes every three months—so that by the time someone has enrolled in Medicaid, they may have moved on already.[69] Texas, California, and Wisconsin are all developing approaches to reciprocity and portability in order to cover migrant farmworkers in stream.

Texas

In May 2001, the 77th Texas Legislature passed HB 1537, which set up a commission to study the feasibility of a Migrant Care Network.[70] The goal would be to create an interstate network to provide health care services to Medicaid or SCHIP-eligible children of migrant farmworkers.[71] If the study shows that a Migrant Care Network is feasible, the U.S. Health and Human Services Department may then develop and implement a pilot program.[72]

California

The California Primary Care Association has recently initiated a demonstration project that focuses on Medicaid availability, affordability, and reciprocity between California, Oregon, and Washington.[73] Information is currently being gathered regarding eligibility requirements, benefits, and provider reimbursement levels for the Medicaid programs in these three states.[74]

Wisconsin

In 1996, the Wisconsin legislature approved a "unilateral" reciprocity program to provide Medicaid coverage for anyone eligible for Medicaid in other states.[75] Currently, Wisconsin's SCHIP program provides coverage for all children under 19, and coverage for parents with incomes up to 200 percent of FPL.[76] Wisconsin is currently using a state planning grant to study the feasibility of covering single uninsured individuals also.[77]

Bi-National Health Plan

One concept which if implemented could have a tremendous impact on the migrant farmworker population is a bi-national health plan with Mexico. In May 2001, the 77th Texas Legislature, recognizing that "the provision of health care coverage in the border area is not conducive to preventive care or prenatal care, or to the provision of a medical home for bi-national families," passed HB 2498.[78] The bill set up a seven-member interim committee to study the prospect of a bi-national health plan in terms of the following objectives:

1. Determine the need for bi-national health benefit plan coverage;
2. Assess the health care needs of the border area and how those needs can be served by various types of providers; and
3. Assess the affordability, cost-effectiveness, economic impact, and improved health status achievable through bi-national health benefit plan coverage.[79]

The committee will report its findings and recommendations to the governor and the legislature by October 1, 2002.

From an economic perspective, one of the strongest arguments in favor of a bi-national health plan is that the Mexican economy receives more money from Mexicans working in the U.S. and sending their earnings back over the border than it makes through its thriving tourism industry.[80] Therefore, it would seem to be in Mexico's best interest to help provide health care coverage for its citizens who are working in the United States.

This proposal is obviously quite controversial. One criticism of such a plan is that Mexico could not afford to pay for health care provided in the U.S.

Colonias

The term *colonia* describes rural and unincorporated subdivisions of U.S. cities located along the Texas-Mexico border.[81] *Colonia* residents, like migrant farmworkers (who are often, in fact, the same), represent an extremely impoverished and underserved segment of the immigrant population in Texas. *Colonias* are communities of substandard housing—often consisting of vans, trailers, or temporary structures set up on rented lots of property. They are characterized by inadequate plumbing and sewage disposal systems, and inadequate access to clean water.[82] Consequently, *colonia* residents are especially likely to have communicable diseases and other diseases seen most often in developing countries.

Although it can be difficult to quantify, it is believed that *colonias* exist in 22 of Texas' 254 counties. Table 3.5 reflects the latest data on *colonias* from the Texas Water Development Board.

Table 3.5
Colonias in Texas by County

County	Number of *Colonias*	Population
Bee	4	2,816
Cameron	53	25,882
Coryell	2	868
Dimmit	3	2,830
El Paso	94	54,514
Frio	1	579
Hidalgo	593	110,789
Hudspeth	1	1,100
Kinney	1	66
Maverick	34	18,815
Newton	4	4,502
Reeves	5	91
Sabine	30	6,919
San Patricio	19	3,669
Starr	81	20,673
Terrell	1	1,143
Uvalde	1	1,264
Val Verde	2	3,437
Webb	34	14,197
Willacy	2	2,728
Zapata	1	1,200
Zavala	6	3,976
Total	**972**	**282,058**

Adapted from: The Texas Water Development Board, "Economically Stressed Areas Program." Online. Available: http://www.twdb.state.tx.us/publications/reports/Colonias/status.pdf. Accessed: March 26, 2002.

Outreach workers called *promotoras* play a large role in educating *colonia* residents about where and how to access health care services.

County-Funded Programs

In Texas, the counties are responsible for providing health care for uninsured individuals with incomes lower than 21 percent of FPL.[83] These county-funded programs serve those who are especially poor and likely to be uninsured, regardless of immigration status. For these reasons, they play a key role in providing health care services to Texas' immigrant community.

Counties are required to provide certain basic services, similar to the mandatory services provided under Medicaid, and may choose to also provide optional services, as listed in Table 3.6.

Table 3.6
Services Provided by County-Funded Programs

Basic Services	Optional Services
Primary and preventive services	Ambulatory surgical center services
Immunizations and medical screenings	Diabetic and colostomy supplies and equipment
Inpatient and outpatient hospital services	Durable medical equipment
Rural Health Clinics	Home and community health care services
Laboratory and x-ray services	Certain counseling services
Family planning services	Services provided by physician assistants, advanced practice nurses, certified nurse midwives, and certified registered nurse anesthetists
Physician services	Dental care
Payment for not more than three prescription drugs per month	Vision care including eyeglasses
Skilled Nursing Facility Services	Services provided by federally qualified health centers

Adapted from: Texas Department of Health, *Indigent Health Care Division*. Online. Available: http://www.tdh.state.tx.us/hcf/ihcp/default.htm. Accessed: January 13, 2002.

Counties achieve this through hospital districts, public hospitals, or County Indigent Health Care Programs (CIHCP).

Hospital Districts

Hospital districts are special property taxing districts created in order to provide health care services to their respective residents. Texas has 130 hospital districts that serve all or part of the 112 counties they cover. Hospital districts are required to provide services to individuals at or below 21 percent of FPL, however some choose to serve people with incomes as high as 200 percent of FPL.

Hospital districts are funded through a combination of tax revenue, state funding, federal funding, patients paying out-of-pocket, private insurance, and public insurance. Approximately 25 percent of the funding comes from property taxes, and goes toward providing free or reduced-cost services.[84] The maximum property tax rate that a hospital district can levy is 75 cents per $100 of property valuation; however, in 1999 the average hospital district tax rate was 21 cents per $100 valuation.[85] The state funds certain hospital districts with unclaimed lottery winnings through the Tertiary Care Fund.[86] Hospital districts may also receive federal money through the Disproportionate Share Hospital (DSH) and Graduate Medical Education (GME) programs.[87]

Can Hospital Districts Legally Serve Undocumented Immigrants?

In July 2001, Attorney General John Cornyn issued an opinion that the Harris County hospital district could not provide medical services to undocumented immigrants unless the Texas Legislature explicitly authorized it.[88] The opinion stems from a provision in the Personal Responsibility and Work Opportunity Reconciliation Act of 1996 (PRWORA), that required state legislatures to actively affirm their intention to provide public benefits to undocumented and other "not qualified" immigrants.

Those who take issue with the Cornyn opinion claim that the Texas Legislature complied with PRWORA in 1997 by amending a statute requiring hospital districts to provide medical care for all indigent residents.[89] The Attorney General's opinion is not legally binding, and the majority of Texas hospital districts have continued their policy of serving residents without regard to immigration status. Nonetheless, Representative Gene Green (D-Texas) has introduced a federal bill that would clarify that state and local governments can provide health care to undocumented immigrants without passing new state legislation.[90]

Public Hospitals

Like hospital districts, public hospitals are also required to serve people at or below 21 percent of FPL, but are given the flexibility to expand services as desired. Currently, 32 counties are served in whole or in part by public hospitals.[91]

Public hospitals are funded in much the same way as hospital districts, and also have access to DSH and, if they have residency programs, GME funding. However, local tax support is not dedicated as it is for hospital districts, so funding for public hospitals is less stable from year to year depending on others needs of the county.[92] Because of this unstable funding mechanism, most counties with public hospitals are attempting to phase them out by selling them to private entities, creating hospital districts, or simply closing them down.[93]

Texas' Emergency Care Crisis

Many Texas counties are facing a crisis in that hospital emergency capacity has reached its limit and emergency patients are being turned away. This crisis as it exists in Harris County has been documented by Guy Clifton, M.D., Chief of Neurosurgery at Hermann Hospital in Houston.[94]

Nationally, 50 percent of emergency room admissions do not involve actual emergencies.[95] This is due in large part to the fact that uninsured and Medicaid patients—often immigrants—know that they will be treated 24 hours a day by hospital emergency rooms, regardless of the severity of their condition or their immigration status.[96] The high percentage of uninsured in Texas has resulted in the overuse of hospital emergency resources for non-emergency health care needs.[97] Consequently, emergency rooms are increasingly unable to deliver the quality of care that patients deserve.

County Indigent Health Care Programs

County Indigent Health Care Programs (CIHCPs), operated by 138 Texas counties, reimburse providers for treating beneficiaries and do not receive federal matching funds.[98] CIHCPs must provide health care for uninsured individuals with incomes lower than 21 percent of FPL.[99]

Counties fund their own CIHCPs until they reach 8 percent of their general revenue tax levy (GRTL). The state will reimburse the county for 90 percent of its expenditures above and beyond the 8 percent GRTL threshold until the state fund for this purpose is exhausted.[100]

Community Health Centers

Community health centers (CHCs)—a specific category within the larger umbrella of federally qualified health centers (FQHCs)—are a crucial piece of the health care network for the immigrant population in Texas.

FQHCs are public or non-profit health care facilities that provide inexpensive primary and preventive care to uninsured individuals.[101] FQHCs function as an essential part of the health care safety net by serving areas designated as Medically Underserved Areas/Populations (MUAs/Ps). FQHCs are supported by federal grants under Section 330 of the U.S. Public Health Service Act, and are also eligible to receive cost-based reimbursement of Medicaid and Medicare funds.[102] They are governed by consumer boards, which must be made up of at least 51 percent consumers of center services.[103] This unique structure allows FQHCs to more effectively define and address the needs of their respective communities. FQHC is essentially a Medicaid provider-type designation that describes several different types of health center services, including:[104]

- **Community Health Centers (CHCs):** CHCs target their services to meet the specific needs of the community and special populations such as the homeless, migrant workers, HIV/AIDS, the elderly, and chemically-dependent.

- **Migrant Health Centers (MHCs):** Linked with other health and social services within the service area. They use *promotoras* and outreach workers to serve migrant and seasonal farmworkers and their families.

- **Rural Health Clinics (RHCs):** RHCs were created to provide enhanced Medicaid reimbursement as well as reimbursement to midlevel practitioners working independent of physicians in rural areas.

- **Federally Qualified Health Center Look-Alikes:** Same as FQHCs except they do not receive Section 330 funds. They still receive Medicaid/Medicare cost-based reimbursement.

Who Is Served?

Of the various types of FQHCs, community health centers (CHCs) play the most crucial role in providing health care services to Texas' poor Hispanic and immigrant populations. Texas does not have designated migrant health centers (MHCs) *per se*, however the CHCs do provide the same services as MHCs.[105] Many uninsured Hispanics in Texas are largely dependent on CHCs for their health care needs. Patients are only required to live within the service area, and are not asked to provide documentation regarding immigration status. For this reason, undocumented immigrants often use CHCs for their health care needs.

There are currently 8.2 million people defined as medically underserved in Texas, and 31 CHCs operating 201 health centers across the state.[106] The total population served by CHCs is 432,047—72 percent of whom are Hispanic.[107] They are quite poor; all of them earning less than 200 percent FPL, and 69 percent earning less than 100 percent FPL.[108] As would be expected, the insurance rate among the CHC population is low: 61 percent are uninsured, 25 percent have Medicaid, 7 percent have Medicare, and 7 percent have private insurance.[109] Of the uninsured people served by CHCs in Texas, 88,492 are children.[110]

As shown in Table 3.7, there are nine CHCs operating a total of 60 service sites in Texas' border counties.

Table 3.7
CHCs Operating in Texas Border Counties

CHC	Counties Served	Sites operated	Patient population (1999)	Percent Hispanic
Brownsville CHC	Cameron	4	15,517	99%
Centro De Salud Familiar La Fe	El Paso	9	17,894	99%
Centro San Vicente	El Paso	3	13,898	99%
Community Action Council of South Texas	Jim Hogg, Starr, Zapata	12	18,064	99%
Gateway CHC	Webb	6	11,182	99%
Nuestra Clinica del Valle	Hidalgo	6	22,022	99%
Su Clinica Familiar	Cameron, Willacy	6	24,199	98%
United Medical Centers	Kinney, Maverick, Val Verde	11	19,383	91%
Valley AIDS Council	Cameron, Hidalgo, Willacy	3	325	87%

Adapted from: Texas Association of Community Health Centers, "Texas Association of Community Health Centers Membership Directory" (Austin, Tex., 2000), pp. 12-142.

Services Offered

The main function of CHCs is to offer a variety of primary and preventive services to people residing within the service area. These typically include:

- Preventive health services, including: well-child services, adult primary care services, immunizations, family planning services, pre- and perinatal services, breast and cervical cancer screening, and children's eye and ear examinations to determine need for vision or hearing correction
- Emergency medical services
- Diagnostic laboratory and radiologic services
- Preventive dental services
- Pharmaceutical services
- Physician, physician assistant, and nurse clinician services
- Transportation services as required for adequate patient care
- Referrals to providers of medical services and other health-related services, including substance abuse and mental health services
- Patient case management services and other assistance in establishing eligibility for and gaining access to federal, state, and local programs that provide or financially support the provision of medical, social, educational, and other related services
- Health education and outreach.[111]

Services are provided at a discount to patients below 200 percent of FPL. [112] Individuals and families at or below 100 percent of FPL are not required to pay for CHC services. Those between 101 and 199 percent of FPL are required to pay discounted rates for services on a sliding-fee scale.[113]

Project Alberto: Covering Kids Initiative

In January 1999, the Texas Association of Community Health Centers (TACHC) was awarded a Robert Wood Johnson Foundation grant to participate in the Covering Kids health access initiative for low-income, uninsured children. TACHC's effort, dubbed Project Alberto, focused on implementing specific outreach strategies and research projects to eliminate barriers to accessing children's Medicaid.[114] As part of the initiative, TACHC undertook the following:

- Designed and conducted training programs for outreach staff, *promotoras,* and volunteers to help uninsured families enroll in Medicaid;
- Developed Medicaid outreach materials to provide information to uninsured families and assist outreach workers;

- Created an Outreach Resource Center and web site to supply information on state and federal Medicaid and SCHIP policy, effective outreach strategies and best practices, and funding;
- Implemented Children's Medicaid Simplified Enrollment pilot programs in Fannin, Hunt, and Cameron counties;
- Implemented Presumptive Eligibility for Children pilot program in Bexar county; and
- Conducted research studies to estimate costs to the state associated with implementing the following policy changes in the Medicaid program: 1) eliminating the assets test; 2) simplifying enrollment by eliminating the face-to-face interview and burdensome and unnecessary verifications; 3) implementing continuous eligibility for children; and 4) implementing presumptive eligibility for children.[115]

Although the assets test was not eliminated nor was presumptive eligibility implemented, this initiative contributed to the successful passage of Children's Medicaid Simplification (SB 43) by the 77th Texas Legislature, which was discussed in more detail earlier.

For the second phase of Project Alberto, TACHC will be conducting a study of Harris County and the Lower Rio Grande Valley with the following three outreach goals in mind: 1) conduct and coordinate outreach programs, 2) simplify enrollment and renewal processes, and 3) coordinate existing health coverage programs.[116]

CHC Efforts to Enroll Children in Medicaid and SCHIP

One of the most important outreach functions performed by CHCs is to educate immigrant parents—including undocumented pregnant women—about enrolling their children in Medicaid or SCHIP. Outreach workers, such as Outstationed Eligibility Workers (OEWs) and *promotoras*, work in cooperation with CHCs to provide families with accurate information and assistance to get the health care coverage they need. As part of Project Alberto, TACHC plans to work with the state to place 50 additional OEWs in community settings around the state.[117] OEWs located in CHCs will be electronically connected to TDHS using the TACHC Telecommunications Network to facilitate faster processing of applications.[118]

Although all citizen children in families below 200 percent FPL are eligible for these programs, their immigrant parents are often reluctant to sign them up for fear of risking their own immigration status. This public misperception surrounding what constitutes a "public charge" is quite prevalent, and is often perpetuated by people in trusted positions of authority, such as immigration attorneys and public notaries.[119] As part of Project Alberto, TACHC will be holding state level meetings with Immigration and Naturalization Services (INS), the Texas Bar Association, and the Texas Secretary of State Office (which regulates public notaries) to clarify INS policy with regard to public charge.[120]

Although the literature unanimously asserts that immigrant parents will not risk deportation by enrolling their eligible children in public programs, it is important to note that some in the Lower Rio Grande Valley feel the reality is quite different.[121] Paula Gomez, executive director of Brownsville Community Health Center (BCHC), reports that on at least one occasion the Border Patrol has come to BCHC looking for a woman who wanted to enroll her children in Medicaid.[122] For this reason, BCHC does not aggressively encourage parents who are fearful of deportation to enroll their children in public programs for which they are eligible.[123]

Barriers to Access for Secondary and Tertiary Care Services

Although CHCs are very good at providing primary and preventive care to their patients, sometimes more advanced or specialized services are required. In these cases, a whole new layer of barriers to access is presented.

"Tin-Cup" Medicine

"Tin-cup" medicine refers to the practice often employed by CHC physicians of essentially begging for advanced care services for their patients. CHC physicians are often required to spend a good deal of their time bartering with other health care providers in order to obtain necessary services for their patients.[124] Dr. Fitzhugh Mullan with the Upper Cardozo Community Health Center in Washington, D.C., describes this practice as he experiences it:

> Medicaid... covers medications, diagnostic tests, and the costs of specialists and hospitalizations. But for the two-thirds of our patients without Medicaid, the only answer is the tin cup. This means resorting to charity services, give-away programs, personal connections, system loopholes, solicited forbearance, and persuasion.... Some days I spend as much time pleading as I do practicing.[125]

The difference between CHCs in Washington, D.C., and the Lower Rio Grande Valley is that Washington has many more resources to tap into, including some of the best teaching hospitals in the world. In Texas' Lower Rio Grande Valley, comparable resources are scarce to non-existent. Still, physicians barter with their colleagues as necessary to obtain the care that their patients require.

It should be noted that plans are currently underway to establish the Regional Academic Health Center (RAHC), which will serve the four counties of the Lower Rio Grande Valley, Cameron, Hidalgo, Starr, and Willacy Counties. The RAHC will be used for undergraduate clinical education, graduate residency training programs, and medical research, thereby providing a much-needed source of advanced medical care for uninsured immigrants in the region. RAHC is expected to begin residency training in July 2002.[126]

Crossing the "Second Border"

Dr. Stanley Fisch of Harlingen Pediatrics Association cites the "second border" as a major barrier to access for the children he treats.[127] Immigrants often come across the U.S.-Mexico border and live in the Lower Rio Grande Valley for years without experiencing any threat to their immigration status. However, individuals requiring advanced medical care that cannot be provided in the Valley are often sent to one of the hospitals in Houston or Galveston. This requires crossing a second border checkpoint, like the Sarita Checkpoint, located 60 miles north of McAllen on US 77. An undocumented immigrant attempting to cross this checkpoint faces a 50 percent chance of deportation.[128] Dr. Fisch often sends a note addressed to INS along with the children he refers to Houston, which he says is usually enough to get the patient through the checkpoint. However, the second border does create a daunting barrier to health care access for immigrants fearing deportation.

The "Gatekeeper" System

Some Texas counties, which cover indigent care over and above that provided by CHCs, require CHCs needing to refer patients out for specialized care to do so through a "gatekeeper" system.[129] The gatekeeper system creates unnecessary barriers for CHC patients in need of secondary care. For example, Cameron County (where BCHC is located) has two gatekeeper physicians who are both family practitioners.[130] If an internist at BCHC believes that a patient needs to see a specialist, he or she cannot refer the patient directly, but must rather refer them to one of the gatekeeper physicians. The gatekeeper is responsible for determining whether specialized care is needed, and then makes the necessary referral. This system is both inefficient and potentially dangerous. Because the physicians at BCHC are internists and the gatekeepers are family practitioners, the BCHC physicians are actually more qualified to determine whether a patient requires specialized care. In addition, under this system patients may have to wait several extra weeks before finally getting in to see a specialist. In cases where a patient's condition requires immediate medical attention, valuable time is wasted and the patient ultimately suffers.

Counties have the power to waive the requirement that CHCs must refer patients to gatekeeper physicians before they may receive secondary health care services.[131] Such a waiver would, in effect, give CHCs gatekeeper authority, allowing them to certify the type of care a patient requires and refer them directly to the services they need.

CHC Expansion

CHCs have recently been enjoying the spotlight as a popular and relatively inexpensive solution for dealing with the problem of the uninsured. In December 2001, a House/Senate Conference Committee approved the Resolution to Expand Access to Community Health Centers (REACH) representing a $175 million funding increase for CHCs for FY2002—the largest ever increase for this program.[132] The National Association of Community Health Centers (NACHC) plans to put this new funding towards its goal of doubling of the capacity of health centers over the next five years.[133]

The Committee also approved $105 million in funding for the Community Access Program (CAP), which helps coordinate services for underserved populations by integrating CHCs with other health care providers.[134] Although this represents a $20 million decrease for CAP from FY2001 appropriations, it is still considered a victory over President Bush's call to eliminate the program completely.[135]

The Statewide Strategic Plan set forth in August 2001 by TACHC outlines a plan to expand access to 325,361 new patients and expand services to 247,993 new and current patients over the next five years.[136] This would involve expansions to 247 new and existing centers, and hiring another 338 providers.[137] TACHC has estimated that these expansions would require $99 million in additional grant support.[138] To meet this goal, TACHC is working with CHCs to develop and submit applications for federal Section 330 funding.

Table 3.8 lists the counties that TACHC has targeted for expansion over the next five years, as well as the types of expansion planned for each year. In other counties, such as Travis or Harris, FQHCs are maintained by the city, county, or the hospital district and are not under the TACHC umbrella.

Table 3.8
TACHC Statewide Strategic Plan

County	2002	2003	2004	2005	2006
Armstrong			New site		
Atascosa	New/expand				
Bailey	Expansion	Expansion		Expansion	
Bexar	New/expand	Expansion	Expansion	Expansion	Expansion
Bosque			New site		
Brewster	New site	Expansion	Expansion	Expansion	Expansion
Briscoe	New/expand				
Caldwell	Expansion				
Cameron		New/expand	New site	Expansion	
Chambers			New site		
Comanche		Expansion	Expansion		Expansion
Coryell					New site
Dallas	Expansion	Expansion	Expansion	Expansion	Expansion
Deaf Smith	Expansion	Expansion	Expansion	Expansion	
Delta		New site			
Donley		New site			
Eastland	New site				
Edwards					New site
El Paso	New/expand	New/expand	New/expand	Expansion	New/expand
Falls	New site				
Fort Bend		New site	Expansion	Expansion	Expansion
Frio					Expansion
Galveston	Expansion	Expansion	Expansion	Expansion	Expansion
Gonzales	Expansion				
Guadalupe		New site			
Hale	Expansion	Expansion	Expansion	Expansion	Expansion
Hidalgo	Expansion	New/expand	New/expand	New site	
Hill		New site			
Hopkins			New site	Expansion	
Hunt Rockwall	Expansion				
Jasper		New site			
Jefferson	New/expand	Expansion	Expansion	New/expand	Expansion
Karnes			New site		New site
Kinney	Expansion	Expansion	Expansion	Expansion	Expansion
La Salle	Expansion				
Lavaca				New site	
Lee					New site
Limestone				New site	
Lubbock	Expansion	Expansion	Expansion	Expansion	Expansion
Maverick	Expansion	Expansion	Expansion	Expansion	Expansion
McLennan	Expansion	Expansion	Expansion	New/expand	
Medina	Expansion		Expansion		
Moore					New site
Motley	Expansion			Expansion	
Nacogdoches	Expansion	Expansion	New site		Expansion
Oldham				New site	
Orange					Expansion

County	2002	2003	2004	2005	2006
Pecos	New site	Expansion	Expansion	Expansion	Expansion
Potter	Expansion	Expansion	Expansion	Expansion	
Presidio	New site	Expansion	Expansion	Expansion	Expansion
Real	Expansion	Expansion	New/expand		
Runnels		New site			
Shelby				New site	
Sherman					New site
Terry		New site			
Tom Green	Expansion	Expansion	Expansion	New/expand	Expansion
Uvalde	Expansion		Expansion	Expansion	Expansion
Val Verde	Expansion	Expansion	Expansion	Expansion	Expansion
Webb	Expansion	Expansion	Expansion	Expansion	Expansion
Wharton					New site
Wichita	Expansion	Expansion	Expansion	Expansion	
Willacy	Expansion				New/expand
Wilson			New site		
Yoakum			New site		
Zavala	New site	Expansion	Expansion		

Adapted from: Texas Association of Community Health Centers, "Texas Statewide Strategic Plan Prepared for BPHC and NACHC" (Austin, Tex., August 22, 2001), Appendix C (draft proposal).

Note: Plans for new site development are denoted by "New site" in the table, plans for expanding services provided by existing sites are denoted by "Expansion," and plans for both new site development and expansion are denoted by "New/expand."

Charitable Organizations

In addition to county-funded programs and CHCs, many of Texas' uninsured immigrants seek health care services from private, not-for-profit charitable organizations. Most of these organizations offer the same services as CHCs, however they receive no public funding. Following are profiles of two charitable health care organizations in Austin.

El Buen Samaritano

El Buen Samaritano (EBS) is an Episcopal mission seeking to "help working-poor Spanish-speaking families secure a productive and meaningful place in the community through healthcare, basic education, advocacy, training in community responsibility, and emergency food and clothing."[139] The health clinic offers many low-cost services including pediatrics, adult services, prenatal care, family planning, and laboratory testing. Fees range from $2 for certain lab tests to $20 for a comprehensive medical consultation. The clinic serves approximately 30-50 clients per day, and is open during regular business hours from Monday through Friday, with extended evening hours on Mondays and Tuesdays. EBS trains *promotoras* to do community outreach, including group facilitation on topics ranging from pregnancy to mental health.

EBS has several funding sources including the United Way, March of Dimes, grants, and private donations. Although there has been past discussion about becoming a Medicaid provider, serious concerns about the additional administrative burden and lack of staff have prevented EBS from pursuing this option. As part of their prenatal care, pregnant clients are taken on a tour of Brackenridge Hospital where they will deliver, and are encouraged to enroll their babies in Medicaid or SCHIP at that time.

People's Community Clinic

People's Community Clinic (PCC) was founded by volunteer doctors and nurses in 1970, and has since become "Austin's largest comprehensive primary health care center serving the uninsured working poor."[140] PCC serves anybody requiring medical care, regardless of their ability to pay. Clinic hours are 8:30 am to 8:30 pm Monday through Friday, and services include: prenatal care, gynecology, family planning, adult primary care, teen prenatal care, pediatric primary care, adolescent health, immunizations, nutrition counseling, HIV testing/counseling, pharmacy services, and social work services. PCC serves a largely Hispanic clientele (57 percent).[141]

PCC is involved in many collaborative efforts within the community. For example, together with LifeWorks, PCC operates the Project Phase Street Outreach program to provide basic health care and education to homeless youth. PCC also provides medical care to adolescents enrolled in the Phoenix Academy's residential treatment program. In addition, PCC works with the St. David's and Seton Health Care Systems to provide aftercare for medically indigent patients discharged from the hospital or emergency room.

General Recommendations

Although immigrants in Texas receive health care services from a wide variety of sources, it seems that emphasis should be placed on expansion solutions which capitalize on federal sources of capital. Considering the crucial role that CHCs play in providing care to Texas' uninsured regardless of immigration status, the recent increase in federal Section 330 funding signifies one of the very few bright spots for expanding access to this underserved population. The following are CHC-focused options for expanding and improving access to health care for Texas' immigrants.

Proceed with TACHC Statewide Strategic Plan: The Statewide Strategic Plan set forth by TACHC outlines a strategy to expand access to 325,361 new patients and expand services to 247,993 new and current patients over the next five years.[142] Since 70 percent of the people served by CHCs are Hispanic, and a large percentage of these individuals are immigrants, this would mean a significant increase in health care access for immigrants in Texas.[143]

Empower CHCs as "Gatekeepers": It is clear that the CHC "gatekeeper" system imposed by certain counties creates unnecessary barriers for CHC patients in need of secondary and tertiary care. This is especially a problem in the Lower Rio Grande Valley, where much of Texas' immigrant population resides. Counties have the power to waive the requirement that CHCs must refer patients to gatekeeper physicians before they may receive secondary health care services. Such a waiver would, in effect, give CHCs gatekeeper authority, allowing them to certify the type of care a patient requires and refer them directly to the services they need.

Increased Outreach Efforts: The success of programs to enroll children in Medicaid and SCHIP is due in large part to the efforts of CHC-based outreach workers, including *promotoras*. These efforts much continue at the highest possible level in order to ensure that every eligible child is enrolled in a public health insurance program. To this end, it will be very important for TACHC to follow through the second phase of Project Alberto, by placing additional outreach workers in communities around the state, and using new technologies to facilitate faster processing of applications.

Notes

[1] U.S. Department of Labor, Bureau of Labor Statistics, *2001 March Current Population Survey.* Online. Available: http://www.bls.census.gov/cps/cpsmain.htm. Accessed: April 8, 2002.

[2] Kaiser Family Foundation, *State Health Facts Online.* Online. Available: http://www.statehealthfacts.kff.org. Accessed: November 9, 2001.

[3] Lyndon B. Johnson School of Public Affairs, *Expanding Health Care Coverage for the Uninsured in Texas*, Policy Research Project Series, no. 141 (Austin, Tex., 2001), pp. 207-228.

[4] U.S. Department of Labor, Bureau of Labor Statistics, *2001 March Current Population Survey* (Online).

[5] Ibid.

[6] Ibid.

[7] Ibid.

[8] Lyndon B. Johnson School of Public Affairs, *Expanding Health Care Coverage for the Uninsured in Texas*, pp. 207-228.

[9] Ibid.

[10] Kaiser Family Foundation, *State Health Facts Online.* Online. Available: http://www.statehealthfacts.kff.org. Accessed: November 9, 2001.

[11] Lyndon B. Johnson School of Public Affairs, *Expanding Health Care Coverage for the Uninsured in Texas*, pp. 207-28.

[12] Ibid.

[13] Ibid.

[14] Ibid.

[15] Lyndon B. Johnson School of Public Affairs, *Expanding Health Care Coverage for the Uninsured in Texas*, pp. 87-102.

[16] Texas Health and Human Service Commission, *Children's Medicaid Simplification-Senate Bill 43 Proposed Implementation Outline.* Online. Available: http://www.hhsc.state.tx.us/chip/SB43/ SB43_Simplification_Intro.html. Accessed: January 27, 2002.

[17] Anne Dunkelberg, *Children's Medicaid Eligibility Simplification Bill, SB 43, Sent to the Governor* (Austin, Tex.: Center for Public Policy Priorities, 2002), p. 1.

[18] Texas Association of Community Health Centers, "Robert Wood Johnson Foundation Grant Narrative" (Austin, Tex., 2001), p. 4.

[19] Texas CHIP Coalition. *What is this new CHIP program?* Online. Available: http://www.main.org/txchip/page3.html. Accessed: October 20, 2001.

[20] Ibid.

[21] Ibid.

[22] U.S. Department of Labor, Bureau of Labor Statistics, *2001 March Current Population Survey* (Online).

[23] Lyndon B. Johnson School of Public Affairs, *Expanding Health Care Coverage for the Uninsured in Texas*, pp. 207-28.

[24] Ibid.

[25] U.S. Department of Labor, Bureau of Labor Statistics, *2001 March Current Population Survey* (Online).

[26] Ibid.

[27] Lyndon B. Johnson School of Public Affairs, *Expanding Health Care Coverage for the Uninsured in Texas*, pp. 207-28.

[28] Ibid.

[29] Ibid.

[30] U.S. Department of Labor, Bureau of Labor Statistics, *1999 March Current Population Survey*. Online. Available: http://www.bls.census.gov/cps/cpsmain.htm. Accessed: April 8, 2002.

[31] U.S. Department of Labor, Bureau of Labor Statistics, *2000 March Current Population Survey*. Online. Available: http://www.bls.census.gov/cps/cpsmain.htm. Accessed: April 8, 2002.

[32] U.S. Department of Labor, Bureau of Labor Statistics, *2001 March Current Population Survey* (Online).

[33] Randy Capps, The Urban Institute, "Hardship among Children of Immigrants: Findings from the 1999 National Survey of America's Families." Online. Available: http://newfederalism.urban.org/html/series_b/b29/b29.html. Accessed: November 8, 2001.

[34] Ibid.

[35] Ibid.

[36] Ibid.

[37] Lyndon B. Johnson School of Public Affairs, *Expanding Health Care Coverage for the Uninsured in Texas*, pp. 207-28.

[38] Anne Dunkelberg, "Immigrants' Access to Benefits in Texas: Five Things to Remember," Presentation given at 25th Annual Texas State National Association of Social Workers (NASW) Conference, Austin, Texas, October 12, 2001.

[39] Leighton Ku and Shannon Blaney, Center on Budget and Policy Priorities, *Health Coverage for Legal Immigrant Children: New Census Data Highlight Importance of Restoring Medicaid and SCHIP Coverage*. Online. Available: http://www.cbpp.org/10-4-00health.htm. Accessed: January 3, 2002.

[40] Interview by Jennifer Eldridge with Anne Dunkelberg, Senior Policy Analyst, Center for Public Policy Priorities, Austin, Texas, November 15, 2001.

[41] Michael E. Fix and Karen Tumlin, The Urban Institute, *Welfare Reform and the Devolution of Immigrant Policy*. Online. Available: http://newfederalism.urban.org/html/anf_15.htm. Accessed: November 8, 2001.

[42] U.S. Department of Labor, Bureau of Labor Statistics, *1999 March Current Population Survey* (Online).

[43] U.S. Department of Labor, Bureau of Labor Statistics, *2000 March Current Population Survey* (Online).

[44] U.S. Department of Labor, Bureau of Labor Statistics, *2001 March Current Population Survey* (Online).

[45] Anne Dunkelberg, Senior Policy Analyst, Center for Public Policy Priorities, Class Presentation, Lyndon B. Johnson School of Public Affairs, Austin, Texas, November 13, 2001.

[46] Texas Association of Community Health Centers, "Texas Statewide Strategic Plan Prepared for BPHC and NACHC" (Austin, Tex., August 22, 2001), p. 1 (draft proposal).

[47] Dunkelberg, "Immigrants' Access to Benefits in Texas: Five Things to Remember" (Presentation).

[48] Maternal and Child Health Bureau, *MCHB Mission*. Online. Available: http://mchb.hrsa.gov. Accessed: January 4, 2002.

[49] Texas Department of Health, *Women's Health in Texas*. Available: http://www.tdh.state.tx.us/women/famsrc.stm. Accessed: January 10, 2002.

[50] Ibid.

[51] Dunkelberg interview.

[52] Ibid.

[53] Ibid.

[54] The Texas Health Access Project, "Random Access: Holes in the Texas Health Care Safety Net: Reports from the Communities" (Austin, Tex., 2001), p. 23.

[55] Center for Public Policy Priorities, *CHIP and Children Who Are Not U.S. Citizens*. Online. Available: http://www.cppp.org/products/policyanalysis/briefingpapers/brpchip3.pdf. Accessed: January 11, 2002.

[56] Ibid.

[57] Center for Public Policy Priorities, *Inclusion of Undocumented Persons by Texas Indigent Health Care Providers*. Online. Available: http://www.cppp.org/products/policyanalysis/briefingpapers/brpHC1100.html. Accessed: January 10, 2002.

[58] The Migrant Clinicians Network, *Farmworker Migration Patterns*. Online. Available: http://www.migrantclinician.org. Accessed: January 20, 2002.

[59] The Migrant Clinicians Network, *The Farmworker Population: Background.* Online. Available: http://www.migrantclinician.org. Accessed: January 20, 2002.

[60] Interview by Jennifer Eldridge with Jana Blaisi, Deputy Director, Texas Association of Community Health Centers, Austin, Texas, January 17, 2002.

[61] The Migrant Clinicians Network, *Farmworker Health Issues*. Online. Available: http://www.migrantclinician.org. Accessed: January 20, 2002.

[62] Ibid.

[63] Ibid.

[64] Ibid.

[65] Ibid.

[66] Lyndon B. Johnson School of Public Affairs, *Expanding Health Care Coverage for the Uninsured in Texas*, pp. 207-228.

[67] Ibid.

[68] The Migrant Clinicians Network, *The Farmworker Population: Background* (Online).

[69] Ibid.

[70] Benjamin Flores, Chief of the HRSA Migrant Health Branch, Presentation given to 11th Annual Midwestern Farmworker Stream Forum, Austin, Texas, December 6, 2001.

[71] Ibid.

[72] Ibid.

[73] Office of State and National Partnerships, Bureau of Primary Health Care, *Current Approaches to Medicaid Reciprocity and Portability*. Online. Available: http://bphc.hrsa.gov/osnp/Medicaid2.htm. Accessed: January 15, 2002.

[74] Ibid.

[75] Ibid.

[76] Ibid.

[77] Ibid.

[78] Texas House Bill 2498, 77th Legislature (2001). Online. Available: http://www.capitol.state.tx.us/tlo/77r/billtext/HB02498F.HTM. Accessed: February 1, 2002.

[79] Ibid.

[80] Interview by Jennifer Eldridge with Elena Marin, M.D., Executive Director, Su Clinica Familiar, Harlingen, Texas, February 1, 2002.

[81] Texas Department of Human Services, *Colonias Factbook*. Online. Available: http://chud.tamu.edu/colonias/factbook.html#health. Accessed: February 1, 2002.

[82] Ibid.

[83] Evan Christman, Scott Atnip, Laura Koenig, and Senator Chet Brooks, Lyndon B. Johnson School of Public Affairs, "Indigent Health Care in Texas" (Austin, Tex., November 2001), p. 1 (unpublished policy brief).

[84] Caton M. Fenz, The Access Project, *Providing Health Care to the Uninsured in Texas*. Online. Available: http://www.accessproject.org/downloads/TEXAS.pdf. Accessed: January 15, 2002.

[85] Ibid.

[86] Ibid.

[87] Ibid.

[88] National Immigration Law Center. *Texas AG Issues Opinion that County Hospitals Not Allowed to Serve "Not Qualified" Immigrants.* Online. Available: http://www.nilc.org/immspbs/health/health012.htm. Accessed: January 22, 2002.

[89] Ibid.

[90] Ibid.

[91] Caton M. Fenz, The Access Project, *Providing Health Care to the Uninsured in Texas.* Online. Available: http://www.accessproject.org/downloads/TEXAS.pdf. Accessed: January 15, 2002.

[92] Ibid.

[93] Ibid.

[94] Guy Clifton, M.D., Hermann Hospital, "Addressing Houston's Emergency Room Crisis," Houston, Tex., October 30, 2001, p. 1 (draft paper).

[95] Ibid.

[96] Ibid.

[97] Ibid.

[98] Christman, Atnip, Koenig, Brooks, "Indigent Health Care in Texas," p. 1.

[99] Ibid.

[100] Texas Department of Health, *Indigent Health Care Division.* Online. Available: http://www.tdh.state.tx.us/hcf/ihcp/default.htm. Accessed: January 28, 2002.

[101] Texas Association of Community Health Centers. *What is an FQHC?* Online. Available: http://www.tachc.org. Accessed: November 14, 2001.

[102] Ibid.

[103] Ibid.

[104] Ibid.

[105] Blaisi interview.

[106] Texas Association of Community Health Centers, "Texas Statewide Strategic Plan Prepared for BPHC and NACHC" (Austin, Tex., August 22, 2001), Table entitled "Growth and Resource Plan (2002-2006) State of Texas" (draft proposal).

[107] Ibid.

[108] Ibid.

[109] Ibid.

[110] Ibid.

[111] Texas Association of Community Health Centers, "Texas Association of Community Health Centers Membership Directory" (Austin, Tex., 2000), p. 6.

[112] Ibid.

[113] Ibid.

[114] Texas Association of Community Health Centers. *Project Alberto/Covering Kids Initiative.* Online. Available: http://www.tachc.org/o_pa_main.htm. Accessed: January 2, 2002.

[115] Ibid.

[116] Texas Association of Community Health Centers, "Robert Wood Johnson Foundation Grant Narrative" (Austin, Tex., 2001), pp. 10-12.

[117] Ibid.

[118] Ibid.

[119] Ibid.

[120] Ibid.

[121] Interview by Jennifer Eldridge with Paula Gomez, Executive Director, Brownsville Community Health Center, Brownsville, Texas, January 31, 2002.

[122] Ibid.

[123] Ibid.

[124] Ibid.

[125] Fitzhugh Mullan, M.D., "Tin-Cup Medicine," *Health Affairs*, vol. 20, no. 6 (November/December 2001), p. 220.

[126] The University of Texas Health Science Center at San Antonio, "Regional Academic Health Center." Online. Available: http://rahc.uthscsa.edu. Accessed: April 10, 2002.

[127] Interview by Jennifer Eldridge with Stanley Fisch, M.D., Physician, Harlingen Pediatrics Association, Harlingen, Texas, January 31, 2002.

[128] Gomez interview.

[129] Ibid.

[130] Ibid.

[131] Ibid.

[132] National Association of Community Health Centers, *Conference Committee Approves Record Increase for Health Center Program.* Online. Available: http://www.nachc.com/Federal_Affairs/2002/Conference_Passage.htm. Accessed: January 4, 2001.

[133] Ibid.

[134] Ibid.

[135] Ibid.

[136] Texas Association of Community Health Centers, "Texas Statewide Strategic Plan Prepared for BPHC and NACHC," p. 3.

[137] Ibid.

[138] Ibid.

[139] El Buen Samaritano, "Mid-Year Report, Project Year 2001-2002" (Austin, Tex., 2001), p. 1.

[140] People's Community Clinic, *About Us.* Online. Available: http://www.pcclinic.org/about.html. Accessed: March 24, 2002.

[141] People's Community Clinic, *2000 Services Report.* Online. Available: http://www.pcclinic.org/report.html. Accessed: March 24, 2002.

[142] Texas Association of Community Health Centers, "Texas Statewide Strategic Plan Prepared for BPHC and NACHC," p. 3.

[143] Ibid.

Chapter 4. Premium Assistance Programs: Reducing the Number of Uninsured Working Texans with Low to Moderate Incomes

by Lisa Ewart

Introduction

In the United States, employer-based health insurance is the most common form of coverage.[1] Nearly two-thirds of Americans receive their health insurance through their employers.[2] Health insurance for employees offers several benefits, including security from financial loss if an employee or a member of their covered family becomes seriously ill, increased worker productivity by helping to keep individuals healthy, and compensation for workers by providing an adequate benefits package that works to recruit and retain workers. Perhaps most importantly, it enables individuals to obtain affordable health care.[3]

According to the Texas Health and Human Services Commission, approximately 12.5 million children and adults in Texas receive their health insurance through their employers. However, many employed individuals are uninsured. Approximately 2 million uninsured individuals in Texas are non-retired, working, individuals ages 18 to 64.[4] They do not have coverage either because they were 1) not offered coverage through their employer, 2) they were ineligible, or 3) they declined coverage.

Many low to moderate-income workers have access to health insurance. Nationally, of the working parents who have been uninsured for at least a year, 18 percent of those falling below 100 percent of the Federal Poverty Level (FPL) have access to employer-based coverage. For uninsured parents earning 100 to 132 percent of the FPL, about 38 percent have access to employer-based coverage, and about 45 percent of uninsured parents with incomes between 133 and 199 percent of the FPL have access to employer-based coverage.[5]

In Texas approximately 693,500, or 8.8 percent, of individuals who have access to employer-sponsored coverage have declined to participate.[6] This 8.8 percent includes the many participants that decline insurance through their employers because they have health insurance through other means such as their spouses' plans; however, it also includes the working population that declines because they are unable to afford the premiums of their employers' plans. This group, who declines because of the prohibitive cost of the employer plan, remains uninsured.

The cost of health insurance premiums rose by 90 percent nationwide between 1987 and 1993, but the wages of these workers rose only 28 percent.[7] It is difficult for low-income workers to afford to pay their own premiums, much less the premiums to cover their families.[8] Additionally, a national study by the Center for Studying Health System Change reported that most individuals who do not "take up" or enroll in available employer-sponsored coverage cite cost as the main reason why.[9] Two-thirds of uninsured worker and nearly three-fourths of low-income uninsured workers stated that cost was the most prominent reason for declining to participate in the employer-sponsored insurance.[10] One way to cover this group of uninsured individuals would be to provide subsidies so they could afford the coverage offered by their employer plan.

Subsidies for Employer-Sponsored Health Insurance

This paper will focus on options for providing public subsidies to individuals to enable them to buy into their employer-sponsored health insurance. These types of programs are aimed at individuals who currently have access to an employer benefits program, but who cannot afford to pay the premiums. States partner with the private-sector employer under an employer buy-in to provide private coverage.

This partnership has the potential to be "a win-win coverage technique for states" for several reasons.[11] First, using public money to subsidize employer sponsored private health insurance allows the state and working individuals to take advantage of private money contributed by the employer to the employee health care plans. Public subsidies also enable an individual to buy into their employer's private insurance rather than receiving benefits through a public program. Participation in a private insurance plan, with the help of public money, reduces the welfare stigma attached to public health insurance programs. In addition, subsidizing employer coverage also provides for family coverage, keeping families together under one insurance plan.[12]

Although there are benefits, there are many problems associated with implementing these programs. Problems include low participation rates due largely to the fact that nationally only 11 percent of the uninsured are eligible for employer group coverage,[13] administrative burdens and cost, and an inadequate number of employer plans that meet the benefit and contribution requirements associated with receiving federal money. Additionally, many employer plans do not meet the cost-effectiveness test imposed by the states and many workers who are eligible for public funds are mobile and are not staying in a particular job long enough to establish the buy-in.[14]

Despite these setbacks, some programs taking advantage of employer-sponsored insurance are succeeding. States have approached the task of providing premium assistance in several different ways. Some states have decided to focus on the working Medicaid-eligible population (including the working population with dependents eligible for Medicaid) by using Medicaid dollars to pay employer health insurance premiums for the individual and their dependents when it is cost effective. Other states have expanded their premium payment programs by using SCHIP funds to cover children and adults in families with a SCHIP eligible family member, and finally, some states finance premium assistance programs solely with state funds. Using state funds can allow for greater flexibility in determining all aspects of the program.[15]

Recently, the federal government has allowed additional flexibility in using federal dollars for public health insurance programs. The United States Department for Health and Human Services under current President Bush developed the Health Insurance Flexibility and Accountability (HIFA) initiative that grants additional flexibility to states in establishing employer buy-in programs in an effort to encourage states to explore ways to use public funds to subsidize private health insurance.[16] Premium assistance programs could be effective when implemented as a part of a HIFA waiver because as states expand public assistance insurance programs to individuals and families at higher income levels, it is likely that many of the individuals who are now eligible for public insurance programs will also be working.

The proposed HIFA waiver presented in the Policy Research Project Report entitled *Expansion through Waivers*[17] is one example of this type of waiver. The report proposes expanding Medicaid coverage to childless adults and parents of SCHIP- and Medicaid-eligible children. By cutting some benefits and requiring additional cost-sharing on the part of the individual in the expanded population, the option proposed in the report would cover from 73,000-560,000 previously uninsured individuals. The cost of this option would run from $91 million to $783 million.[18] The state might be able to lower some of these costs by implementing a premium assistance program. The cutting of benefits and the greater cost-sharing for expansion populations, as discussed in the report, would enable more employer plans to be eligible for the program and cost effective. As more plans become eligible, more individuals will enroll in these plans, reducing the cost of the public program to the state and encouraging private health insurance options.[19]

The new national focus and the expanded eligibility for public insurance programs make public subsidies for employer-based insurance coverage a viable option for states in the implementation of their public health insurance programs.

Subsidies Using Medicaid Funds: The HIPP Program

In 1990, the Health Insurance Premium Payment (HIPP) Program was created as part of the Medicaid program that required states to subsidize the cost of employer-based health insurance for eligible individuals when it was cost effective to do so. This program was authorized under Section 1906 of the Social Security Act. States had difficulty meeting this requirement because of difficulties identifying eligible individuals and gaining cooperation from both the employer and the employee.[20] The program was ultimately made optional, and a small number of states have started aggressive programs. One such aggressive program is the Iowa HIPP program (see Appendix B for information regarding this program).

The HIPP program allows states to use federally matched Medicaid funds to pay the costs associated with employer-sponsored health insurance including premiums, deductibles, and coinsurance on behalf of Medicaid recipients when the state determines it to be cost effective.[21] Cost effective means that it costs the state less to pay for the employee's part of the employer health insurance than to enroll the family in the state Medicaid program. In determining cost-effectiveness, states must also consider any "wrap-around" services that states are required to provide when the employer-based insurance is not as comprehensive as the Medicaid package.[22]

Premium assistance programs such as the HIPP program save the state money because they cost the state less to pay for the individual's share of the employer-sponsored coverage than to provide for the individual through Medicaid, and programs encourage individuals who have access to employer coverage to participate in the private insurance market. Programs also allow the state to expand to additional uninsured populations by providing subsidized insurance to many non-Medicaid family members. This arrangement occurs when it is necessary to subsidize health insurance for the non-eligible member in order for the eligible member to participate in the employer-sponsored program. In this situation, the cost-effectiveness test still applies, but it is modified by testing whether it costs less for the state to subsidize the premiums for both the non-Medicaid and Medicaid eligible individuals than it costs to pay the health care costs of only the Medicaid eligible individual under the state Medicaid plan. If this cost-effectiveness test is met, the HIPP program offers states an avenue to expand employer-sponsored health coverage to low-income workers, while simultaneously saving money, receiving federal matching funds, and encouraging family health insurance.[23]

The HIPP Program in Texas

The HIPP program in Texas started on September 1, 1994, and it saves the state approximately $4 million annually. Today around 2,500 families are covered under the HIPP program.[24] To be eligible for this program, the individual must have access to employer based coverage, he/she must be Medicaid-eligible or the parent/guardian of a Medicaid-eligible child, and enrollment must be cost effective for the state. HIPP pays the coverage for the entire family, not just the Medicaid individual, but it will not pay any co-pays or deductibles for the non-Medicaid eligible family members.[25]

The National Heritage Insurance Company (NHIC), the insurer of the Texas Medicaid program, determines cost effectiveness by establishing the Medicaid expenditures for the past year of the entire household, taking into consideration the specific health-related circumstances of the household. The past Medicaid payments for the household are compared to the cost of the premiums and other cost-sharing expenditures for the most comprehensive employer sponsored policy. If the cost of that insurance is less than the Medicaid payments, then the policy is deemed cost-effective. When NHIC decides that it is cost-effective for the family to enroll, the individual is required to enroll in the HIPP program and the employer-based coverage as a condition of Medicaid eligibility.[26]

Procedurally, the premium for health insurance is deducted from the HIPP enrollee's paycheck. The individual sends a copy of the pay stub to NHIC, and the individual is reimbursed for the cost of the premium.[27]

The benefits of the HIPP program are evident. The state saves money and is able to provide insurance for family members who are not Medicaid-eligible. The individual has access to family coverage, and in some instances access to insurance with a better benefit package than Medicaid. If the package does not cover all the services that Medicaid does, the state will pay for those extra services. Additionally, if the individual becomes ineligible for Medicaid—for example, an eligible child ages out of Medicaid—then the family still has private insurance coverage. Under these circumstances, the family would be expected to pay the entire cost of their share of the premiums.

The employer also benefits. Having health benefits for the entire family encourages individuals to continue to work which means less turnover and training costs for the employer. Finally, providers might also benefit because many private insurance carriers offer higher payments to medical providers than the public Medicaid reimbursements.

Problems Facing HIPP: Private and Public Solutions

One major problem facing HIPP programs throughout the nation is the open enrollment period. The open enrollment period for employer-based insurance coverage prevents individuals from taking advantage or terminating employer-based coverage except during designated enrollment times. Qualifying events such as divorce and loss of spouse suspend this rule and allow individuals to register. Prior to the last legislative session, enrollment or termination from the HIPP program was not a qualifying event. Individuals who became eligible for HIPP often had to wait to enroll, and individuals whose HIPP eligibility ended often found themselves paying the entire cost of the employee premium until they were able to terminate coverage. Legislation recently alleviated this problem in Texas. House Bill 3038 mandated that enrollment in or termination from the HIPP program is considered a qualifying event and open enrollment periods do not apply.[28]

Another problem for the HIPP program seems to be a difficulty in obtaining information. Many eligible individuals do not know about the program. The lack of individual knowledge about the HIPP program can be partly attributed to the lack of an extensive outreach program in the state, which means that unless the individual hears about the program through the limited outreach that does occur, the only people who learn of HIPP are those who come in to apply for Medicaid for themselves or for their children.[29]

Although efforts should be geared to recruiting individuals who are working in low-income jobs, who are uninsured, and who do not know that they or their family members are eligible for Medicaid, limited effort is made to conduct outreach through the employer. Few of these efforts have not been institutionalized. Additionally, there is a lack of information-sharing concerning the employer plans. The state could conduct extensive research into employer plans to determine if a plan is acceptable for HIPP purposes, though this information can be difficult to collect from the employers.[30]

Finally, even if the state decided to conduct extensive outreach campaign, the state has no efficient way of identifying potentially eligible individuals. For example, Wal-mart is one of the largest employers in Texas.[31] The single cashier with two children might be eligible for Medicaid and therefore the HIPP program. However, little data-sharing exists to get that information to the administrators of Medicaid or the HIPP program. A federal rule mandates employee information-sharing, but that information, by law, can only be used by the Texas Office of the Attorney General to enforce child support. One suggestion might be to look into amending this regulation to enable health departments to obtain new employee information as well.[32]

Oddly enough, programs in other states do not conduct extensive formal outreach either. Occasionally, HIPP staff members from other programs give presentations to community groups, and a HIPP brochure is included in Medicaid application packets.[33] It seems that other HIPP programs will not offer much guidance as to the outreach of individuals eligible for public assistance who have access to employer-based coverage.

A state might decide that it does not want to conduct more extensive outreach because at that particular point in time, the state is not able to expand the Medicaid program. Whether a state seeks to expand enrollment is a policy decision that legislatures must make. The main question is the following: is the state looking to use premium assistance as a method to reduce the number of uninsured, or is it looking to a premium assistance program as a cost-saving measure? In difficult economic times, the state might attempt only to cut costs, but in stronger economic times, perhaps the state should look at the outreach portion of premium assistance programs as a way to decrease the number of uninsured and expand the Medicaid program.

Subsidy Programs for Employer-Based Coverage Using State Funds Only

While a federal match is beneficial, it often comes with strict guidelines that prohibit the states from covering the desired individuals or providing the desired services. These restrictions include a number of requirements regarding benefits, cost-sharing, employer contribution levels, and crowd-out.[34] To achieve greater flexibility in program eligibility and implementation, some states are choosing to entirely fund parts of their public insurance programs.

In recent years, the federal government has granted Medicaid and SCHIP waivers and allowed states to have more flexibility in structuring their programs, so state-only programs have become less viable options to expand coverage. Today, only a handful of states have an extensive state-only funded health insurance program, and it appears that a few of them are trying to obtain federal funding for parts of the program because the federal government has loosened many of the restrictions it placed on the receipt of federal funds by allowing states to apply for a waiver such as the HIFA.[35] For example, Oregon is currently pursuing avenues to take advantage of federal matching dollars. The Oregon plan, called Family Health Insurance Assistance Program (FHIAP) is a state-funded plan that provides for subsidies to be paid for the employee's share of the premium for working individuals up to 170 percent FPL. This program offers subsidies based on a sliding income scale. By not allowing the parents to use the subsidy strictly for themselves, the program encourages coverage for children.[36]

Subsidy Programs for Employer-Based Coverage Using SCHIP Funds

The State Children's Health Insurance Program (SCHIP) allows states to use SCHIP funds to subsidize employer-sponsored health insurance premiums for uninsured eligible families and children. A premium subsidy program can be established either through an amendment to the state's SCHIP plan or as a part of an expansion waiver. Regardless of how the plan is developed, there are a number of federal requirements in place for the states to follow:[37]

1. Benefits of programs must meet the SCHIP "benchmarks." Benchmark plans are the state employee plan, the federal Employees Health Benefit Plan, or the commercial HMO plan with the largest enrollment. Programs can provide the benchmark plan or offer coverage which is equivalent.
2. Coverage must meet the same cost-sharing requirements as coverage provided under regular SCHIP programs.
3. Policies must be established to prevent crowd-out including, for example, a minimum contribution amount by employers.
4. The plan must be cost effective, meaning the cost of enrolling the SCHIP-eligible child does not exceed the cost of enrolling the child in the public program.
5. Children must not be receiving employer coverage for at least six months before they can become eligible for the premium assistance program.

Subsequent guidelines published by the Centers for Medicare and Medicaid Studies (CMS) have loosened these requirements. The requirement for 60 percent minimum contribution from employers has been removed, and states may establish reasonable exceptions to the six-month waiting period.[38] Additionally, the HIFA waiver, which encourages public/private partnerships in providing insurance, allows for greater flexibility in calculating cost-effectiveness and in determining cost-sharing and benefits for optional and expansion populations.[39]

SCHIP Premium Assistance Program in Texas

Currently Texas does not have a premium assistance program available to eligible SCHIP families. In the 77th Texas Legislature, House Bill 3038, which was signed by the governor, allows for the implementation of a program that would provide subsidies to SCHIP-eligible children whose working parents have access to employer-sponsored insurance coverage. The legislation stipulates that the department may provide coverage for the eligible child's family if the child is not eligible to be enrolled, unless the working parent is enrolled and the cost of covering the family in employer sponsored coverage costs less than covering only the child in the public SCHIP plan.[40] The Health and Human Services Commission is currently setting up a premium assistance program in Texas. There are several issues that Texas should consider when implementing a premium assistance program. Additionally, Texas should look to other state examples when developing their program (see Appendix B for information on individual state premium assistance programs).

Issues to Examine when Developing a Premium Assistance Program in Texas

Target Population: Cutting Costs or Expansion to Uninsured Populations

The decision that the implementing state must make is whether this is an expansion effort or a cost-saving effort. There are three potential target groups for premium assistance. In a cost-saving effort, one might target eligible individuals who are already enrolled in SCHIP. Contacting the parents of the enrolled child to see if that parent has access to employer-sponsored coverage or including a question about access to coverage on the renewal form would be avenues to identify this cost-saving population. The state could also screen new SCHIP eligible/enrolled children for access to employer-sponsored coverage by including a question about access to employer insurance on the application or renewal form.

If the state is looking to expand coverage to uninsured parents of SCHIP-eligible children, then the state could conduct outreach in the workplace. They could target low-income working individuals who work for employers that offer employer-sponsored coverage in an effort to get them to apply for the SCHIP program for their children and possibly the premium assistance program.

Finally, if the state is considering a massive expansion effort, they could consider applying for a SCHIP Section 1115 waiver or a HIFA waiver and include either a feasibility study to address the issue of premium assistance programs or plans to implement a premium assistance program.

Given the current budgetary constraints, Texas might consider implementing the premium assistance program as a cost-saving measure. However, the implementation of a premium assistance program lays the groundwork for a program that in the future might be a part of an expansion effort.

Voluntary or Required Participation

The question of the voluntary participation of the program arises with both the employer and the eligible individual. Many states mandate that the individual enroll in the employer-sponsored insurance if the employer plan is deemed cost-effective and the benefits are comparable. Virginia is an exception to this participation requirement. The Texas HIPP program is mandatory for individuals if their employer plans qualify (see Appendix B for information on individual state premium assistance programs).

Voluntariness also applies to the employer who is sponsoring the insurance plan. It is questionable as to whether Texas Health and Human Services Commission can mandate that an employer participate in the program. In fact, many administrators of premium assistance have found that the employers are not very helpful when it comes to finding out information about employer plans. Because the state does not have a right to compel an employer to share details of the plan, the individual often is relied on to obtain the information.

Who Pays Whom for the Employee's Share

States must decide whether they will pay the employer directly for the employee's share of the program costs or whether they will pay the employee back after the employee has paid the premium. Iowa, for example, gives the individual a choice as to whether they pay the employer or the employee.[41]

Making the payment directly to the employee is the only policy that does not breech confidentiality. The employer never knows that the employee is receiving the public subsidy and this helps in the reduction of the welfare stigma. There is a potential problem with this procedure because it requires the individual to pay out-of-pocket until the state can reimburse the individual, usually upon proof of payment to the employer.

Making payments directly to the employer may solve the cash flow problems, but there will be a host of other problems that arise. For example, the employer may consider this process administratively burdensome. Additionally, the employer will then know that the employee is receiving public assistance, which violates that employee's privacy.

Cost-Effectiveness

As stated above, in order for a state to take advantage of federal funds for its premium assistance program, enrolling the child in the employer-sponsored plan must be cost effective. If the state is planning on using SCHIP funds—and it has not been granted a waiver that allows it to expand SCHIP coverage to parents—the cost-effectiveness test only compares the cost of covering the individual children in the public program to the cost of enrolling the children and the parent (if necessary) in the employer program. Employer-sponsored insurance programs might only allow the family to enroll if the worker is also enrolled. If this is the situation, the state must also enroll the parent in the employer-sponsored coverage in order to enroll the child.

If the state has an expansion waiver, then the cost-effectiveness test expands and compares the cost of covering both the parent/working adult and the child in the public plan to the cost of covering the family in the employer-sponsored insurance program. The additional cost on the public side might enhance the possibility that the employer-sponsored coverage will be cost-effective. (For an example of a state that assesses cost effectiveness in this manner, see the section on New Jersey in Appendix B.)

The cost to the state of enrolling the child and/or the parent into the employer-sponsored plan should also take into account administrative costs, wrap-around services if the benefits of the employer plan are not as rich as the public program, and any cost-sharing requirements involved in the plan.[42] (See Appendix B for specific state examples of their cost-effectiveness tests.)

Results in running a preliminary cost-effectiveness test suggest that the employer plan for a family with several SCHIP eligible children is more cost effective than the employer plan for a family with only one or two SCHIP eligible children. Most employer-sponsored insurance is either an individual policy or a family policy. Therefore, the price does not tend to increase with the addition of more children. However, the states' cost to cover a family does increase with the addition of a new child.

In the included example, the following formula was used to estimate the state's cost of enrolling the individual in the employer-sponsored coverage:

Administrative Cost + Employee Contribution – Cost Sharing Requirement

If this amount is less than the amount paid by the state for the cost of covering the child, then the plan is cost-effective.

Table 4.1
Evaluating Cost-Effectiveness

Number of children per family	Premium for SCHIP	Cost to state for employer sponsored coverage	Difference	State cost per child in SCHIP	Admin-istrative Cost	Employee Contribution for family policy	Cost-sharing requirements
1	$110	$296	-$186	$110	$29	$285	18
2	$220	$325	-$105				
3	$330	$354	-$24				
4	$440	$383	$57				
5	$550	$412	$138				
6	$660	$441	$219				
7	$770	$470	$300				
8	$880	$499	$381				
9	$990	$528	$462			Cost of Plan	Employer Contribution
10	$1,100	$557	$543			$500	$215

Adapted from: Interview by Lisa Ewart with Trey Berndt, Special Assistant, Medicaid/CHIP Operations, Health and Human Services Commission, Austin, Texas, February 15, 2002; and Elizabeth Shenkman and Jana Col, *Children's Health Insurance Program in Texas: The New Enrollee Survey Report* (Gainesville. Florida: Institute for Child Health Policy, January 2001), p. 29.

Note: This model does not include the cost of wrap-around services or the amount of cost-sharing imposed by the employer-sponsored plan on the employee.

The formula used in this model to estimate the state's cost of enrolling the individual child in employer-sponsored coverage is only one option for determining cost-effectiveness. Rhode Island recently implemented a new way to determine cost-effectiveness. The state assesses cost-effectiveness at the program level and bases it on the average family rate rather than calculated for each individual family. Using an average might cut down on some of the administrative costs associated with determining cost-effectiveness.[43]

Benefit Package

Benefits must be comparable, and if they are not, the state must develop a mechanism to provide wrap-around services. The additional funds required to provide these services should be included in the cost-effectiveness test. Under the HIFA waiver, benefits can be reduced for optional populations, but not for the children who would otherwise be eligible for the SCHIP public program. By allowing for a less comprehensive benefit package for optional populations, more employer plans might be eligible for participation in the premium assistance program.

Cost-Sharing

There are cost-sharing provisions associated with the use of SCHIP funds:

1. No cost-sharing for well-baby, well-child, and immunizations.
2. Families of eligible children can pay no more than 5 percent of their income on health care costs including both premium contributions and cost-sharing at the point of service.[44]

The HIFA waiver removes restrictions on cost-sharing provisions for expansion populations. With the exception to the nominal levels of contribution for mandatory populations and the 5 percent cap on cost-sharing for optional Medicaid and SCHIP children, no specific limitations exists in regards to cost sharing under HIFA.[45]

Texas House Bill 3038 stipulates that the "department may not provide for the payment of any deductible, co-payment, coinsurance, or other cost-sharing obligation for the child or another individual enrolled in a group health benefit plan" under a previous section.[46] While it is not necessary for the department to pay for the cost sharing of the adult, in order to access the federal SCHIP match, the cost-sharing requirements for the eligible child must not exceed those stipulated by the federal SCHIP legislation.

Crowd-Out

In developing a premium assistance program, states need to consider the extent to which public funds as subsidies may substitute or "crowd-out" private funds. Policies and rules designed to prevent crowd-out are collectively known as "firewalls."[47] Firewalls include the following: look-back periods (a period that an individual must be uninsured before obtaining health insurance through the public program), minimum employer/employee contribution (the employer must contribute a certain amount to the cost of the health insurance), and monitoring changes in employer contributions (extensive survey and evaluation as to whether contributions by employees are changing).[48] Several examples of specific state measures implemented to prevent crowd-out are mentioned in Appendix B.

COBRA Coverage

Federal COBRA (Consolidated Omnibus Budget Reconciliation Act of 1985) legislation requires that employers allow former workers to continue health insurance coverage through their employer's groups health plan for a specific time period.[49] The employee must pay for the full cost of the coverage. The former employee can receive COBRA coverage for herself as well as for her family. While the federal legislation applies only to firms with more than 20 employees, many states have passed legislation to extend COBRA-type legislation to smaller firms. Texas has passed legislation stating that firms with six to 19 employees offer coverage for up to six months and firms with more than 20 offer coverage for up to 18 months.[50]

States can continue to cover individuals who are enrolled in premium assistance programs in COBRA coverage if it is cost-effective.[51] Often it will not be cost-effective because the state will now have to subsidize both the employer and the individuals' portion of the health care insurance plan.

Notions of Fairness

In an effort to prevent crowd-out, most states impose some period of no insurance before SCHIP funds can be used to subsidize employer-based coverage. Therefore, only working individuals who have not been paying for their child's health insurance can participate in the subsidy program. This seems inherently unfair to individuals at similar income levels who work to pay for health insurance even though it puts a strain on their budget. This problem could be addressed by the state. In 1999, New Jersey proposed legislation to use state funds for a program similar to the SCHIP premium assistance program, but it would be available for currently insured children in the same income bracket.[52] However, this program never passed to become law.[53]

Premium Assistance Programs as an Option to Reduce the Number of Uninsured

Premium assistance programs are just one small part of an extensive program that could be implemented to reduce the number of uninsured in Texas. The problems with premium assistance programs—the administrative cost and labor intensity associated with implementing the program—account for the low enrollment and modest success. However, even modestly successful programs can save the state money and help bridge the gap between public and private insurance coverage.

Premium assistance programs have been modestly successful in other states when they are a part of a larger expansion. For example, in Massachusetts the public insurance program covers families at or below 200 percent (see the section on Massachusetts in

Appendix B). As of January 2002, this program had close to 12,000 participants. Massachusetts expanded through an 1115 waiver; another way to expand might be through a HIFA waiver. When expanding in this manner to optional populations—such as the option presented to expand to parents and childless adults—premium assistance programs could also have a modest impact. Because the federal government allows for flexibility in benefit packages and cost sharing for optional populations, many of the limitations of premium assistance—difficulty finding employer plans that meet benefit criteria and cost effectiveness—might be less of a hindrance. When the expansion population enrolls, the state could aggressively seek out these individuals to inquire about their access to employer sponsored plans and attempt to enroll them and their children into the appropriate premium assistance program, including either the established Texas HIPP program or the future SCHIP premium assistance program.

Notes

[1] Paul Fronstin, *Small Employers and Health Benefits: Findings from the 2000 Small Employer Health Benefits Survey*, SR 35 (Washington, D.C.: Employee Benefit Research Institute, October 2000), p. 1.

[2] Kaiser Commission on Medicaid and the Uninsured, "Key Facts" (Washington D.C.: Kaiser Commission, February 2002), p. 1.

[3] Ibid.

[4] Class Presentation by Edli Colberg, Demographer/Program Specialist, Research and Forecasting, Texas Health and Human Services Commission, at the Lyndon B. Johnson School of Public Affairs, Austin, Texas, November 13, 2001.

[5] Ibid.

[6] Texas Department of Insurance, "Characteristics of Texas With and Without Health Insurance" (Austin, Tex.: Texas Department of Insurance State Planning Grant Division, January 2000), p. 21.

[7] Laura A. Tollen, *Purchasing Private Health Insurance through Government Health Care Programs: A Guide for States* (Washington D.C.: Institute for Health Policy Solutions, Inc., June 1999), p. 2.

[8] Ibid.

[9] Peter J. Cunningham, Elizabeth Schaefer, and Christopher Hogan, *Who Declines Employer-Sponsored Health Insurance and is Uninsured* (Washington D.C.: Health System Change, 1999), p. 1.

[10] Ibid., p. 2.

[11] State Coverage Initiatives, "State of the States" (Washington, D.C.: Academy for Health Care Services Research and Health Policy, 2002), p. 14.

[12] Tollen, *Purchasing Private Health Insurance*, pp. 4-5. Individuals would be eligible to receive the premium assistance if they are eligible for Medicaid or SCHIP or they have dependents who are eligible for Medicaid or SCHIP.

[13] Presentation by Michael Miller, Community Catalyst/ Health Care for All, at the Families USA Conference, Washington, D.C., January 17, 2002.

[14] State Coverage Initiatives, "State of the States," p. 14.

[15] Sharon Silow-Carrol, Stephanie E. Anthony, and Jack A. Meyer, *State and Local Initiatives to Enhance Health Coverage for the Working Uninsured* (New York, NY: The Commonwealth Fund, November 2000), pp. 2-3.

[16] Leslie Jackson Conwell and Ashley C. Short, *Premium Subsidies for Employer-Sponsored Health Coverage* (Washington, D.C.: The Center for Studying Health System Change, December 2001), p. 1.

[17] Lyndon B. Johnson School of Public Affairs, *Expansion through Waivers,* Policy Research Report Working Paper (Austin, Texas, 2002), pp. 33-41. (draft)

[18] Ibid.

[19] Conwell and Short, *Premium Subsidies for Employer-Sponsored Health Coverage*, p. 2.

[20] Ibid.

[21] Silow-Carrol et al., *State and Local Initiatives,* p. 20.

[22] Ibid.

[23] Ibid.

[24] Interview by Lisa Ewart with Terry Cottrell, Project Director, Texas HIPP Program, Health and Human Services Commission, Austin, Texas, November 14, 2001.

[25] Texas Department of Health, *The Health Insurance Premium Payment (HIPP) Reimbursement Program for Texas Medicaid Recipients and Family.* Online. Available: http://www.tdh.state.tx.us/cshcn/hipp.htm. Accessed: November 19, 2001.

[26] Ibid.

[27] Terry Cottrell, "Health Insurance Premium Payment Program (HIPP)" (Austin, Tex.: Health and Human Services Commission, March 2001), p. 1.

[28] Texas House Bill 3038, 77th Texas Legislature, regular session (2001).

[29] Cottrell interview, November 14, 2001.

[30] Ibid.

[31] Ibid.

[32] Ibid.

[33] Silow-Carrol, et al., *State and Local Initiatives,* p. 21.

[34] Tollen, *Purchasing Private Health Insurance,* pp. 13-15.

[35] Institute for Health Policy Solutions, *Coordinating State Children's Health Insurance Programs with Employer-Based Coverage: Design and Implementation of Premium Assistance Programs* (Washington, D.C., October 1999), p. 7.

[36] Ibid., pp. 7-8.

[37] Tollen, *Purchasing Private Health Insurance,* pp. 13-15.

[38] Jennifer M. Ryan, *Health Insurance Family Style: Public Approaches to Reaching the Uninsured,* (Washington, D.C.: National Health Policy Forum, September 2001), p. 5.

[39] Ibid., p. 7.

[40] Texas House Bill 3038, 77th Texas Legislature, regular session (2001).

[41] Presentation by Anita Smith, Manager, Health Insurance Purchasing Unit, Iowa Department of Human Services, at the Effective Coverage Expansions for Uninsured Kids and Their Working Parents: Links to Job-Based Coverage Conference, Washington D.C., May 18, 2001.

[42] Tollen, *Purchasing Private Health Insurance,* p. 27. See Appendix B for specific state examples of their cost-effectiveness tests.

[43] State Coverage Initiatives, "State of the States," p. 14.

[44] Ibid.

[45] Ryan, *Health Insurance Family Style,* pp. 5-7.

[46] Texas House Bill 3038, 77th Texas Legislature, regular session (2001).

[47] Tollen, *Purchasing Private Health Insurance*, p. 20.

[48] Ibid.

[49] Families USA, "More than 725,000 Laid-Off Workers Have Lost Health Coverage Since the Recession Began in March" (Washington, D.C.: Families USA, 2001), p. 2.

[50] Ibid.

[51] Presentation by Beth Waldman, Acting Director of Program Implementation, Massachusetts Division of Medical Assistance, at the Effective Coverage Expansions for Uninsured Kids and Their Working Parents: Links to Job-Based Coverage Conference, Washington D.C., May 18, 2001.

[52] Institute for Health Policy Solutions, "Coordinating State Children's Health Insurance Programs with Employer-Based Coverage: Design and Implementation of Premium Assistance Programs" (Washington, D.C.: Institute for Health Policy Solutions, 1999), p. 14.

[53] Telephone interview by Lisa Ewart with Dennis Doderer, Deputy Assistant Director, Premium Support Program, Division of Medical Assistance and Health, New Jersey Department of Human Services, Trenton, NJ, January 15, 2002.

Chapter 5. SCHIP Full-Cost Buy-In Programs

by Jie Zhou

Overview

The uninsured population of the United States is disproportionately comprised of lower-income workers and their families whose employers offer no health benefits. In most states, these workers are not eligible for Medicaid, even if their children are. Although employer-sponsored health insurance remains the foundation for coverage of working families, a few states are exploring ways to allow those uninsured with higher income an opportunity to pay the full premium associated with a state-run insurance program like SCHIP. These eligibility expansions are referred to as full-cost buy-ins.[1]

SCHIP Full-Cost Buy-Ins

The State Children Health Insurance Program (SCHIP) differs from Medicaid programs in that SCHIP receives a higher federal match than Medicaid, and SCHIP eligibility was originally limited to low-income children. In recent years, the federal government has begun to allow states more flexibility in expanding their programs to children at higher income levels. A few states have taken advantage of the SCHIP enhanced federal match, implementing some strategies like employer buy-in programs and full cost buy-in programs.

Four states, Connecticut, Florida, New York, and North Carolina, allow moderate-income families to purchase coverage for their children through SCHIP at no state subsidy. These moderate-income families generally have access to the same benefits and health plans as SCHIP-eligible children, but they pay the full cost of the premium and may have cost-sharing when accessing services.

The rationale behind the SCHIP full-cost buy-in program is that when public programs become larger and more solid, administrative efficiencies and purchasing power can help people receive lower premiums than what they could receive in the private market. However, the main objective of the full-cost buy-in programs is not to constrain the insurance price, but to provide an additional opportunity for affordable access to insurance.[2]

The following sections describe the experiences of the four states mentioned above regarding their full-cost buy-in programs for the purpose of exploring the feasibility of developing a similar model in Texas.

Connecticut Experience: Healthcare for Uninsured Kids and Youth

Design Issues

On January 15, 1998, Connecticut submitted a Title XXI State Plan to expand coverage for uninsured children through the combination of a Medicaid expansion for children and the creation of a separate children's program. State legislation authorized the Healthcare for Uninsured Kids and Youth (HUSKY) Plan Part B and the HUSKY Plus Plan Part C programs.

Connecticut makes a buy-in option available to children in families with incomes above 300 percent of FPL with no federal or state subsidy. No federal monies are received for coverage or services delivered to this population.

By March 2000, 5,006 children had been enrolled in HUSKY B. Of this total, only 2 percent of enrollees have household income exceeding 300 percent FPL, and the remaining 98 percent of enrollees are subsidized by SCHIP.[3]

There is 12-month continuous eligibility. A shorter version of the original application is mailed to the renewing family, with information originally supplied pre-printed on the form. Some documentation is required, but some eligibility exists for substitution of documentation. (In January 2001, Medicaid expanded to include relative caretakers with income levels up to 150 percent FPL of children. The asset limit was also dropped as an eligibility criterion.)

Benefits Package

Connecticut is using a benchmark coverage benefit package based on the state employee coverage. The coverage is based on the most generous benefits offered under the three state employee options, which are Blue Cross, MD Health Plan, and Kaiser Permanente.

HUSKY Part B benefits includes the following services: hospital inpatient and outpatient, physician, surgical, clinic, health center, ambulatory, prescription drugs, laboratory, x-ray, prenatal care, family planning and supplies, inpatient mental health, outpatient mental health, durable medical equipment, disposable medical supplies, home and community-based services, nursing care, abortion (to save life, rape, or incest), dental, inpatient and outpatient substance abuse, enabling, and emergency transportation.[4]

There was great concern that adverse selection would develop, especially among the first batch of children to enroll in the new program. Advocates who had supported a pure Medicaid expansion expressed special concern about the adequacy of the state employee benefit package to deal with children with special needs.

In response to these concerns, the HUSKY Plus program was created to provide a supplemental benefit for children with special needs. The program was designed in two parts. HUSKY Plus Physical was an expansion of the existing Title V program for children with special needs. Eligibility for both Title V and HUSKY Plus was expanded up to 300 percent FPL and the diagnostic/functional criteria were liberalized. In addition,

HUSKY Plus Behavioral was created to provide supplemental benefit for children with special needs with behavioral health insurance. Nevertheless, eligibility for both programs was limited to children with family incomes up to and including 300 percent FPL. In other words, children under the full cost buy-in program are not entitled to the benefits provided by HUSKY Plus.[5]

Cost-Sharing

The HUSKY Plan has no deductibles and coinsurance. Although there is a $1,250 maximum for children with household gross incomes exceeding 235 percent of the FPL before income disregards, HUSKY imposes no such limits for children in the full-cost buy-in program.[6] The state officials believe that eliminating the upper limit emphasizes the responsibility on the part of the parent and reduces the stigma of being on a state-sponsored program for many families.[7]

Crowd-Out

A child is not eligible for HUSKY Part B if he/she has been covered by employer-sponsored insurance within the last six months. This may be extended to 12 months if the commissioner determines that six months is insufficient to deter applicants or employers from discontinuing employer-sponsored dependent coverage. However, an application may be approved if the reason for loss of employer-sponsored insurance is unrelated to the availability of the HUSKY Plan B or any of ten other reasons, which include the loss of employment. The exceptions to this six-month waiting period include self-employment, loss of employment, death of parent, and financial hardship (as defined as a family paying more than 10 percent of gross income on health insurance premiums).

During FY 2000, 624 children were denied HUSKY B eligibility due to either having employer-sponsored insurance at the time of application (587) or having dropped it within six months of application (7).[8] Some parents are frustrated because their current employer-based coverage is expensive and offers limited benefits. They find themselves in a dilemma of not being able to access an extensive and affordable program like HUSKY B. They are essentially penalized for having a certain income and a certain health benefit, however limited. In this light, crowd-out accomplishes the goal of discouraging the substitution of public coverage for private coverage.

Florida Experience: Healthy Kids Program

Design Issues

In 1990, the Florida Legislature established a non-profit Florida Healthy Kids Corporation (FHKC) to administer a comprehensive health insurance program—Healthy Kids Program—for uninsured children. It was incorporated under the Kidcare umbrella with 1998's Florida Kidcare Acts. Healthy Kids is the only program that does not have a maximum income eligibility requirement. Healthy Kids serves children ages 5 through 18 and currently has over 225,000 children enrollees.

The full-cost buy-in program starts at 200 percent FPL. Families that exceed the income level to qualify for subsidy may buy into the program and pay the full-priced premium based on the county in which they live. Currently, 2.76 percent of the families enrolled in Healthy Kids are under full-cost buy-in programs.[9]

Benefit Package

The Healthy Kids benefit package is the existing program benefit package that was cited in the Title XXI legislation as an accepted child health coverage program (Title XXI of the Social Security Act established SCHIP, allowing states to receive $24 billion in matching funds over five years for children's healthcare expansion). This benefit package includes a full range of inpatient and outpatient services. Limitations are placed on psychiatric, rehabilitation, and physical therapy inpatient admission; alcohol and drug services; chiropractic services; podiatry services; outpatient rehabilitation services; and durable medical equipment and remedial devices. The 2000 Florida State Legislature directed Healthy Kids to implement a comprehensive dental benefit and provided funding to enroll 160,000 children who reside in counties that contribute a local match, including full-cost buy-in enrollees.[10]

Cost-Sharing

Co-payments are charged for a number of services and reflect Title XXI requirements in the Healthy Kids program. The state plan states that cost and utilization rates will be monitored on a quarterly basis to ensure that costs associated with utilizing health care services do not exceed the 5 percent maximum.[11] If the family spends in excess of 5 percent of their annual income, it will be notified by the state that it is no longer responsible for cost-sharing and will be reimbursed for excess expenses by Florida Healthy Kids Corporation. There are no different co-payment schedules for full-cost buy-in enrollees. It only requires minimal co-payments for mental health outpatient services and unauthorized use of emergency services.[12]

Crowd-out

Studies in 1999 demonstrated that access to employer-based coverage varies significantly by income, with families above 185 percent FPL reporting increased access when compared to those with lower incomes.[13] Thus, families at the upper end of the income cutoff for government subsidized insurance coverage may have greater access to employer-based dependent coverage than families at the lower end of the income range. Parents that have access to employer-based coverage report it is unaffordable. Without a subsidized insurance option, the majority of these children would be uninsured. According to Florida officials, the care for these children is not being shifted from the private sector to the public sector. Rather, these children are receiving insurance coverage and health care when they might have had no coverage at all and limited health care.[14]

According to a recent Healthy Kids program evaluation, only 11 percent of all Healthy Kids enrollees, including those in the unsubsidized component, had employer-based coverage in the year preceding enrollment, compared to 17 percent for Medicaid beneficiaries who have lower incomes.[15] Despite some concerns on crowd-out, Florida Healthy Kids program does not impose any waiting period policy except that it requires children be uninsured at the time of application and they must not have received employer-sponsored coverage in the previous 12 months. Besides this, there is an eligibility renewal process that consists a letter sent to each family every six months, containing all of their account information. Families make corrections to the form and return it to Healthy Kids, or they can call the program.

However, attempts to expand a full-cost buy-in program to younger children (ages 1 to 5 above 200 percent FPL) have raised fears of crowd-out, and policymakers have delayed expansion until further studies on crowd-out are conducted.[16]

New York Experience: Child Health Plus Program

Design Issue

The Child Health Plus program (CHPlus) in New York commenced in 1990. The program is based on a partnership between government and private insurers through the subsidization of private health insurance coverage. An application must be completed for every child applying for Child Health Plus in New York. Children who are not eligible for Medicaid (and the other federal exclusions) and under 19 years of age are eligible for the program at a subsidized level. Those meeting the above criteria but having income above 250 percent of FPL can purchase the product at full price.

Enrollment in the CHPlus program as of September 30, 2000, was approximately 539,000 children (including full cost buy-in enrollees). This is a 150,500 increase over the September 1999 enrollment of approximately 388,500, or a 39 percent increase in CHPlus enrollees.[17] The full-cost buy-in enrollees reached 9,000 at its peak.[18]

Benefit Package

Initially, the package of services for the Title XXI program was the same comprehensive benefit package offered by the state-only program. The state's second amendment on Title XXI program, which was approved in September 1998, expanded the CHPlus benefit for durable medical equipment, inpatient and outpatient mental health, speech therapies, and provides coverage for non-prescription medications authorized by a professional licensed to write prescriptions.

There is no difference in benefit package between families with incomes above 250 percent FPL and other enrolled families in the Child Health Plus Program.

Cost-Sharing

The premium is developed at full cost by the insurance plans participating in the program. Some families may have to contribute $9 or $15 per child per month depending on their incomes. All other children are fully subsidized by the state or they fully pay the premium.[19] The full premium will vary, depending on the insurer selected. It is probably much less than one would pay for other private insurance. An additional premium of $630 will paid for each extra child enrolled in the full cost buy-in program.[20]

There are no co-payments on the health care services received from participating providers. The state has not studied the possible effects of nominal premium contributions on participation in the program. The majority of the enrolled CHPlus population is fully subsidized, and the full-cost buy-in program enrollees receive a different treatment on co-payments.[21]

Crowd-Out

The CHPlus program is designed to prevent crowd-out. Only those children in families who have a net income above 250 percent FPL but do not have access to employer-based coverage are eligible for unsubsidized insurance. An evaluation of the CHPlus program has shown that crowd-out has not been an issue for New York State.[22]

The state established a policy that if, on average, over a nine-month period the crowd-out percentage equals or exceeds 8 percent, a waiting period may be imposed.[23] Since the approval of New York's State Plan under Title XXI, the crowd-out percentage over a nine-month period has been below 6 percent.[24] According to a recent program evaluation, crowd-out is not occurring to a significant degree since the implementation of the CHIPlus program.[25] The state does not feel they have a crowd-out problem and has yet to impose any waiting period. However, they are currently monitoring it through the application process.[26] Should crowd-out occur in 8 percent or more of enrollees, one of two options will be implemented: children with access to employer-based coverage will be deemed ineligible for CHPlus, and/or a required period of uninsurance will be imposed.[27]

North Carolina: NC Health Choice for Children

Design Issues

In 1998, North Carolina created a separate state health insurance program to provide coverage to uninsured children whose family incomes do not exceed 200 percent FPL. Enrollees whose annual incomes increase above 200 percent of the FPL to 225 percent of the FPL will be allowed to buy into the program for one year at full cost.

The North Carolina full-cost buy-in program essentially acts like a COBRA program. A family who has been on North Carolina Health Choice's (Title XXI) subsidized program for one full year or more but whose family income has gone up at the one-year renewal period so that their children are no longer eligible for the program may elect to purchase for one year their North Carolina health choice benefits at the per-member per-month rate for each child affected. [28]

Benefit Package

The benefit package is the state employee coverage provided through the North Carolina Teachers and State Employees' Comprehensive Major Medical Plan (TSECMMP), plus

Medicaid-equivalent benefits for Special Needs Children. Dental, optical, and hearing services are also provided. Children are guaranteed 12 months of continuous enrollment, unless the child receives other insurance coverage during this time period.[29]

Cost-Sharing

Currently, one child would cost $120.84 a month, two children $241.68 per month, and three children $362.52 a month.[30] The payment schedule and mechanism must be worked out with Blue Cross. It is in effect a Blue Cross product designed on the NC Health Choice model.

Crowd-Out

Children are eligible for North Carolina's Health Choice program (Title XXI program) if they are uninsured. The state initially defined uninsured as not having coverage under any private or employer-sponsored creditable health insurance plan for the six-month period immediately preceding the date the Title XXI program became effective. Six months after the state implemented the program, the definition of the term was modified to mean that the applicant has not had coverage for 60 days immediately preceding the date of the child's application. Exceptions are made if the child has lost Title XIX eligibility due to a change in family income or if the family has lost employer-sponsored coverage due to the termination of employment, cessation by the employer of employer-sponsored coverage, cessation of the employer's business, or for a special needs child if health insurance benefits have been terminated due to a long-term disability or substantial reduction in or limitation of lifetime medical benefits or benefit category.[31] According to the Coordinator of NC Health Choice for Children, they have no evidence that there is any crowd-out in North Carolina to the point that they dropped their two-month waiting period for regular programs.[32]

Since the children must meet income requirements before enrolling in North Carolina Health Choice (Title XXI), and must have been enrolled in this for one year before being eligible for the full-cost buy-in, it does not compete with any high-risk pools.[33]

Summary of State Experience

Since concerns about substitution of private coverage have risen due to the higher-income target population; the current active full-cost buy-in programs do not include adults (see Table 5.1 for a summary of the full-cost buy-in programs of the four states that have them). In general, targeting children might cause less competition with private insurance products. Because states do not receive federal funding to operate the full-cost buy-in programs, these programs can be designed with greater flexibility than Medicaid and SCHIP. This is why states have different income limits for subsidized coverage.

Table 5.1
Summary of SCHIP Full-Cost Buy-In Programs

Program Name	Year Implemented	Population Targeted	Eligibility Range	Time limit (if any)
Connecticut HUSKY	1998	Children	300% FPL	--
Florida KidCare	1992	Children ages 5 to 9	>200% FPL	--
North Carolina Health Choice for Children	1998	Previously enrolled children	200-225% FPL	1 year
New York Child Health Plus	1991	children	>230% FPL	--

Adapted from: State Coverage Initiatives, Robert Wood Johnson Foundation. *SCHIP Full-Cost Buy-In.* Online. Accessible: http://www.statecoverage.net/fullcost.htm. Accessed: January 14, 2002.

Full-cost buy-in programs are viable in that states are able to provide a lower premium utilizing administrative efficiencies. According to the New York state officials, New York's Child Health Plus Program created economies of scale by using the administrative framework already in place, allowing the state to process the unsubsidized enrollees at marginal costs.

Flexibility is also part of the reason that some states choose to define a narrower benefit package to reduce the likelihood of adverse selection. For instance, HUSKY Plus, Connecticut's supplemental coverage option for children with intensive physical or behavioral health needs is only available for children in the state's subsidized HUSKY program. The exclusion of full cost buy-in program enrollees from this component of the benefits package was designed as a deterrent for less healthy individuals' enrollment.

There is no evidence of substantial crowd-out, regardless of whether programs required minimum spells without insurance for new enrollees. HUSKY, Connecticut's full-cost buy-in program, requires new enrollees to have completed a six-month waiting period and audits 20 percent of enrollee applications by contacting the benefit managers of parents' employees. According to state officials, the current waiting period is effective in preventing crowd-out. Florida's Healthy Kids and New York's Child Health Plus impose no waiting period on enrollees, and the crowd-out appears to be minimal.

Full-Cost Buy-In Options for Texas

It is estimated that there are 1.4 million uninsured children in Texas.[34] The Texas SCHIP program is currently targeting children with household gross income up to 200 percent FPL. The challenge in addressing the situation for families with income above roughly $33,400 annually for a family of four (above 200 percent FPL) is how to offer them the opportunity to buy into affordable coverage while not undercutting the employer market of which many people in this income group are already part.[35]

Despite the fact that only four states have implemented it, a SCHIP full-cost buy-in still can be considered as an option to expand the coverage of uninsured children.

Design Issues

Target Population: Children with Household Gross Incomes above 200 Percent FPL

Since the buy-in program would focus on families with higher incomes, it is extremely important to structure the program in a way that will not lead to an erosion of the employer market.

Owing to the absence of private insurance products for children only, targeting children might cause less competition with the private market. With children as the target population, the full-cost buy-in option could be integrated into Texas CHIP.

Adverse Selection Minimization

This program will be subject to the risk of adverse selection, like any insurance product in a voluntary market. One possible policy response is to erect barriers to keep high-risk children from shifting into the program. Waiting periods, or exclusions from the program if other sources of coverage are available, could address some of the selection problem. Such policies have been employed in other government programs, and could apply here. Another form of barrier is to scale back the benefit package or use tightly managed care to control the cost and make the full cost buy-in program less attractive to high-cost population.

Competition with the Private Section

Conditions of Participation: No employer-sponsored coverage at the time of application and at least six-month waiting period. As public programs expand eligibility up the income scale, the state's coverage product begins to compete with private insurance products. Families at a higher income may face a choice about whether to purchase private coverage for their children or join in the SCHIP full-cost buy-in program.

The requirements on applicants' pre-existing conditions address the concern of competing with private insurance market. In effect, as moderate-income families decide to purchase a state-sponsored program like full cost buy-in for their children, it may be harmful to private insurance markets. In this sense, it is necessary to ensure that a candidate is not covered by employer-sponsored health insurance at the time of application. A longer waiting period could also prevent the inflow of unhealthy people that might raise premium levels.

Limited benefits coverage: The full cost buy-in program assures that moderate-income children have access to the full range of medically necessary services, guaranteed in a "defined benefit" package, and that they have a variety of health plan choices. The children should not be forced into a few segregated plans. While the benefit package is supposed to include a full range of inpatient and outpatient services, limitations could be placed on certain fields like psychiatric, rehabilitation, durable medical equipment and remedial devices, and the like. The purpose is to avoid the possibility of blending state high-risk pools with full-cost buy-in programs.

Cost Sharing

In order to make an aggregate estimate of premium and cost co-payment for a full-cost buy-in option for Texas, it is important to look first at the current SCHIP premium rates and co-payment. Then, assuming the same risks spread over as SCHIP full cost buy-in enrollees, we will make a rough estimate on the average monthly amount that can be paid to plans per child.

Milliman USA conducted a similar research on Texas SCHIP premium costs in 2002. They concluded that a child currently enrolling in Texas SCHIP costs a premium of approximately $115 per month. Ignoring state costs to administer, Milliman estimate that the adjusted monthly premium per child is approximately $90 for a Texas CHIP full-cost buy-in option excluding dental coverage.[36] They also estimate the full-cost buy-in co-payments as follows:

- Office visit: $15
- Emergency room: $40
- Prescription drugs: $8/$15
- Per hospital admission: $150
- Per outpatient surgery: $0.[37]

Policy Implications

SCHIP full-cost buy-in programs are targeted for children in moderate-income families who receive inadequate medical attention for quite a long time, have no access to employer-sponsored plans, and have income levels above eligibility thresholds for enrollment into public programs.

In theory, taking advantage of administrative efficiencies and the purchasing power generated from pooling with subsidized SCHIP programs, full-cost buy-ins can offer some children a lower-cost coverage alternative than what is available in the private insurance market. However, the program designers have to strike a balance between the premiums charges for buyers and the premiums paid to providers. As part of a public program, a SCHIP full -cost buy-in cannot raise the premiums beyond enrollees' affordability. On the other hand, the program cannot reduce the prices paid to SCHIP providers, who complained that they have reached maximum capacity to serve paying patients.[38] This Catch-22 adds to the difficulty in the implementation of the SCHIP full-cost buy-in program in Texas.

There are also several other concerns associated with a SCHIP full-cost buy-in program. One is competition with the private insurance market products. This is the main reason why the full-cost buy-in options in other states are designed to target children. A second issue is the possibility of the influx of unhealthy populations. As mentioned earlier, some ways to address this concern could include a longer waiting period, medical underwriting, pre-existing condition exclusions, and low benefit levels.

Lastly is the potential for blending the state high-risk pool with SCHIP full-cost buy-in programs. It is of important to ensure that a full-cost buy-in does not perform in the function of a high-risk pool. This can be addressed by either directly banning migration from a high-risk pool to a full-cost buy-in program, or by placing some disincentives to switch. Limiting benefits and avoiding premium capping have proved to be effective in some states.

The full-cost buy-in option is not a panacea. Part of reason is that its principal goal is access to insurance, not necessarily affordability. Enrollment in the SCHIP full-cost buy-in component of a state expansion has typically been less than 5 percent of total program enrollment.[39]

Although the study of these four states cannot fully prove the effectiveness of a full-cost buy-in program in reducing the number of uninsured, the evidence suggests that with the right blend of objectives and design features that reduce the chances of crowd-out and adverse selection, the full-cost buy-in program may be an option to expand coverage without using public funds. Considering full-cost buy-in programs in other states as a percentage of the enrollment of SCHIP, we should also be aware that full-cost buy-in is only a moderate option for expansion. Since the majority of children above 200 percent FPL have parents who are employed, considerable efforts should be made to work with health plans, businesses, and others in the private sector to make health insurance more accessible and affordable to these working families and their children.

Notes

[1] Robert Wood Johnson Foundation, "Full-Cost Buy-Ins: An Overview of State Experience," State Coverage Initiative Issue Brief (Washington, D.C., August 2001), p. 1.

[2] Ibid.

[3] Connecticut Department of Social Services, *Framework for State Evaluation of Children's Health Insurance Plans Under Title XXI of the Social Security Act*, by Linda J. Mead (Hartford, Conn., 2000), p.8.

[4] Connecticut Department of Social Services, *Connecticut State Health Plan Under Title XXI of the Social Security Act*, by Linda J. Mead (Hartford, Conn., 1998), p. 22.

[5] Health Care Financing Administration, *Connecticut Title XXI State Plan Amendment Summary*. Online. Available: http://www.hcfa.gov/init/chpfsct.htm. Accessed: January 14, 2002.

[6] Connecticut Department of Social Services, *Connecticut State Health Plan Under Title XXI of the Social Security Act,* p.24.

[7] Ibid., p. 91.

[8] Connecticut Department of Social Services, *Framework for Annual Report of State Children's Health Insurance Plans*, by Adele Kusnitz, and James Gaito (Hartford, Conn., 2000), p. 16.

[9] Florida Healthy Kids, *Florida Healthy Kids Program Annual Report 2001.* Online. Available: http://www.healthykids.org/overview/annual_reports/2002/2002_annual_report.pdf. Accessed: December 16, 2001.

[10] Health Care Financing Administration, *Florida Title XXI Program Fact Sheet.* Online. Available: http://www.hcfa.gov/init/chpfsfl.htm. Accessed: December 16, 2001.

[11] Ibid.

[12] Health Policy Tracking Service, *Florida State SCHIP Plan Summary*. Online. Available: http://state-serve.hpts.org/hpts. Accessed: December 20, 2001.

[13] Institute for Child Health Policy, *Crowd Out: Evidence From the Florida Healthy Kids Program*. Online. Available: http://www.ichp.edu/Publications/default.htm. Accessed: April 23, 2002.

[14] Ibid.

[15] Institute for Child Health Policy, *Florida KidCare Program Evaluation Report, 2000.* Online. Available: http://www.ichp.edu/FloridaKidCare/1999Reports/FlaKCAppendices.pdf. Accessed: April 30, 2002.

[16] Michael Birnbaum, *Full-Cost Buy-Ins: An Overview of State Experience* (Washington D.C.: State Coverage Initiatives, August 2001), p. 3.

[17] New York State Department of Health, *State Annual Report of State Children's Health Insurance Plans Under Title XXI of the Social Security Act: State Children's Health Insurance Program*, by Dennis P. Whalen (New York, NY, 2000), p. 6.

[18] Michael Birnbaum, *Full-Cost Buy-Ins: An Overview of State Experience*, p. 3.

[19] Email from Ralph M. Bielefeldt, Coordinator, New York Children Health Plus, "Full Cost Buy-In Program", to Jie Zhou, January 14, 2002.

[20] New York State Department of Health, *New York Child Health Plus.* Online. Available: http://www.health.state.ny.us/nysdoh/chplus/cplus-1.htm. Accessed: January 9, 2002.

[21] New York State Department of Health, *New York Child Health Plus Promotion.* Online. Available: http://www.health.state.ny.us/nysdoh/chplus/brochure.htm. Accessed: January 9, 2002.

[22] New York State Department of Health, *State Child Health Plan Under Title XXI of the Social Security Act: New York State*, by Dennis P. Whalen (New York, NY,1998), p. 4.

[23] New York State Department of Health, *Framework for Annual Report of State Children's Health Insurance Plans Under Title XXI of the Social Security Act: New York*, by Dennis P. Whalen (New York, NY, 2000), p. 13.

[24] Ibid.

[25] Ibid.

[26] Email from Ralph M. Bielefeldt, Coordinator, New York Children Health Plus, "Full Cost Buy-In", to Jie Zhou, January 14, 2002.

[27] Health Care Financing Administration, *New York Title XXI Program Fact Sheet.* Online. Available: http://www.hcfa.gov/init/chpfsny.htm. Accessed: January 14, 2002.

[28] Email from June Milby, Coordinator, NC Health Choice for Children, "Full Cost Buy-In Program", to Jie Zhou, January 15, 2002.

[29] Ibid.

[30] Ibid.

[31] Health Care Financing Administration,. *North Carolina Title XXI Program Fact Sheet.* Online. Available: http://www.hcfa.gov/init/chpfsnc.htm. Accessed: January 14, 2002.

[32] Milby email.

[33] Ibid.

[34] Cleveland Public Power, *Texas CHIP Fast Facts.* Online. Available: http://www.cppp.org/products/fastfacts/CHIP.html. Accessed: January 14, 2002.

[35] Ibid.

[36] Sue Hart, Milliman USA, *Options for Expanding Health Insurance in Texas—CHIP Full Cost Buy-In* (paper presented at Texas State Planning Grant Conference, Houston, Texas, January 31-February 1, 2002), p. 6.

[37] Ibid., p. 7.

[38] "Transition to the Market," Focus Group at "Investing in Texas: Financing Health Coverage Expansions" Conference, Lyndon B. Johnson School of Public Affairs, Austin, Texas, March 22, 2002.

[39] Robert Wood Johnson Foundation, "Full-Cost Buy-Ins: An Overview of State Experience," p. 4.

Chapter 6. Assessing the Impact of Medicaid and SCHIP Reimbursement Rates on Access to Care in Texas

by Yolanda Davila, Elizabeth Kaufman, and Sarah Stout

Adequacy of the provider network in the Medicaid program has been a longstanding area of concern to policymakers, program administrators, and providers. Dissatisfaction with Medicaid has deterred some providers from participating in Medicaid and has pushed others to limit their Medicaid clientele. Most providers cite low reimbursement rates offered by Medicaid relative to Medicare and the commercial market as the most significant problem limiting provider participation. As rates in the State Children's Health Insurance Program (SCHIP) are similar to Medicaid rates, there is also concern that reimbursement rates in this program also may not be high enough to ensure adequate levels of provider participation.

In implementing SCHIP, Texas has taken steps to expedite enrollment into the new program through an extensive marketing campaign. Texas has also attempted to reduce barriers to care through the simplification of Medicaid enrollment procedures. These outreach efforts are important to insure Texans and should be continued. However, to ensure access to care for an increased client base, the current provider network needs to be expanded, or at minimum, retained. If reimbursement rates and administrative complexities involved in participating in these programs prevent a sufficient number of providers from participating, people enrolled in the programs may be insured, but will not be able to obtain consistent health care services. With a growing Medicaid population, a shrinking provider base could limit the viability of any future expansions in the public health arena. This paper examines reimbursement rates and methodologies in the Texas Medicaid and SCHIP programs and evaluates their impact on provider networks and access to primary and acute care.

The Importance of Reimbursement Rates

Provider reimbursement rates in the Medicaid program have historically been lower than reimbursement rates in the Medicare program and in the private market. SCHIP rates are only slightly higher than Medicaid managed care rates. According to the Texas Department of Health, Texas Medical Association, Texas Health and Human Services Commission, and the Texas Department of Insurance, providers are reportedly dissatisfied with payment rates. There are conflicting points of view on whether dissatisfaction with reimbursement levels actually leads to an insufficient network of providers in the Medicaid and SCHIP programs.

However, even if there is not sufficient evidence to demonstrate that Medicaid and SCHIP reimbursement rates are a barrier to provider participation in the programs, this issue merits serious consideration by policymakers and program administrators. The adequacy of reimbursement rates in Medicaid and SCHIP is important because rates may deter physician participation in the programs and thus reduce client access to care. Also, providers who do participate in the Medicaid and SCHIP networks may be supplementing their practices with their own personal funding or shifting costs to their other non-Medicaid and SCHIP clients. Consequently, the increased cost in the private sector may further exacerbate the growing problem of health care inflation.

The Texas Medicaid Model

As of September 1, 2001, Medicaid rates are set by the Texas Health and Human Services Commission (HHSC). Prior to this date, rates for the Medicaid program were set by staff at the Texas Department of Health (TDH), the Department of Human Services (DHS), HHSC, and the Texas Department of Mental Health and Mental Retardation (TDMHMR). It is hoped that centralizing this function at HHSC will "Improve coordination and consistency of rate-setting process."[1] In Texas, physicians' fees under Medicaid vary by service delivery model. There are currently three reimbursement models being used in the state. Traditional Medicaid (fee-for-service) dominates the Medicaid marketplace, accounting for over 70 percent of Medicaid clientele. Medicaid managed care has also been incorporated into the state and has quickly become the new model for any rollouts. Two reimbursement delivery models exist under Medicaid managed care: HMOs and a Primary Care Case Management (PCCM) model. Under traditional Medicaid, physicians are paid on the fee-for-service (FFS) schedule.

Under Medicaid managed care, providers are paid through their HMO or PCCM broker (National Heritage Insurance Company) in Texas. HMOs and the PCCM broker receive capitated payments per member enrolled per month and are responsible for paying their own providers. These models are discussed in detail in this paper but are outlined briefly below.

Table 6.1
Medicaid Service Delivery Models in Texas

	Traditional Medicaid	**HMO**	**PCCM**
Structure	• Clients may choose any Medicaid provider. • The state contracts directly with providers. • Risk is shared between the state and the claims administrator.	• HMO provides a "medical home" to clients. • HMO delivers and manages health services on a risk basis. • HMO receives a monthly capitation payment for each member enrolled.	• Combination of FFS and managed care. • State sets up a network of physicians (Texas Health Network). • Providers receive FFS reimbursement. • PCPs provide a "medical home" and receive a monthly fee

	Traditional Medicaid	HMO	PCCM
		• HMO is at risk for additional costs. • Profits are shared between the HMO and the state (in FY1999, the state retained 24% of profits and the HMO retained 76% of profits).	per member per month in addition to the billing for services provided. • The state is at risk for all costs.
Provider Network	Any provider enrolled in Medicaid accepting Medicaid patients.	Network of providers developed by the HMO.	Network of providers developed by the state plan administrator.
Administration	• TDH contracts with providers. • NHIC enrolls providers and administers claims.	• TDH contracts with HMOs. • HMO contracts with providers. • NHIC enrolls providers.	• TDH contracts with providers. • National Heritage Insurance Company enrolls providers and administers claims.
Reimbursement	Physicians and other providers are paid at discounted rates.	• HMO is capitated for all Medicaid services. • HMO pays network providers on a FFS or capitated basis.	• Physicians and other providers are paid at discounted rates. • PCP receives $3.00 case management fee per member per month.

Adapted from: Texas Department of Health, *Texas Medicaid Managed Care Report: Fiscal Year 1997* (Austin, Tex., December 1998), pp. 6-10.

Traditional Medicaid: Fee-for-Service Payment Methodology

Under FFS, states pay physicians for services under a standard fee schedule that reimburses physicians at the same rates across the state. Most of the fees are based on Medicare's Resource Based Relative Value Scale (RBRVS), which compares the amount of physician work involved in providing one service with the amount of work required to provide other services. Other fees are based on the Accessed-Based Fee system, which fills in some gaps in the RBRVS system.

Medicare RBRVS

RBRVS, the payment methodology for physician services under Medicare, also serves as the basis for many states' Medicaid FFS payment schedules and also many commercial payers. In fact, according to the American Academy of Pediatrics, more than 63 percent of public and private payors use a variation of RBRVS.[2] RBRVS was implemented as the payment methodology for Medicare in January 1992, replacing the historical charge payment methodology under which providers were compensated for the "customary, prevailing and reasonable" charge for each service.[3]

The RBRVS assigns weights to services based on the relative physician work required to provide the service in comparison with other services. This *relative value* takes into account average practice and malpractice expenses associated with each service, and is then adjusted for geographic area. It is interesting to note that the geographic adjustments for Texas reflect malpractice expenses in Beaumont, Brazoria, Galveston, and Houston that are significantly higher than the national average. For Texas, Medicare makes adjustments for eight regions: Austin, Beaumont, Brazoria, Dallas, Fort Worth, Galveston, Houston, and Rest of Texas.[4] For each area, the relative expenses of work, practice, and malpractice are calculated and applied to the base relative value to reach the total value for each RVU.

The geographically adjusted value is multiplied by a *conversion factor* to determine the payment to the physician. The conversion factor is a dollar amount. Under Medicare, there is one national conversion factor as determined by the Balanced Budget Act of 1997, which is updated annually. Under Medicaid, each state that employs the RBRVS sets its own conversion factor, which is typically lower than the Medicare conversion factor. In 2002, the Texas Medicaid conversion factor is $27.276[5] and the Medicare conversion factor is $36.1992,[6] which represents a 5 percent decrease from 2001.

RBRVS in Texas

In Texas, the RBRVS was implemented for Medicaid physician services on April 1, 1992. Texas policymakers adopted the RBRVS system because of two concerns about the method of basing payments on historical charges: 1) the usual charge method had resulted in relatively lower payments for primary care services; and 2) the fees paid to physicians were not related to the resources required to perform the services for which they were being reimbursed.[7]

Like many states, Texas did not adopt the RBRVS system in full. As described below, a significant number of services are reimbursed under the Access-Based Fee System. Texas also evaluates and adjusts the weights assigned to procedures under Medicare. The Texas Legislature made between 700 and 1,000 adjustments to the weights assigned to procedures in state fiscal year 2000-2001.[8]

Unlike the Medicare program and some other state Medicaid programs, the Texas Medicaid program does not geographically adjust the relative value units. Therefore, under Medicaid, providers operating under the FFS system in one part of the state will receive the same reimbursement as providers in other parts of the state.

Texas does adjust the payment under the RBRVS system by reimbursing at different levels based on the place of service. For services performed in a hospital facility, an overhead fee is included in the payment, but if the service is performed in an office, a separate overhead fee is paid to the physician.[9]

Access-Based Fees

When Texas implemented the RBRVS system for Medicaid physician services in 1992, it created a separate system of payment for approximately 800 pediatric and obstetric/gynelogic procedures. The state determined that payments for these procedures would have decreased by more than 35 percent under RBRVS because they were undervalued in the Medicare program. These fees account for 50 percent of physician payments made under the Texas Medicaid program.[10] Access-based fees are uniform throughout the state.

Evaluating Texas Fee-for-Service Medicaid Rates

While there are not data available linking provider participation in the Medicaid program to reimbursement rates, there are several ways to gain some sense of the adequacy of the rates. First, the rates could be compared to the actual cost to the provider to perform the procedures, which would indicate whether providers can afford to perform the service. This approach was beyond the scope of this report.

Another approach to evaluating the adequacy of the rates is to compare the fees paid under the Medicaid program to the fees paid by other payors, such as other state Medicaid programs, Medicare, and commercial payors. Overall, Texas Medicaid FFS rates appear to be fairly average when compared to other state Medicaid programs. As Medicaid traditionally pays rates lower than other programs and is in fact limited from paying rates higher than Medicare (in the aggregate per state), this is probably the fairest comparison. It is interesting to note though that while Texas ranks roughly in the middle of the states in terms of payments overall, one study found that of the ten largest states, Texas has the highest Medicaid FFS reimbursement rates.

Comparing Texas Medicaid FFS rates to non-Medicaid payors paints a different picture. In Texas, Medicaid FFS rates are significantly lower than Medicare and commercial payors. This is typically true across the nation, but this should still be a concern for Texas policymakers.

This section draws on data from a variety of sources to compare Texas Medicaid FFS fees to those of other states, the Medicare program, and selected commercial data. The data presented in this section have limitations, but taken together they draw a fairly complete picture of how Texas Medicaid reimbursement compares to other payors. It should be noted that this section only compares FFS rates. The data and methodology for comparing Medicaid managed care rates are more complex and are discussed in the Medicaid managed care section below.

Comparing Texas to Other States

In a 2001 report for the Medi-Cal Policy Institute, PriceWaterhouse Coopers selected commonly used Current Procedural Terminology (CPT) codes across a range of services and ranked the states by payment for each code. This study was unusual in that it factored utilization into the weighted ranking, making this data more meaningful than most available data comparing rates across states. Incorporating utilization into the rankings is important because it ensures that commonly used procedures are weighted more heavily in the rankings than less commonly used procedures.

The rankings from the Medi-Cal Policy Institute study are separated by specialty and listed below. A ranking of 1 would indicate that Texas had the highest reimbursement rates, on average, within that specialty. A ranking of 51 would indicate that Texas had the lowest reimbursement rates.

Table 6.2
Texas Medicaid FFS Rankings by Service Type

Service	Weighted Average Ranking
Lab/Pathology	5
Psychiatry	7
Surgical Services	18
Vision/Opthamology	19
Radiology	21
Maternity	27
Medicine and Testing	27
Evaluation and Management	31
Dental	36

Adapted from: Joel Menges, Chris Park, Jennifer Babcock, Lisa Chimento, Randall Haught, Silver Ho, The Lewin Group, *Comparing Physician and Dentist Fees Among Medicaid Programs* (Oakland, CA: Medi-Cal Policy Institute, June 2001), Appendix 4, p. 22. Online. Available: http://admin.chcf.org/documents/mcpi/ComparingPhysicianAndDentistFees.pdf. Accessed: January 31, 2002.

In 2001, the American Academy of Pediatrics (AAP) released a report comparing FFS Medicaid payments for selected procedures by state and to the U.S. Medicaid and Medicare averages. The report included payments by state for 142 CPT codes across a broad spectrum of services. For example, for CPT Code 99222 (Inpatient Hospitalization—moderate complexity), the report provides the Texas payment ($82.65), the U.S. Medicaid average payment ($75.08) and the U.S. Medicare average payment ($117.45).

This report is extremely helpful in understanding how Texas compares to other states with respect to Medicaid payments. However, there are limitations in using this report. Though the methodology used to select the 142 CPT codes analyzed is not provided with the report, it is clear that the selection is not a random sample and that the study includes a higher proportion of procedures related to the care of children. Though the selected procedures were not chosen at random, they do appear to include some of the more commonly billed procedures across a broad array of medical settings (see Appendix C for a list of procedures included in the study).

Of the 142 procedures included in the AAP study, we selected 104 for comparison of Texas's rates to the Medicaid average. We excluded 38 codes for which there was missing data for Texas or a significant number of other states. Of the codes examined, Texas pays below the national Medicaid FFS average for 53 procedures and above the national average for 49 procedures (see Figure 6.1).

Figure 6.1
Texas Compared to U.S. Medicaid FFS Payment

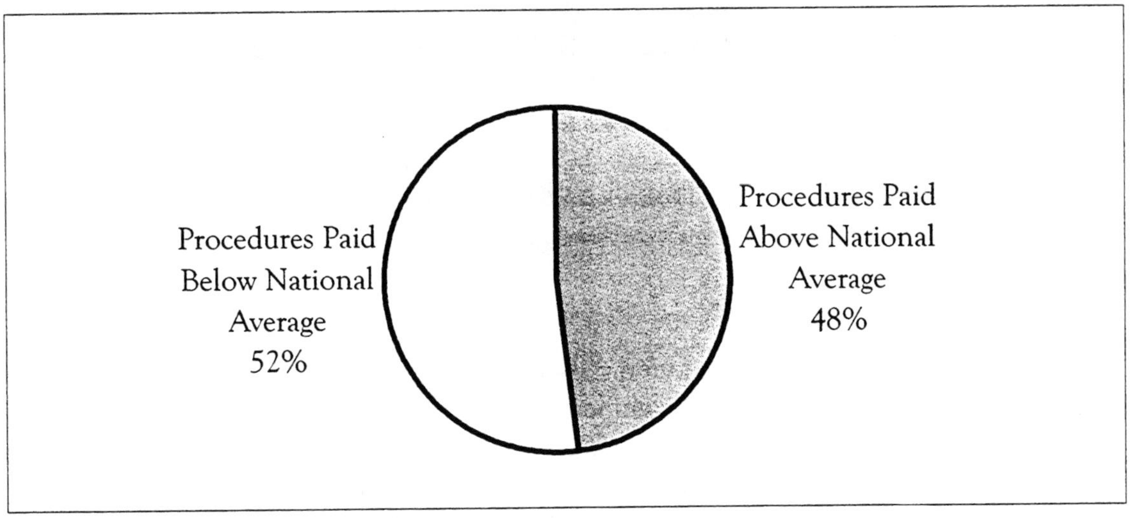

Adapted from: American Academy of Pediatrics, *Medicaid Reimbursement Survey, 2001: 50 States and the District of Columbia.* Online:.http://www.aap.org/research/medreimPDF01/all_states.PDF. Accessed: November 13, 2001.

For most of the codes included in the study, the Texas Medicaid FFS payment was within 25 percentage points of the national average (see Figure 6.2). While for most codes, the Texas payment was fairly close to the national average, there were some significant outliers. For example, the Texas reimbursement for the EPSDT hearing test is 438 percent of the national average while the state's reimbursement for an echocardiography procedure is only 34 percent of the national average.

Figure 6.2
Comparison of Texas Fee-for-Service Medicaid Payments to U.S. Average Payments, 2001

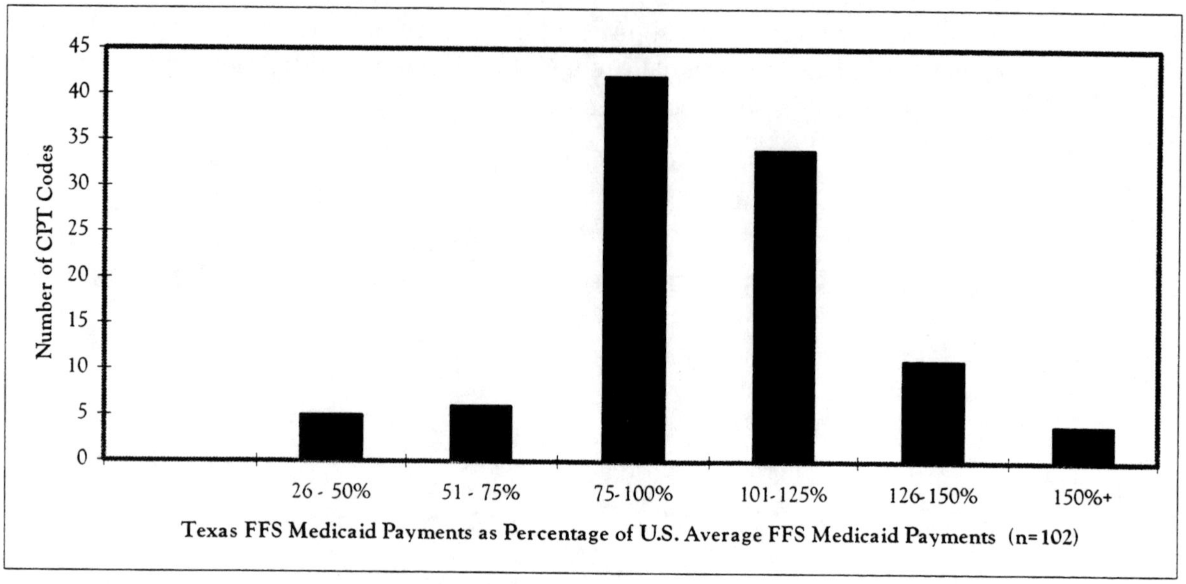

Adapted from: American Academy of Pediatrics, *Medicaid Reimbursement Survey, 2001: 50 States and the District of Columbia*. Online: http://www.aap.org/research/medreimPDF01/all_states.PDF. Accessed: November 13, 2001.

These findings are consistent with the results of a study conducted by the Urban Institute in 1998. The authors report examined payments for selected commonly used procedures and determined a national average for each group of procedures and a Medicaid-to-Medicare fee ratio for each state. Unfortunately, because Texas misreported the payment for one of the codes, many of the findings of the report with respect to this state are unusable. But, for four commonly used procedures, the report shows that reimbursements in Texas are fairly close to the national average (see Table 6.3).

Table 6.3
Comparison of Texas Fee-for-Service Medicaid Payments to National Average for Selected Procedures, 1998

Texas	Office Visit, New Patient, 30 minutes	Office Visit, Established Patient, 15 minites	Vaginal Delivery	Ceasarean Section
National Average	$47.57	$26.87	$700.00	$700.00
Texas as % of National Average	$40.01	$26.46	$695.89	$775.30

Adapted from: American Academy of Pediatrics, *Medicaid Reimbursement Survey, 2001: 50 States and the District of Columbia*. Online: http://www.aap.org/research/medreimPDF01/all_states.PDF. Accessed: November 13, 2001.

While these studies indicate that Texas was an average to above-average payor relative to other states, a 2001 Lewin Group study for the Medi-Cal Policy Institute that among the ten largest states in the country, Texas has the highest Medicaid FFS rates. This study compared the average percentage of Medicare-allowed charges in each of the ten states and found that Texas paid, on average, 77.6 percent of the Medicare-allowed charge (see Figure 6.3). The national average was 80.8 percent.[11]

Figure 6.3
Average Percentage of Medicare-Allowed Charge, Ten Largest States

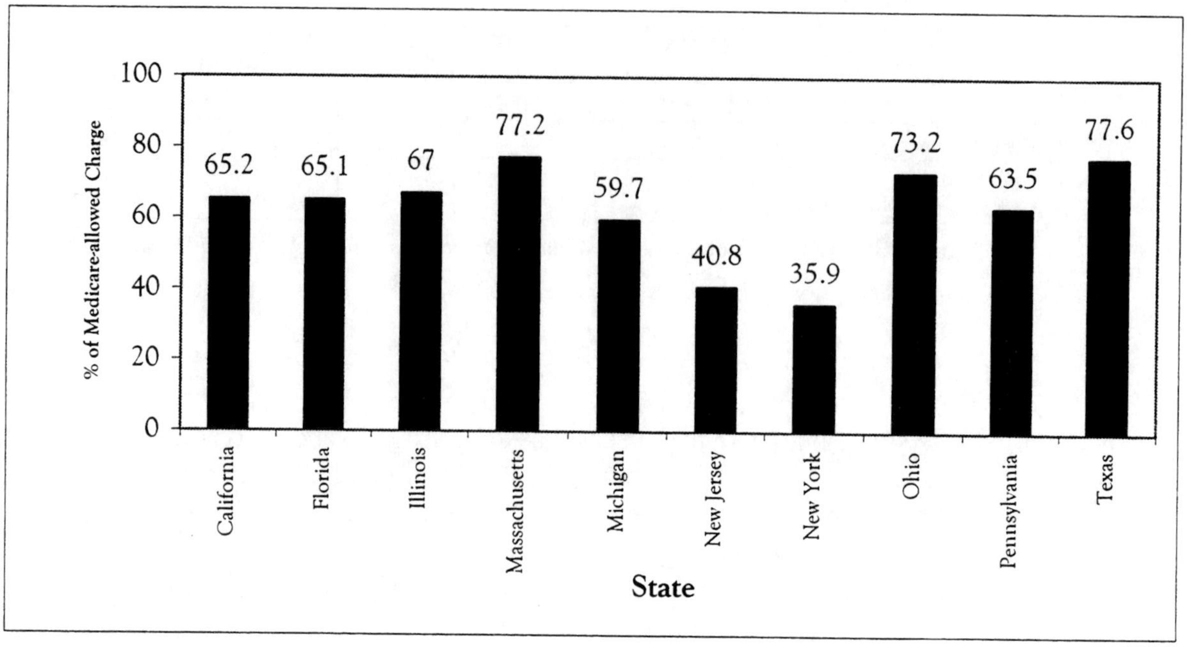

Adapted from: Joel Menges, Chris Park, Jennifer Babcock, Lisa Chimento, Randall Haught ,Silver Ho, The Lewin Group, *Comparing Physician and Dentist Fees Among Medicaid Programs* (Oakland, CA: Medi-Cal Policy Institute, June 2001). Online. Available: http://admin.chcf.org/documents/mcpi/ ComparingPhysicianAndDentistFees.pdf. Accessed: January 31, 2002.

Texas's rank nationally for the average percentage of Medicare-allowed charge is 27th, which is consistent with the state's rankings in other state-by-state comparisons.

Comparing Texas Medicaid to Medicare

Payments to providers under the Medicaid program are traditionally lower than payments to providers under the Medicare program. The Texas Medicaid physician reimbursement system is partially based on Medicare's RBRVS. In 2001, the Texas Medicaid payment was, on average, 60 percent of the payment under Medicare for those Medicaid services included in the RBRVS system.[12] However, 50 percent of Medicaid's physician fees are Access-Based fees, which are typically higher than they would be under the RBRVS.[13]

The weight for the procedure is multiplied by a conversion factor to determine payment. Under the Medicaid program, each state sets its own conversion factor. As established by the Balanced Budget Act of 1997, under the Medicare program, there is only one conversion factor for the whole country.[14]

Under the RBRVS, a relative weight is assigned to each procedure. Payments are determined by multiplying the total weight assigned to the procedure by a conversion factor. In 2001, the conversion factor for Texas Medicaid program was 27.261[15] while the conversion factor for Medicare is 38.2581[16] for most services. The higher Medicare conversion factor results in typically higher payments for procedures under the Medicare program than under the Medicaid program in Texas. Because the state sometimes adjusts the weight assigned to certain procedures under the Medicaid program, payments for some procedures under the Medicaid program in Texas exceed the Medicare payment or are significantly lower. These adjustments account for some of the variability across procedures in Medicaid and Medicare payments.

Example 1. CPT Code 99395, Preventive Medicine, Preventive Visit, Established Patient, Age 18-39

	RVU		Conversion Factor		Total Payment
Medicare	2.15	x	38.2581	=	$82.25
Medicaid	2.15	x	27.261	=	$58.61
				Difference	$23.64

For more complicated procedures, the difference in payment between the two programs is even more significant.

Example 2. CPT Code 93530, Right Heart Catheterization, Congenital

	RVU		Conversion Factor		Total Payment
Medicare	24.12	x	38.2581	=	$922.79
Medicaid	24.12	x	27.261	=	$657.54
				Difference	$265.25

A 1999 study by the Urban Institute examined Medicaid to Medicare fee ratios by state for 19 selected primary care, obstetric, and other services and found that for these services, on average Medicaid pays approximately 64 percent of Medicare nationwide.[17] Because Texas significantly over-reported one of its fees, this number may be slightly lower.

Comparing Texas Medicaid to Commercial Payers

Many commercial payers also use the RBRVS or a variation on the system to formulate their reimbursement fees for providers, which facilitates comparisons between Medicaid, Medicare, and commercial payors.[18] A study conducted by Milliman Associates of RBRVS in Texas compared the conversion factor for Medicare and commercial payers across seven specialties. In this study, the conversion factor for Medicare was compared to the commercial median conversion factor for each specialty. As a percentage of the commercial median, the Medicare conversion factor ranged from 47 percent for pathology services and 90 percent for evaluation and management services. On average for the seven specialty areas, the Medicare conversion factor was 60 percent of the commercial median.

Of course, as the Medicaid conversion factor is lower than the Medicare conversion factor, the Medicaid conversion factor as a percentage of the commercial median is even lower (see Figure 6.4).

Figure 6.4
Comparison of Medicaid, Medicare, and Commercial Conversion Factors

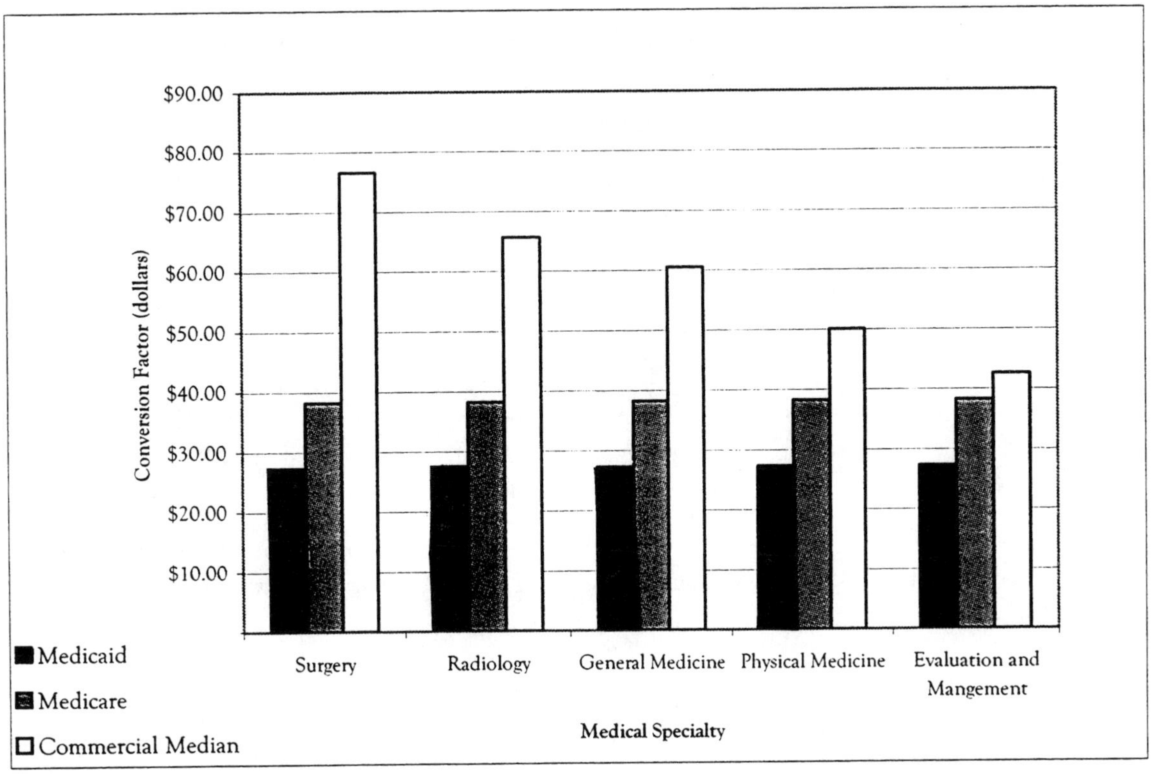

Adapted from: Milliman Associates, *Medicaid Comparative Price Analysis*, report to Texas Medical Association (Austin, Tex., 2000), p. 1.

Though this chart does not take into account commercial payers using other reimbursement methodologies than the RBRVS, it does demonstrate a clear difference between commercial payers and Medicaid. The disparity in payments is supported by the findings of a 1998 study conducted by TMA comparing Texas Medicaid FFS fees to commercial payers in San Angelo and Houston, Texas.

As Figure 6.5 shows of the 107 CPT Codes examined, for the majority of codes (63 percent), the payment under the Texas FFS Medicaid program falls within 26 to 50 percent of the average commercial payer in Houston.

Figure 6.5
Texas Medicaid Fee-for-Service Payments Compared to Average Houston Commercial Payments for Selected CPT Codes, 1998

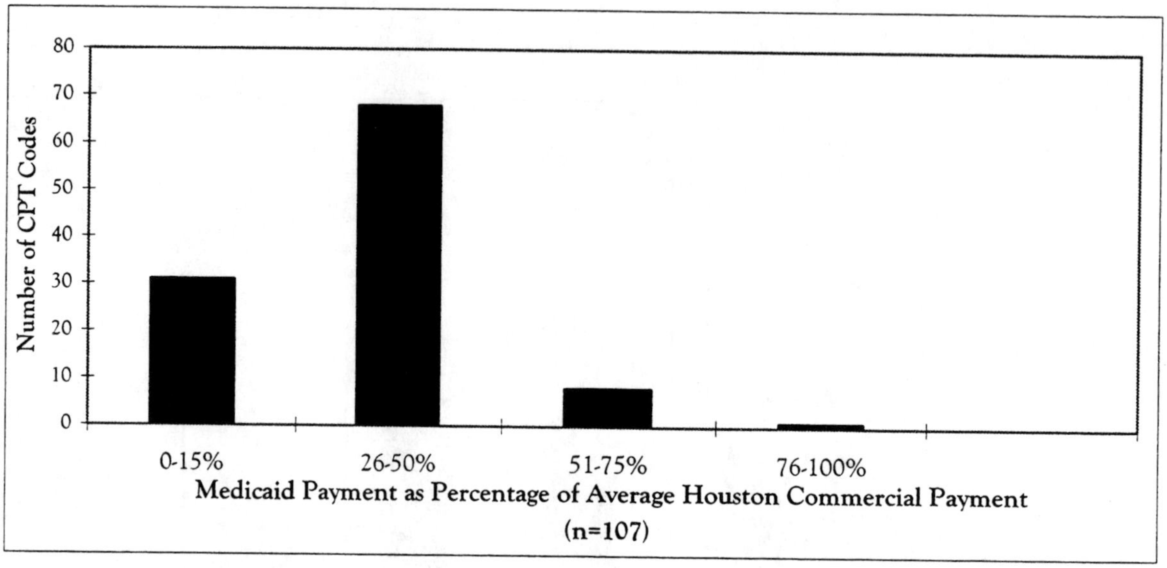

Adapted from: Milliman Associates, *Medicaid Comparative Price Analysis*, report to Texas Medical Association (Austin, Tex., 2000), p. 1.

It should be noted that according to TMA, commercial payments in Houston are among the highest in the state, meaning the difference between Medicaid and commercial payments may be higher than the average for the state. To draw comparisons between Medicaid payments and payments in rural areas, TMA also compared Medicaid FFS fees for the same procedures to the average commercial payments in San Angelo (see Figure 6.6).

Figure 6.6
Texas Medicaid Fee-for-Service Payments Compared to Average San Angelo Commercial Payments for Selected CPT Codes, 1998

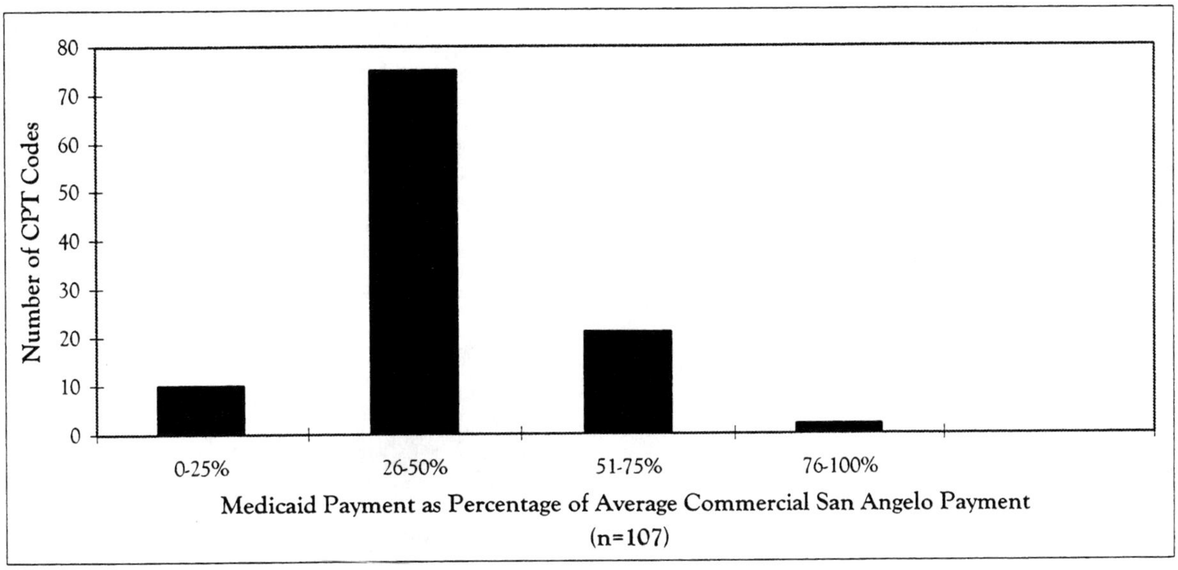

Adapted from: Milliman Associates, *Medicaid Comparative Price Analysis*, report to Texas Medical Association (Austin, Tex., 2000), p. 1.

As Figure 6.6 shows, Medicaid payments are also significantly lower than the average commercial payments in San Angelo, Texas. Compared to Houston, there are fewer codes for which the Medicaid payment is below 25 percent of the commercial payment and more codes for which the Medicaid payment is above 51 percent of the average commercial payment. However, like Houston, the majority of Medicaid payments (70 percent) fall within 26 to 50 percent of the average commercial payment in San Angelo.

Though this study was limited in scope, this ratio of Medicaid to commercial payments is very similar to the findings of a PriceWaterhouseCoopers report released in 2001 comparing payments under Medi-Cal (California's Medicaid program) to Medicare and commercial payors. The study found that for the majority of codes examined, payments under Medi-Cal ranged between 35 to 60 percent of payments by commercial PPOs.[19]

Hospitals

There is a base of approximately 500 hospitals in Texas, including 450 general/acute care and rehabilitation hospitals, eight children's hospitals, 25 psychiatric hospitals and 15 state-owned hospitals.[20] The adequacy of the hospital network is a concern to policymakers. In the 1990s, Texas led the nation in hospital closures, which has a particular impact on rural areas. As Figure 6.7 shows, 32 percent of rural counties in Texas have no hospitals while 53 percent have only one hospital.

For public and safety-net hospitals, the Medicaid program is a significant source of revenue. Hospitals receive Medicaid funds both as reimbursement for services and through disproportionate share hospital funds.

Figure 6.7
Number of Hospitals per Texas Rural County

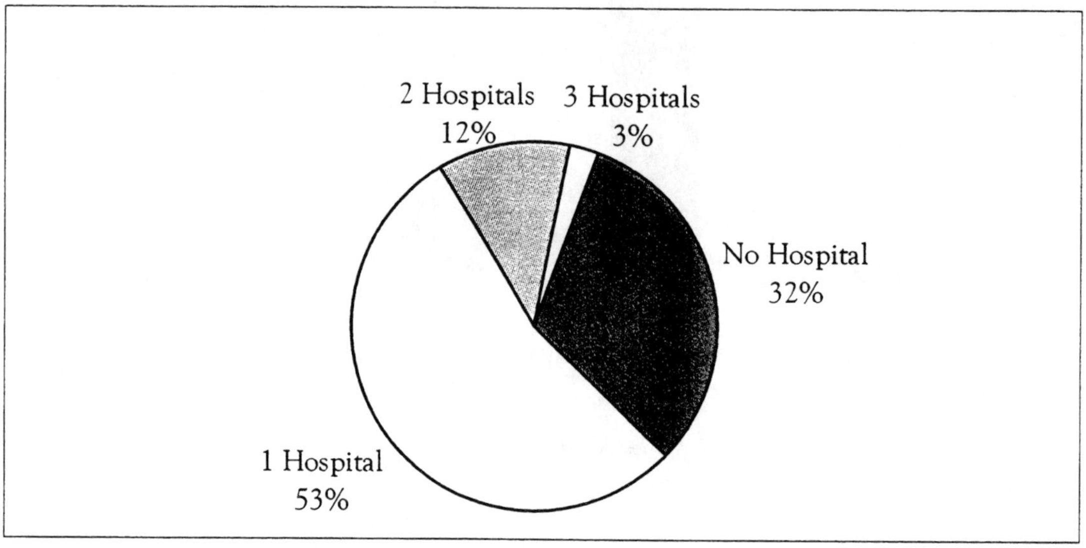

Adapted from: Texas Health and Human Services Commission, *Selected Medicaid Rate Methodologies,* Budget Brief (Austin, Tex., November 2001), p. 1.

Inpatient Hospital

In Texas, inpatient hospital services account for 16 percent of Medicaid spending.[21] Approximately 500,000 people per year are admitted to a Texas hospital for inpatient services.[22] Inpatient hospital reimbursement rates are calculated by multiplying a DRG weight by a hospital's SDA rate, as described below. This methodology is based on Medicare's prospective payment system.

Payment Methodology for General/Acute Care Hospitals

Texas uses a prospective payment system to reimburse providers for inpatient services. The prospective payment system, which is also used in the Medicare program, reimburses hospitals a fixed amount per patient based on diagnosis. Inpatient reimbursement rates are based on the Diagnosis Related Grouping payment methodology. The DRG system organizes all possible diagnoses from the *International Classification of Diseases, 9th Revision, Clinical Modification (ICD9-CM)* system into 523 "medically meaningful groupings."[23] Each grouping is assigned a weight that reflects that amount of hospital resources required to care for patients in that grouping.

The DRG weight is then multiplied by the hospital Standard Dollar Amount weight to determine payment. Every hospital is assigned a Standard Dollar Amount (SDA) that is based on its standardized average cost of treating a Medicaid patient. The SDA is calculated specifically for each hospital by the National Heritage Insurance Company using methodologies left over from the retrospective reimbursement system used prior to September 1, 1986. The average adjusted SDA for Texas hospitals in FY 1998 was $3,335.16.[24] The following is an example of how to calculate a hospital's payment for treating a normal newborn on an inpatient basis.

SDA x Relative Weight DRG 391 (normal newborn) = total payment[25]

$3400 x .1357 = $461.38

Hospitals may qualify for additional outlier payments in cases of especially high-cost hospitalization.

The SDA largely determines how much individual hospitals receive as payment per service. The methodology for determining a hospital's SDA is complicated. For each hospital, dollars spent per case are adjusted and standardized and then further adjusted to take the average relative weight per case (case mix index) and to account for inflation.[26]

Outpatient Hospital

In Texas, outpatient hospital costs account for five percent of total Medicaid spending.[27] At the approximately 500 hospitals and satellite facilities in the state, there are approximately 4,000,000 outpatient encounters per year.[28] Unlike for inpatient and physician services, reimbursement for outpatient services is based on cost not resources.

High volume providers are reimbursed at 84.48 (an increase of 5.2 percent from last year) percent of cost while low volume providers are reimbursed at 80.3 percent of cost.[29] Under this system, hospitals are paid at an interim payment rate throughout the year. At the end of the year, when they submit their cost reports to the state, their final reimbursement rate is determined and the difference is settled retrospectively.[30]

The Disproportionate Share Hospital Program

The Medicaid Disproportionate Share Hospital Program (DSH) is a vital part of the safety net for the uninsured. Accounting for 12 percent of total Medicaid spending nationally,[31] the DSH program reimburses hospitals that serve a disproportionate number of Medicaid and uninsured patients. As part of Medicaid, DSH is a federal-state matching program.

DSH was established by the Omnibus Budget Reconciliation Act of 1981, but most states did not participate significantly in the program until 1987. Between 1989 and 1992 the

DSH program grew from $600 million to $17 billion. This tremendous growth was primarily due to 1) increased state participation in the program, 2) the swelling of the Medicaid rolls as a result of the declining economy, and 3) general health care inflation.[32] In 1992, the DSH program accounted for 15 percent of total Medicaid spending.

Concerned about the unrestrained growth of the DSH program, in 1991 Congress established an aggregate national limit on DSH of 12 percent of total Medicaid spending and established DSH caps for each state.[33] The cap on federal DSH funds for Texas for 2001 and 2002 is $765 million.[34]

With the third largest DSH program in the country, Texas has a long history of taking full advantage of this program, drawing down 100 percent of available federal matching funds. Despite a steady decline in federal DSH funds over the last few years, DSH still accounted for 15 percent of the state's Medicaid funds in Fiscal Year 1998.[35]

In Texas, the state portion of the DSH program is funded through intergovernmental transfers from state and locally-owned public hospitals. Rather than appropriating money for the state portion of the program, the state requires public hospitals to make intergovernmental transfers of funds to the state. The state pools these funds and draws down the federal match. The funds are then redistributed to all DSH eligible hospitals, including both the public hospitals that contributed to the state match and private and not-for-profit hospitals that are not required to contribute.

Eligibility

In FY 1998, of 451 hospitals in the state, 166 Texas hospitals qualified for DSH funding.[36] Of these, 98 were public hospitals, 39 were private not-for-profit hospitals and 29 were private for-profit hospitals.[37] Texas automatically deems the three University of Texas Teaching Hospitals and all children's hospitals as DSH hospitals. For all other hospitals, eligibility is determined by the number of inpatient Medicaid or inpatient low-income days a hospital reports.

There is a hospital-specific, federally-imposed cap that limits the amount of DSH funding that a hospital can receive. Under the hospital-specific cap, DSH funding for a facility cannot exceed the facility's costs of providing inpatient and outpatient services to Medicaid and uninsured patients less payments received from Medicaid and uninsured patients.[38] The cap for each hospital is determined by HHSC based on annual financial reports submitted by the hospitals to the state.

Distribution of Funds

Texas has structured the DSH program to enhance payments to state-owned facilities, which, in theory, allows the state to reduce its appropriations to those facilities. State-owned facilities receive the maximum amount allowed under their hospital-specific caps. The University of Texas Hospitals, which are obligated to return at least their federal DSH payment to the state, are an exception.

Facilities not owned by the state receive about 40 percent of the DSH pool.[39] The formula for determining how much DSH funding each non-state facility in Texas receives is based on the volume of care provided to Medicaid and low-income patients (Medicaid days + low-income days/Total Medicaid days + low-income days for all eligible DSH hospitals).[40]

Table 6.4 breaks down the distribution of Texas DSH funds by ownership and type of care for Fiscal Year 1997.

Table 6.4
Texas DSH Allocations

	Acute	Mental	Totals
Private	263,000,000	5,000,000	268,000,000
Local/County Public	615,000,000	-	615,000,000
State	236,000,000	394,000,000	630,000,000
Totals	1,140,000,000	399,000,000	1,513,000,000

Adapted from: Teresa Coughlin, Leighton Ku, Johnny Kim, *Reforming the Medicaid Disproportionate Share Hospital Program in the 1990s* (Washington, D.C.: The Urban Institute, January, 2000), pp.16-17.

Conditions for Receiving DSH Payments

Texas places minimal restrictions on how DSH funds can be used. In Texas, DSH hospitals must 1) advise patients of the availability of charity and low-cost care, 2) submit annual reports to the state on the use of DSH funds, 3) conduct an "annual assessment of the health needs of the community", and 4) participate in the development of a regional trauma network.[41]

According to a report on the DSH program profiling the Texas program, these conditions are not strongly enforced and there is some question to whether DSH funds are being used as effectively as possible.[42]

The Texas Medicaid DSH program has been criticized for the following things:

- **Penalizing public hospitals.** While the state's base DSH formula is modified to provide additional funding to institutions that make intergovernmental transfers to the state, these adjustments do not offset the full amount of money the hospitals transferred. Critics of the Texas DSH program point out that because private hospitals are not burdened with contributing to the state's share of the program, they often fare better than public hospitals under this system. Several for-profit hospitals are reimbursed for over 90 percent of their costs of providing uncompensated care.[43] In contrast, eight public hospital districts received net

DSH funds that covered only 38 to 53 percent of their uncompensated care costs.[44]

- **Retaining funds for the state.** A controversy surrounding the DSH program has been that many states retain a portion of their DSH funds and allocate them to general revenues or other health programs. These funds, known as "residual funds" are not well accounted for. Texas retains a relatively high percentage of its DSH funds for the state's general revenues. In FY 1997, of the total $1.5 billion Texas DSH funds, the state gained $394,533,000 (or 26 percent) in residual funds, the majority of which was used to fund the state's mental health institutions.[45]

- **Diverting funds to mental health institutions.** Texas, like many other states, uses DSH funds to finance state-owned institutes for mental diseases (IMDs). In Texas, 24 percent of DSH funds are used for IMDs. Because Congress views support for mental health institutions to be a traditional responsibility of the states, it acted in 1997 to limit the amount of DSH money that states can divert to IMDs.[46]

- **Discouraging outpatient care.** Because the DSH formula is based on inpatient days, some have argued that it discourages hospitals from transferring patients to outpatient care when appropriate. As inpatient care is more costly than outpatient care, the formula encourages higher costs.

Recent Increases

A number of legislative increases in provider reimbursement rates were approved and implemented in 2001. Table 6.5 presents a list of rate increases authorized by SB 1.

Table 6.5
Recent Legislative Rate Increases: Medicaid PPS/FFS

Specialty	Rate and Procedure	Effective Date	Appropriated Funds for SFY 02-03
Professional fees	EPSDT (fee increased to $70)	9/1/2001	$31 million
	Additional office-based, primary care/preventive, volume and geographic adjustments		$19 million
Dental fees	13.5% increase 33 high-volume procedures	10/1/2001	$20 million
Outpatient hospital discount factor	5.2% increase to high-volume providers along the border and in MSAs.	10/1/2001	$35 million
Community care	Various rate increases for attendant wages in selected programs	9/1/2001	$50 million
Nursing facility rates	An average 11.5% increase plus other specific adjustments	9/1/2001	$175 million
Home and community-based waiver services	1.2% increase over FY01 rates	9/1/2001	$2.5 million
HMOs	Varies according to SDA and risk group	9/1/2001	$35 million
STAR-Plus	Under negotiation	1/1/2002	$4.5 million
SCHIP	19.7% average increase[1]	10/1/2001	$292 million[2]

Adapted from: Don Gilbert, Commissioner, Texas Health and Human Services Commission, Presentation to Senate Finance Committee, Austin, Texas, October 24, 2001.

[1] This is the average increase of payments made to managed care plans serving SCHIP beneficiaries.

[2] This amount represents the legislative increase for the total state SCHIP budget and not reimbursement increases in particular.

Medicaid Managed Care

Medicaid managed care (MMC) has not penetrated the Texas market as significantly as it has the rest of the country. By the beginning of 2001, 31.64 percent of Texas Medicaid clients were enrolled in Medicaid managed care, including most of the clients in the state's major urban areas. Nationally, more than 56 percent of all Medicaid beneficiaries are enrolled in some form of managed care.[47]

In Texas, both an HMO and a PCCM model dominate the managed care delivery system. Under the HMO system, Texas Health and Human Services Commission contracts out to managed care organizations that are paid a capitated rate per member enrolled per month. The HMO is at full-risk for any additional costs incurred above the total capitation payments and is responsible for establishing and paying their own provider network. All profits are shared between the state and the HMO. With the PCCM model, the state contracts with Birch and Davis to enroll providers and serve Medicaid clients. NHIC is responsible for payment and billing procedures but the state assumes all financial risk.

Providers are paid on a fee-for-service basis with primary care providers receiving an extra $3 stipend per client per month.

The contracting network is geographically divided up into eight different service delivery areas (SDA) as follows: El Paso, Lubbock, Dallas, Tarrant, Travis, Harris, Bexar, and a Southest Region. The first pilot programs began in 1993 in Travis County and in the Southeast region. These pilot programs established the framework for the new Medicaid delivery system in Texas. From September 1996 through December 1999, MMC was rolled out into the other delivery areas. Most areas include a combination of PCCM and HMOs, except for Tarrant and Travis which are HMO only and the Southeast Region which is PCCM only. As of November 1, 2001, there were 606,944 total clients in Medicaid managed care: 59.3 percent were enrolled in HMOs and 39.9 percent were enrolled in the PCCM network. Another .8 percent were enrolled in a Preferred Health Plan (PHP).[48] There are currently 13 HMOs serving Medicaid clients in Texas and three to four plans per delivery area. All of the Medicaid plans also serve commercial accounts except for Superior and Americaid (now called Amerigroup), which are strictly for Medicaid and SCHIP beneficiaries.[49]

Medicaid managed care in Texas is known as the State of Texas Access Reform (STAR) program. STAR was implemented in Texas with several important goals: 1) control rising costs, 2) reduce inappropriate utilization of health services, 3) improve quality of and access to care, 4) increase provider satisfaction, and 5) improve accountability.[50]

STAR serves the largest number of Medicaid clients in managed care. The Texas Health and Human Services Commission is responsible for its operation and management. In FY 1998, Medicaid managed care was extended to the elderly and disabled beneficiary population who qualify through SSI or Medical Assistance Only (MAO). This program is known as STAR+PLUS and is operated by the Texas Department of Human Services (DHS). STAR+PLUS is currently operating in the Harris delivery area. STAR+PLUS currently has 57,000 enrollees with 8,100 in PCCM and the remainder in two HMOs. In July 1999, Medicaid managed care began a pilot program in the Dallas delivery area to expand mental health and chemical dependency benefits. This program is known as NorthSTAR and is operated by the Texas Department of Mental Health and Mental Retardation (TDMHMR) and the Texas Commission on Alcohol and Drug Abuse (TCADA).[51] Because STAR+PLUS and NorthSTAR are currently pilot programs and use different rates, risk groups, and methodologies than STAR, evaluations of MMC in this paper will examine the STAR program.

The STAR program is under intense scrutiny at this time. While managed care is controversial at many levels, the Medicaid element adds additional components to the managed care debate. HMOs are reluctant to participate in MMC due to the lower reimbursement rates, and thus profitability, and the cost of Medicaid administrative requirements. HMOs also feel burdened by the extensive contractual requirements that exceed those of commercial contracts. Providers appear hesitant to become involved with Medicaid at all levels, but perceive the managed care entities with even more suspicion.

Legislators and policy analysts are concerned that managed care does not work in rural areas and are also concerned about the success in meeting the five goals. Recently, a moratorium has been placed on any form of HMO rollout in Texas. The planned rollout of the PCCM model in April 2002 will be delayed while evaluations are completed.

Medicaid Managed Care: Provider Network

Findings from a Texas Department of Health survey on Medicaid managed care has established that providers are, in general, dissatisfied with MMC. The TDH survey found that 71 percent of physicians participating in Medicaid managed care were dissatisfied with reimbursement levels. In addition, 71 percent of physicians reported being dissatisfied with the amount of paperwork required and 77 percent reported being dissatisfied with the amount of phone work required.[52] Many physicians also appear to retreat from Medicaid managed care due to the state requirements for Medicaid HMO and PCCM primary care networks. These requirements include around-the-clock availability of PCPs and appointment and wait time standards, among other extra responsibilities.

Despite physician dissatisfaction with the program, both TDH and HHSC report that the actual number of providers is sufficient to ensure access. The Texas Department of Health reported in its Texas STAR Medicaid Managed Care Report that in all of the service delivery areas in which Medicaid managed care had been implemented in 1998, there was a sufficient number of primary care providers participating in the Medicaid program. However, this report did not include the El Paso service delivery area because Medicaid managed care had not yet been established in that area.[53] More recently, HHSC has claimed that the HMOs are meeting the state provider network requirements. These requirements ensure that the provider base of the HMOs be sufficient enough to serve at least 45 percent of the managed care eligibles in each service area.[54] Yet, while there are documented decreases in physician participation within certain HMOs, there is evidence that for 1998 to 1999, there was a 2 percent statewide increase in physician participation overall.[55] This increase may reflect a state recruitment effort of providers that started in 1998.

In contrast, recent surveys conducted by TMA suggest a decrease in the number of physicians in Texas willing to accept Medicaid patients. In a 2000 survey of physicians, it was found that 61 percent of physicians will accept all Medicaid patients for treatment (versus 68 percent in 1998), while 16 percent of physicians limit the number of Medicaid patients they will accept (versus 10 percent in 1998), and 23 percent of physicians will not accept any Medicaid patients (versus 22 percent in 1998).[56] This survey reflects both FFS and MMC Medicaid providers and may reflect a decrease in the number of physicians participating in FFS, rather than just managed care. Specifically, a survey-study by TDH and the Texas Health Quality Alliance shows that 71 percent of physicians in MMC report that Medicaid patients make up less than 50 percent of their practice.[57]

In an HHSC comparative study, member to provider ratios were assessed for both traditional Medicaid and Medicaid managed care in August 2000. In four categories (family practice, internal medicine, ob/gyn, and pediatrics) it was found that the ratio was generally smaller for STAR managed care in most counties. For example, in the Harris SDA there are 184 members per general practice provider in MMC while there are 283 per general practice provider in traditional fee-for-service. The difference is even more noticeable for pediatrics, with 297 per pediatrician in MMC while there are 596 per pediatrician in traditional Medicaid.[58] In Travis SDA, on the other hand, the ratios are approximately the same. However, it must be noted that providers participating in a Medicaid managed care health plan may not necessarily be taking Medicaid clients or may limit the amount of clients that they take in. This is especially so in a commercial managed care organization that may not take as many Medicaid clients overall. Providers in traditional Medicaid usually have higher concentrations of Medicaid patients in their practice. In Harris County, 11 percent of traditional providers showed more than 1,000 clients in their practice compared to only 1.5 percent of Medicaid managed care providers with more than 1,000 members.[59]

STAR + PLUS primary care provider (PCP) to client ratios also presented ratios that are lower than the traditional program ratio. The traditional program ratio for Harris County was one PCP to 125 members. For Americaid this ratio was one PCP for every 57 Medicaid clients but with HMO Blue this number dropped to one PCP for every 26 clients.[60] These numbers again should be interpreted cautiously as HMOs such as Blue have large provider networks, but not all providers accept new Medicaid patients and many providers limit the amount of Medicaid clients in their practice. Also, these numbers point out that even within the same SDA, the provider ratios can alter substantially depending on the MCO.

There are also major problems in some counties. In El Paso, for example, legislators and stakeholders are troubled over the appropriateness of the network. As of 2000, there were only 302 PCPs for 68,508 members. In the Bexar SDA, there are 198 pediatricians available to serve 67,256 children ages 0 to14 in MMC; 781 of these children do not have access within 30 miles to a pediatrician.[61] However, both Bexar and El Paso delivery areas include large rural counties that were underserved even before MMC implementation. Hudspeth County, for example, has only one full-time traditional Medicaid provider. This problem of provider proximity is beyond the scope of just Medicaid and needs to be placed in the context of the larger health care market.

There is no definitive conclusion to make on patients access to care in Medicaid managed care. Measuring access has proved difficult in the complex network systems that exist in Texas. Since it is the beneficiaries that face the consequences of accessibility to care, it is important to mention that current MMC members are generally satisfied with the provider network. Texas Health Quality Alliance (THQA) found that 70 to 71 percent of STAR clients and 73 to 80 percent of STAR + PLUS clients reported having a personal doctor in their MCO in state FY 2000. In addition, 58 to 65 percent of STAR clients and 51 to 54 percent of STAR + PLUS clients reported having no problem finding a usual source of care in SFY 2000. However, this is a notable decrease from SFY 1999, when 63 to 73 percent of STAR clients and 52 to 62 percent of STAR + PLUS clients reported having no problem finding a doctor.[62] According to this study, it has become more burdensome for clients to find a usual source of care. It is unclear whether the reduced ease stems from a smaller provider base or a provider base more unwilling to see Medicaid patients.

Medicaid Managed Care: Rate Setting Methodology

Under managed care, a plan is paid a uniform capitated amount for each person served on a monthly basis. In Texas, capitation rates vary by service delivery area and are updated on an annual basis. Capitation rates approximately amount to 95 percent of the FFS for a given area.

Capitation rates are computed and distributed for seven risk groups: 1) TANF adult, 2) TANF children, 3) pregnant women, 4) newborns, 5) expansion children, 6) federal mandated children, and 7) SCHIP Phase I children.[63]

In Texas, managed care capitation rates are set in a three-stage process: 1) determining the base rates 2) adding on legislatively appropriated funds; and, 3) making a budget-neutral risk adjustment.

Establishing the Base Rates

Like many other states, Texas uses a reduced FFS model to determine base rates. Managed care capitation rates are based on FFS data of historical costs and utilization in a service delivery area. The FFS estimates use data from before managed care and projects the cost forward, taking into account statewide trends.[64]

The state's methodology for projecting costs includes applying area factors to the statewide FFS cost data. Area factors adjust a service delivery area's average cost relative to the statewide costs for each risk group. Area factors are determined using data from 1994 to 1996, before managed care rollouts, except for in the Travis SDA because this was part of the pilot program. Travis therefore uses area factors calculated from 1992 to 1993. For example, the Harris SDA has an average area factor of 1.153, because 1996 costs in that area were higher than statewide averages. El Paso, on the other hand, has the lowest average area factor of .844, because historical costs were lower than the state.[65]

Setting the base rate also includes applying delayed enrollment factors to the statewide FFS costs. The delayed enrollment factor adjusts the base rate to reflect the typical two-month delay in enrollment in Medicaid managed care. Many people enrolling in Medicaid do so because they have an immediate health care need and their first two months in Medicaid, which will be spent in FFS, will tend to be more expensive than the period they spend in managed care.[66] The delayed enrollment factors are accounted for by risk group within each county and display the average cost for managed care members relative to all members. In Harris SDA, the TANF Children group has a delayed enrollment factor of 0.971 because this risk group costs less relative to the other risk groups.

The base rates are therefore established by multiplying the FFS projected costs to the area factor and then multiplying this number by the delayed enrollment factor. To establish a base rate for TANF children in Harris SDA, the projected FY 2001 statewide incurred claims of $98.636 is multiplied to the area adjustment factor of 1.153, and then multiplied again to the delayed enrollment factor of 0.971. A 12 percent managed discount factor is then taken into account, to amount to a premium rate of $97.18 before taking into account legislative increases.

Legislative Increases

For the 2002-2004 biennium, the legislature increased funding available to HMOs by $35 million in general revenue (GR), or $87.5 million with the federal match (all funds). For FY 2002, the state is using 47.27 percent of this funding as caseloads are expected to be higher in FY 2003.

Physician fees have been increased by $20.90, for a total of $70 per Early and Periodic Screening, Diagnosis and Treatment Planning (EPSDT) screen, at current caseloads. The amount added varies by risk group because of the different screening rates. Outpatient hospital increases are $87.5 million in all fund dollars; 20.76 percent of this funding is available to HMOs for two years. Cost increases were also added for medical policy changes and increase capitation rates by approximately 14 cents per member per month.[67] After accounting for legislative increases, Harris SDA's base rate of $97.18 per TANF child is increased to $105.79 per child per month.

Budget-Neutral Risk Adjustment

In computing capitated rates, federal regulations mandate that states not pay managed care organizations more than what it would pay had there been no managed care. States are therefore constrained by the upper payment limit used in traditional FFS payments. The rates that are set must be cost effective and actuarially sound.[68]

Medicaid Managed Care: Provider Reimbursement

Managed care organizations are responsible for paying their providers. With 71 percent of Medicaid managed care providers expressing dissatisfaction with reimbursement levels,[69] it is imperative to assess the rates for adequacy and equity. Unfortunately, payments to physicians are not public records and therefore difficult to obtain. It is also difficult to assess the rates to providers when providers participate in several different networks and use different payment arrangements. A study by TDH and the Texas Health Quality Alliance found that 38 percent of primary care providers (PCP) participating in Medicaid managed care were paid on a fee for service basis by their plans. Another 19 percent of PCPs held capitated contracts, and 33 percent had a combination of arrangements. Most HMOs reimburse specialists on a fee for service basis (72 percent).[70]

According to a Medicaid managed care evaluation by the Texas Health and Human Services Commission, most providers are paid at traditional Medicaid rates.[71] However, as each provider, or group of providers, has unique contracts with the HMOs, rates to providers fluctuate around the state. HMOs, however, cannot afford to pay their providers below the traditional Medicaid rates since they compete for providers with the PCCM and FFS models in addition to the Medicare and commercial market.

Medicaid Managed Care: Rate Comparisons within Texas

Examining the reimbursement rates to HMOs may help explain the variations in provider reimbursements around the state. The capitated rates per risk group for the seven service delivery areas with HMOs are listed in Appendix D. The average payment across the state for all risk groups is currently $184.79 per member per month. Across the state, the average rate ranges from $135.20 in the El Paso delivery area to $207.78 for the Harris delivery area.

For all risk groups, the Harris and Tarrant delivery areas receive the highest capitated rates, with the exception of TANF adults. The Lubbock delivery area currently receives the highest rate for TANF adults. As is historically true, El Paso and the Texas/Mexico border region receive the lowest average rates even with a 15 percent increase in payments (in accordance with HB 2896).[72] These lower rates can be explained by several factors including historical utilization rates. These utilization rates are used to help determine the FFS projected rates that are applied when calculating the HMO rates. Some areas, particularly the border areas, tend to have historically lower utilization rates than other areas. These utilization rates lower the FFS projections and thus reduce the capitated rates. This applies regardless of the current area utilization rates under managed care. This trend will be further discussed in the Border Area section of this paper.

There are large ranges of payments within each risk group as well. Payments for pregnant women range from $512.10 per member per month (PMPM) in Lubbock to $614.23 in Harris. Payments for newborns range from $450.99 in El Paso to $634.21 in Harris. It is also clear that risk groups for children pay much lower than for adults (over 18 years of age).

It is difficult to assess what the capitated payments pay for, as it must cover administrative expenses as well as provider payments. However, it is clear that rates vary widely around the state but administrative expenses tend to be equivalent throughout the delivery areas. Therefore, it is likely that reduced rates across the border area may lead to lower payments to providers, which would help explain the increased dissatisfaction with managed care in that area. On the other hand, it is not necessarily the case that increased capitation rates translate into increased physician reimbursement rates. It is possible that some HMOs place a cap on provider reimbursement at traditional fee-for-service levels.

Medicaid Managed Care: Texas Rate Comparisons with the Nation

Comparing managed care payment rates across the states is difficult because states are not required to submit their rates to any centralized agency. Collecting information is therefore a more difficult process. There are also other limitations on comparing capitation rates.

First, Medicaid managed care benefits to recipients vary across the nation. Some states include dental, mental health, prescription benefits, amongst other services while others states carve these services out. Rates fluctuate according to the benefit package. Second, risk groups are different in each state. Some states, such as Tennessee, have twenty risk groups while other states do not have any. Texas, for example, does not differentiate between genders like some states do. Third, many states, like Texas, will add a supplemental payment for pregnant women or newborns. However, many times these extra stipends are not calculated into the capitated rates. DSH payments are also sometimes included in the capitated rates but not consistently throughout the nation. Finally, the commercial market varies throughout the U.S. which affects what level of payments will attract and maintain a sufficient HMO base.

Despite these limitations, a 1998 study of Medicaid managed care payment rates performed by the Urban Institute is helpful in assessing how Texas compares to other states. This study evaluated rates for TANF and poverty-related children and pregnant women across 41 states. It did not include SCHIP expansion children, the elderly and disabled, or the medically needy clients of managed care. Rates were adjusted for disproportionate-share hospital, graduate medical education payments, and services carved out for capitation. To standardize the payment rates, the study uses 1990 census data on the population below 200 percent of the federal poverty line to create weights so that data could be aggregated into common risk groups across the nation and within each state. This is a necessary step in order to calculate and compare statewide averages.[73]

At the time of this report, 13 percent of Texas' Medicaid population was enrolled in Medicaid managed care, with 7 percent in HMOs and 6 percent in the PCCM plan. Although Texas did not have a large percentage in MMC, it was found that Texas had some of the highest average capitated rates. Texas ranked higher than the 75th percentile for four of the six risk groups studied. Adjusted capitated rates for males and females age one to thirteen was below the 50th percentile. For 45 to 64 year olds, Texas also was lower than the national average. Other states that had high average rates at the time of this study were Connecticut, Hawaii, Kentucky, and Massachusetts. California, Florida, Georgia, Indiana, and Tennessee had the lowest rates.[74] However, since Medicaid managed care was still relatively new to Texas at the time of this study, it is possible that these higher rates reflect an attempt to attract and encourage health plans to participate.

As the Urban Institute concludes from this survey, the data help to make rate comparisons but should not solely be used to determine the adequacy of rates. The entry and exits of plans from the Medicaid arena reflect a variety of issues. Other factors need to be taken into consideration including the history of managed care in the state, plans' ability and willingness to adapt to the Medicaid environment, the excess provider capacity in the state, and the degree of managed care regulation.[75] All of these factors will affect the adequacy and equity of the rates. For a more thorough evaluation of capitation rates, more data needs to be collected using current figures and input from the plans and providers. It would be useful for CMS to collect rate data on a yearly basis for future trend analysis on national rates.

State Children's Health Insurance Program in Texas

SCHIP was established in Texas in two phases. Phase I began on July 1, 1998, and expanded the state Medicaid program to children ages 15 to 18 years of age. Phase II created a separate SCHIP program that became available on May 1, 2001. Currently, there are 512,048 children in Texas enrolled in the program.[76]

With the intention of differentiating SCHIP from a state welfare program, the SCHIP provider base has been privatized through contracting with managed care organizations while still being funded by the state. The medical provider base for these recipients is an essential component in the functioning of SCHIP. The state must depend on the health care organizations to supply enough providers and benefits to meet the needs of the SCHIP recipients. Without this solid base, recipient access to care is limited.

Health plans for SCHIP were selected by the state based on the extensiveness of their provider network and the cost of the plan. The HMO bidding process did not draw in many commercial health plans such as HMO Blue because as a new program, there was no history to draw upon and therefore was a risky investment. Plans reluctant to take on a government entitlement program were further discouraged as Medicare rates began to decline. The plans that were inclined to work with the state to insure SCHIP participants were mostly hospital-owned and non-profit HMOs.

One of the biggest challenges in the implementation of the SCHIP program was the establishment of a health care system to serve the rural areas of Texas. An Exclusive Provider Network (EPO) was created to cover these large areas. An EPO is a managed care organization that resembles a Preferred Provider Organization (PPO) in that patients can see any provider in their network without going through their primary care physician (PCP). Administratively, the EPO functions much like the Medicaid PCCM model. It was difficult for HHSC to find one indemnity carrier to take on such a geographically large entity. Clarendon Health Care was eventually contracted out as the SCHIP EPO at a higher cost than the HMO's were to receive (see Appendix E).

The provider network in Texas is geographically divided up into 11 SCHIP Service Areas (CSA). There are one to three SCHIP HMO contractors per CSA. Rural counties that are not part of the HMO network are covered by the EPO. Each health care plan is responsible to contract with hospitals, specialists, and PCP's to ensure access to care for their geographic region's SCHIP recipients. The CSA counties and health plans, along with the enrollment figures and rates, can be found in Appendix E.

In the first period of the SCHIP Phase II program, May 1, 2000 through September 30, 2001, aggressive outreach efforts produced enrollment figures exceeding all expectations. It was also found that during this period, the SCHIP population of children who entered into care in the first year had more health care needs than the average child. This higher rate of utilization coupled with the increased enrollment frustrated HMO's during the first period. A few HMOs threatened to withdraw from the program but despite these threats, all 12 HMOs and the EPO remained in the program for the second year.

SCHIP: Provider Base

SCHIP PCPs reduce costs to HMOs by reducing inappropriate utilization of hospital services and performing preventive services such as immunizations. PCPs, as "gatekeepers" to other providers, also have the most contact with SCHIP recipients. Thus, a strong PCP base is essential to maintain sufficient access to care and the viability of the program.

With SCHIP enrollment rolls unexpectedly exceeding enrollment goals in a short period of time, health plans have expressed concern that their networks are being stretched to their limits. Although there are no formal studies documenting network adequacy, health policy analysts have claimed that that the provider base is increasingly becoming weaker.

It is difficult to determine SCHIP beneficiaries' access to providers. Evaluating beneficiary to primary care provider ratios is not always trustworthy because many network providers limit their SCHIP client base. Also, as many physicians are a part of several health plan networks, provider counts may be misleading. Even in areas with only one plan, provider counts should be interpreted cautiously. For example, Seton Health Plan lists 153 primary care providers in their network to serve 20,111 SCHIP beneficiaries. On average, this means there are 132 SCHIP beneficiaries for every primary care provider. Yet in Travis County, Seton's most populous region, there are only 28 pediatricians. All pediatricians listed as holding offices in Travis County were called on January 31, 2001 and were asked if they were taking new SCHIP patients. Only seven pediatricians reported that they were currently taking new SCHIP patients. Perhaps the best determinant of provider accessibility is to evaluate recipient opinions on access.

In an enrollee survey performed by the Institute for Child Health, only 13 percent of parents in Texas reported having difficulty in obtaining a usual source of care for their children as opposed to 23 percent who reported this before enrolling in SCHIP. Before SCHIP, 54 percent of parents reported no difficulty in obtaining a usual source of care for their children. This figure increased to 67 percent post-SCHIP enrollment.[77]

Policy creators, in Texas, anticipating provider needs based on Medicaid experience, were purposeful in developing SCHIP to modify certain aspects of the system to ensure provider satisfaction. SCHIP, as opposed to Medicaid, has 12-month continuous coverage for beneficiaries. Providers with SCHIP do not have to frequently update their client base or call to see which of their clientele is still in the program. Another innovation in the SCHIP program for providers is the elimination of the traditional Medicaid fee-for-service payment program. SCHIP providers are alleviated from much of the paper work and administrative cost associated with fee-for-service.

Despite the improvements made in the creation of SCHIP, many providers are still ambivalent about participating in the program. Providers' perception of the program does not appear to differ from Medicaid even with the emphasis on privatization. In both programs, providers site administrative burdens and client noncompliance (such as missing appointments) as major sources for frustration. However, providers primarily point to low reimbursement levels to explain their hesitation to participate.

A survey of pediatricians in Texas performed by the American Academy of Pediatricians helps to explain physician reluctance to participate in Medicaid. This survey, done before the Phase II expansion in 2000, may help to assess the SCHIP provider sentiment since SCHIP reimbursement rates are only slightly higher than that of Medicaid. In this study, 62 percent of private office-based primary care pediatricians in direct patient care rated "low reimbursement" as a "very important" reason for limiting participation in Medicaid. This is higher than the U.S. statistics in which only 56.3 percent of doctors reported that low reimbursement was the reason for limiting participation.[78] Since reimbursement levels are most likely deterring providers from participating, it is important to evaluate reimbursement rates.

SCHIP: Reimbursement to Health Care Plans

Available funds for the SCHIP health plan reimbursement are allocated by the Texas Legislature. In its budget, Texas has allocated $302.6 million of the $343.6 million in funding for the benefits aspect of the SCHIP Phase II program for FY2001. Of this funding, cost-sharing by SCHIP recipients accounts for more than $15 million. The FY 2002 budget allocates an additional $292 million for benefits in anticipation of more SCHIP beneficiaries.[79] As there are limited federal regulations for financing the health plans providing services, the state bases their funding on actuarial estimates of enrollment and cost. The Center for Medicare and Medicaid Services only requires that if the program utilizes managed care services, the program must be cost-effective. This means that the rates to the providers cannot exceed what would be given to the providers if there had not been managed care.

There have been two financial periods within the Phase II program thus far. The first premium rates covered the period from May 1, 2000 through September 30, 2001. These original premium rates were developed by HHSC with consultation from an external actuary, David Wilkes. Since there was no SCHIP historical experience to base rates on, the rate setting methodology used Medicaid children FFS data with adjustments for the four age risk groups, region, services offered, and cost sharing contribution. The four risk groups are as follows: children ages 0-1, ages 1-5, ages 6-14, and ages 15-18.[80] The resulting premium rates created by this methodology were published in the bid process as the Target Premium Rates. Health plans used these rates as a base to bid for contracts. The rates, as shown in Appendix E, were established based on this bid process conducted in 1999 and early 2000. Capitation rates to each HMO ranged from an average of $63.53 PMPM for Texas Universities Health Plan in the El Paso area to $86.97 PMPM for Texas Children's Health Plan in the Houston area. This reflects the trend of this original Phase II period in which border areas such as El Paso received rates at a much lower level than that of the Houston or Dallas areas. The EPO also was paid capitated rates and like the HMO, took on full-risk of its clients. Clarendon Health Plan, the EPO serving the rural areas of Texas, was paid higher capitated rates than any other plan during this period (see Appendix E).

Each health plan renegotiated their capitated payment rates with HHSC over the summer of 2001. This second period covers the time from October 1, 2001 through September 30, 2002. HHSC used the plans' actual experience in the first period of Phase II to develop the second period rates in order to more accurately predict future costs. 13 of the 14 HMOs reported losses of $33 million during the first period of operation and requested an average increase of 45.9 percent or $64.8 million in General Revenue.

SCHIP managed care plans claim that their losses were due to several factors. Most importantly, SCHIP HMOs were not informed that Children with Special Health Needs would be able to enroll in the program and therefore did not factor in this cost component into their capitation bid.[81] Premiums were therefore insufficient to cover the expenses of these higher cost children.

HHSC offered the plans an average increase of 10.5 percent or $14.8 million, based on the already established appropriation act assumptions for FY 2002.[82] Under the final agreement, reimbursement rates were increased at different rates ranging from 0 percent for Americaid to 29.4 percent for Texas Children's Hospital Health Plan. The average increase was 19.7 percent. The increased rate for Texas Children's Hospital amounts to a capitated payment increase from $93 PMPM to $120 PMPM. Even with this dramatic increase, Texas Children's Hospital still projects that it will face a loss up to $10 million for this period.

The difference in rate increases depends mostly on the experience of the plans in the first period. In CSAs with more than one HMO, certain risk groups are more inclined to enroll in one plan over others. This disproportionate share of higher cost patients into one HMO incurs greater overall risk and cost. These HMOs therefore received a higher rate increase.[83]

Some HMOs claim that the unequal capitated payment to HMOs in the same service area makes it difficult to maintain their provider network and thus reduces access to care. To resolve this issue, the HMOs would have to collectively bid, by geographic region, with HHSC to ensure equal payments for each risk group. To accommodate for the disproportionate share of higher-cost children in some HMOs, the state could add a subsidy (or another risk-group) for each child with established special health care needs. With the consistency of these equalized payments, competition between HMOs for providers may decrease and providers may feel more stable within the network. With a more consistent provider base, access to care can be increased. This type of bidding process would probably cost the state more money that it would with individual HMO bargaining.

Clarendon, the EPO for the rural areas of Texas, chose not to be financed on a capitated PMPM basis for the second period of SCHIP. Instead, the state will contract with Clarendon for a contracted amount for the entire year. If Clarendon's costs exceed this contracted amount, Clarendon will pay a penalty to the state and the state will pay the extra costs incurred. Essentially, this puts the state at full-risk for all SCHIP beneficiaries in rural areas.

SCHIP: Reimbursement to Physicians

HMOs participating in SCHIP reimburse their PCPs on either a capitated or fee for service basis. HMOs that have contracted with SCHIP do not have legal limitations on the level of their physician reimbursement or on the equity of their rates. Theoretically, two doctors performing the same service for the same HMO could be paid different rates. However, in order to keep an adequate network, HMOs must reimburse at a competitive level relative to the private marketplace. As HMOs are private organizations, their payment rates to doctors are not public records. Obtaining this information is therefore difficult. Most policy experts assume that HMOs are paying at traditional Medicaid rates.

SCHIP: The Harris Service Delivery Area

SCHIP Service Area number six encompasses Harris County and the surrounding area. As the second most populous urban area with over 125,000 SCHIP beneficiaries, the need for an expansive provider base is essential to the success of SCHIP. There are currently three HMO's serving this service area as follows: Amerigroup, UTMB Health Care System (Choice 1), and Texas Children's Health Plan. Together, the three HMOs have 982 PCPs. The provider count does not account for duplication of providers across networks. Consequently, the actual PCP count is probably slightly lower than this number. For every PCP available, there are 128 children in need of services. The capitated payment rate to each health plan for the first period was the highest in the state with an average of $86.60 per member per month. This high payment reflects the inflated cost of services in the Houston area.

For the second period, Americaid, which finished the first period with positive returns, was not granted any increase in funding from the state.[84] Texas Children's Health Plan (TCHP), which reported high losses in its first period, received the highest rate increase in the state at 29.4 percent above its first period rates. As a result, TCHP now has the highest PMPM rate in the entire state (see Appendix E). Reported losses are due, in part, to the increased cost HMOs face in contracting with Houston area hospitals, which have raised rates over the last few years. Since HMOs are not able to negotiate with the hospitals or raise the premium rates to their members, the plans can incur losses. During this first period, five major Medicare HMO providers withdrew from the Houston market citing decreased governmental reimbursements and administrative burdens. Since SCHIP rates are much lower than Medicare rates, additional commercial managed care organizations will most likely stay out of the SCHIP marketplace.

SCHIP: Future Outlook

There are currently an estimated 127,541 children eligible for SCHIP in the state who are not yet enrolled. With a decrease in employment and a slow-down of the economy, this number may increase dramatically and SCHIP rolls may reach unexpected heights. With the state government anticipating a major revenue shortfall in the coming biennium, access to medical care has become a critical and pressing issue. The current provider base can only stretch so far. It is therefore important to expand the network and to do so may mean increasing reimbursement rates and reducing administrative burdens to providers.

Border Issues

SB 1053 Advisory Committee: Border Rate Workgroup on Medicaid and SCHIP

While low rates are cited as contributing to the weak Medicaid provider base everywhere within the state, the border region, made up of 43 counties (Appendix F), appears to be plagued with additional problems unique to the area.[85] To study this phenomenon, the 77th Texas Legislature created a committee through Senate Bill 1053. The Health and Human Services Commission was asked to convene a 20-member workgroup made up of health economists, physicians, and public officials.[86] They are expected to have final recommendations by November 2002.

Rate Increases

A few recommendations by the first workgroup, regarding Medicaid rates, have recently come into effect. A 16 percent rate increase has been finalized with HMOs and the EPSDT fee has risen from $49.01 to $70 for an estimated cost of $31 million in general revenue for the biennium. High volume providers in the border and medically underserved inner city areas were given a 5.2 percent increase in payment rates. Only hospital outpatient, ambulatory surgical centers and birthing center services are eligible for this particular increase. This increase applies to an estimated 95 percent of total outpatient services provided.[87]

Border Demographics

Twenty-one percent of the Texas population can be found in the border counties. Of these 4,289,000 people, 1,178,000 people below the age of 66 are uninsured.[88] This figure tells us that 20 percent of the uninsured in Texas below the age of 66 live in the border counties. According to the Texas Health and Human Services Commission, in 2000, approximately 1,065,000 people lived in poverty within the border counties. This means that one in four of border county inhabitants lived in poverty, while one in seven did throughout the rest of Texas.[89] Border counties also have a greater percentage of their population enrolled in Medicaid compared to the state as a whole (see Appendix G).

Barriers to Utilization

The border area, because of its proximity to Mexico, has a demographic makeup of a disproportionate number of both documented and undocumented immigrants, overwhelming poverty rates, and high unemployment. In 2000, for example, border counties had a higher average unemployment rate of 7 percent than did the rest of the state at 4.2 percent unemployment.[90] A significant number of the border population is eligible for Medicaid, but enrollment and utilization numbers indicate that not all take advantage of this opportunity.

Several reasons have been cited as to why Medicaid eligible people do not enroll and why enrollees do not utilize many services in the program. Some argue that immigrants waiting to be naturalized choose not to enroll in Medicaid because they believe their immigration status will be negatively affected if they are part of this public health program. Another argument set forth is one that claims that some Medicaid eligibles do not want the welfare stigma often associated with Medicaid.[91]

Another unique healthcare issue that the legislature-appointed task force on reimbursement rates in the Texas border area identified in its report to the legislature in May 2000 was that of poor transportation infrastructure found in the *colonias*. Lack of an adequate transportation system makes it difficult for Medicaid clients in *colonias* to access, much less utilize, services. However, even if the poor infrastructure were to be improved, the problem of access and utilization would not be solved since the problem of a disproportionately low number of health care providers compared to the rest of the state would still exist in the region.[92] The lack of providers in this medically underserved region includes PCPs, specialists, and nurses. The utilization of outpatient hospitals (FFS) is also affected by the lack of providers. This causes different services to be delivered and thus, utilized by the Medicaid population. Because specialty providers are not available, utilization for inpatient hospitals services, outpatient hospital services, and professional services tend to be lower in border areas than in other areas in the state.[93]

Capitation Rates Lower along the Border

Importance of Utilization

It is believed that the low rate of utilization is further exacerbated in the Texas-Mexico border by the easy and inexpensive access to physicians, specialists and medications available to this border population in Mexico.[94] Reasons for low utilization in the border area is of great significance because of the effect that access and utilization has on capitation rates for HMOs.[95] While Fee For Service (FFS) rates are uniform throughout the state, capitation rates vary from county to county based on the base period FFS average paid out to a particular county. Therefore, the higher the FFS average paid out to each county, the higher the subsequent capitation rate for HMO's within that county. Since Medicaid managed care capitation rates are constrained by federal limitations regarding cost-effectiveness, capitation rates cannot exceed what FFS would cost without managed care. [96]

Effects of Utilization

Because of this rate setting methodology, total FFS payments for each person on average to each county becomes crucial in determining capitation rates for HMO's. According to the Border Rate workgroup, "on average, border counties received a lower payment PMPM."[97] The workgroup also provided a summary of the rate differences found between the border communities and statewide averages. According to the Border Rate workgroup, border rates were lower than the rest of the state.

- Inpatient Hospital (FFS): This area is considered to have the most significant difference in utilization between the border region and other areas in the state. Counties with children's hospitals or other specialty hospitals have higher rates. Furthermore, the type of services provided in specialty hospitals have higher reimbursement rates than do typical professional services. Houston, for example, has a number of specialty hospitals. High reimbursement rates, coupled with high utilization rates result in a higher average payment for Houston and other areas like it. Border counties, already disadvantaged by other problems, receive lower average payments.

- Outpatient Hospital (FFS): Again, the low utilization of these services in the border region as compared to other areas, especially Houston, results in similar low average payments.

Conclusions

Provider surveys have revealed a general dissatisfaction with Texas reimbursement rates both in the traditional and managed care Medicaid program. Though the Medicaid reimbursement rates appear average in comparison to the rest of the country, they are significantly lower than rates of other payers within the state. Whether these relatively low reimbursement rates deter providers from participating in the Medicaid program has not been established. Presumably, however, reimbursement rates are a primary factor in providers' decisions about participating in any health program.

Currently, the Medicaid provider network appears to be stable in most of the state's delivery areas. Yet, there is concern that in rural areas, especially near the Texas-Mexico border, the provider network is inadequate and may limit access to care. Enrollment in the Texas Medicaid program is expected to grow at an increasing rate reflecting the downturn in the economy. The anticipated increase in enrollment coupled with proposed expansions of the program could strain the existing provider network. If Medicaid rates remain uncompetitive, the network may not be sufficient to accommodate future increases in enrollment.

As Texas is entering the next biennium with a $5 billion deficit, there is concern about how much money will be available to finance health care programs. In the current biennium, there have been relatively substantial increases in provider reimbursement rates. Given the state of the economy, it is unlikely that there will be strong support for further rate increases using general revenue. Currently, $2,985,159,031 in general revenue is allocated to HHSC for acute Medicaid service related expenditures. If additional funding were sought specifically to increase reimbursement rates, it would take $149,257,951 million dollars to increase the aggregate service expenditures by five percent.[98] To increase aggregate service expenditures by 10 and 15 percent, an additional $298,515,903 million and $447,773,854 million would need to be raised respectively.

Suggestions for Future Research

It is difficult to find current data about reimbursement rates and methodologies in Texas and throughout the nation. Easier access to this information would enhance the capacity of researchers and policymakers to evaluate reimbursement under the Medicaid program. Creating a central depository of reimbursement data would allow for comparisons of rates across and within states. With the managed care rates, in particular, a comprehensive index of state rate-setting methodologies and standardized capitation rates would allow for easier and more current evaluations. This depository could be located at the federal Center for Medicaid and Medicaid Services.

In addition to creating this central source of information, there is a need for additional studies to evaluate Medicaid reimbursement rates and methodologies. Three such studies are recommended:

- An investigative study to determine what percentage of capitation rates are passed through to providers. The study could include a comparison of the pass-through rates of Medicaid-only and commercial managed care organizations.

- A quantitative study to examine the effects of Medicaid reimbursement rates on provider participation in the program. The study could include a comparison of rates and participation under different service-delivery models.

- An analysis of the impact of making geographic adjustments to the Texas FFS rates for malpractice and other differing expenses.

This information would help Texas policymakers make better-informed decisions about how to use limited funds to enhance provider reimbursement rates.

Notes

[1] Texas Health and Human Services Commission, Advisory Committee for Senate Bill 1053 and Senate Bill 1299, *Fee-for-Service Physician and Outpatient Hospital Fee Methodology* (Austin, Tex., October 25, 2001), p. 1.

[2] American Academy of Pediatrics, *2002 RBRVS. What Is It and How Does It Affect Pediatrics?* Online. Available: http://www.aap.org/visit/pedrbrvs.htm. Accessed: February 1, 2002.

[3] Ibid.

[4] American Academy of Pediatrics, *2002 RBRVS* (online).

[5] Interview by Sarah Stout with Donna Kinney, Manager, Regulatory Advocacy, Texas Medical Association, Austin, Texas, December 6, 2001.

[6] American Academy of Pediatrics, *2002 RBRVS* (online).

[7] Sandra Hunt, Susan Maerki, Doug Porter, Janice Fang, PriceWaterhouseCoopers, *Applying RBRVS to Medi-Cal: Case Studies in Seven States* (Oakland, CA: Medi-Cal Policy Institute, June 2001), p. 23. Online. Available: http://admin.chcf.org/documents/mcpi. Accessed: January 31, 2002.

[8] Ibid, p. 32.

[9] Ibid.

[10] Ibid, p. 31.

[11] Ibid, p. 22.

[12] Sandra Hunt, *Applying RBRVS to Medi-Cal*, p. 31 (online).

[13] Ibid.

[14] American Academy of Pediatrics, *2002 RBRVS* (online).

[15] Kinney interview.

[16] American Academy of Pediatrics, *2001 RBRVS. What Is It and How Does It Affect Pediatrics?* Online. Available: http://www.aap.org/visit/2001RBRVS.pdf. Accessed: February 1, 2002.

[17] Stephen Norton, "Recent Trends in Medicaid Physician Fees, 1993-1998," discussion paper no. 99-12 (Washington, D.C.: Urban Institute, September 1999), p. 9. Online. Available: newfederalism.urban.org/html/discussion99-12.html. Accessed: November 15, 2001.

[18] American Academy of Pediatrics, *2002 RBRVS* (online).

[19] Sandra Hunt, Susan Maerki, Rob Tompkins, PriceWaterhouseCoopers, *Comparing CPT Code Payments for Medi-Cal and Other California Payers* (Oakland, CA: Medi-Cal Policy Institute, June 2001), p. 2. Online. Available: http://admin.chcf.org/documents/mcpi/ComparingCPTCodePayments ForMedi-CalAndOtherPayers.pdf. Accessed: January 31, 2001.

[20] Texas Health and Human Services Commission, *Selected Medicaid Rate Methodologies,* Budget Brief (Austin, Tex., November 2001), p. 1.

[21] Class presentation by Edli Colberg, Demographer/Program Specialist, Texas Health and Human Services Commission, at the Lyndon B. Johnson School of Public Affairs, Austin, Texas, November 13, 2001.

[22] Texas Health and Human Services Commission, *Selected Medicaid Rate Methodologies,* p. 1.

[23] William O. Cleverley, *Essentials of Health Care Finance, 4th Edition* (Gaithersberg, MD: Aspen Publishers, 1997), p. 19.

[24] Email from Dr. David Warner, Professor, Lyndon B. Johnson School of Public Affairs, "Standard Adjustment Amount for Texas Hospitals," to Sarah Stout, January 24, 2002.

[25] Texas Health and Human Services Commission, presentation to SB 1053 Workgroup, Austin, Texas, October 26, 2001.

[26] Ibid.

[27] Colberg presentation.

[28] Texas Health and Human Services Commission, *Selected Medicaid Rate Methodologies,* p. 1.

[29] Ibid.

[30] Texas Health and Human Services Commission, presentation to SB 1053 Workgroup.

[31] Jocelyn Guyer, Andy Schneider, and Michael Spivey, *Untangling DSH: A Guide for Community Groups to Using the Medicaid DSH Program to Promote Access to Care* (Boston, MA: The Access Project, 2000), p. 22.

[32] Jean Hearne, *Medicaid Disproportionate Share Payments* (Washington, D.C.: Congressional Research Service, 2001), p. 4.

[33] Ibid.

[34] Texas Health and Human Services Commission, *Texas Medicaid in Perspective* (Austin, Tex., February 1999), p. 66.

[35] Jocelyn Guyer, *Untangling DSH,* p. 42.

[36] Texas Health and Human Services Commission, *Texas Medicaid in Perspective*, p. 65.

[37] Ibid.

[38] Jean Hearne, *Medicaid Disproportionate Share Payments*, p. 7.

[39] Jocelyn Guyer, *Untangling DSH*, p. 43.

[40] Interview by Sarah Stout with Henry Welles, Program Specialist, Texas Department of Health, Austin, Texas, January 30, 2002.

[41] Jocelyn Guyer, *Untangling DSH,* p. 44.

[42] Ibid.

[43] Ibid.

[44] Ibid.

[45] Teresa Coughlin, Leighton Ku, and Johnny Kim, *Reforming the Medicaid Disproportionate Share Hospital Program in the 1990s* (Washington, D.C.: The Urban Institute, January 2000), p. 20.

[46] Jocelyn Guyer, *Untangling DSH,* p. 44.

[47] Center for Medicaid and Medicare Services, *Managed Care Entities* (2000). Online. Available: http://www.hcfa.gov. Accessed: November 13, 2001.

[48] Texas Department of Health, *Texas Medicaid Managed Care Update: July 24, 2001*. Online. Available: http://www.tdh.state.tx.us/hdf/mc/reports. Accessed: January 3, 2002.

[49] Texas Department of Health, *Participating Plans* (2001). Online. Available: http://www.tdh.state.tx.us/hcf/mc/plans/particip.htm. Accessed: November 16, 2001.

[50] Texas Health and Human Services Commission, *Medicaid Managed Care Report* (November 1, 2000). Online. Available: http://www.hhsc.state.tx.us/Medicaid/MMCR_Main/MMCR_html_frontpage.htm. Accessed: January 10, 2002.

[51] Texas Department of Health, *Texas STAR Medicaid Managed Care Report: Second Edition, Fiscal Year 1998* (Austin, Tex., May 2000), p. iii.

[52] Texas Department of Health, *January 2000 Provider Satisfaction Survey for Medicaid Managed Care: Final Executive Summary* (Austin, Tex., July 27, 2000), pp.3-5,10.

[53] Texas Department of Health, *Texas STAR Medicaid Managed Care Report*, pp. 23.

[54] Texas Health and Human Services Commission, *Medicaid Managed Care Report* (online).

[55] Ibid.

[56] Walt Borges, "Managing Medicaid: Medicaid Managed Care Leaves Physicians, Patients, and Legislators Frustrated," *Texas Medicine*, vol. 11, no. 96 (1996), pp. 34-41.

[57] Texas Department of Health and Texas Health Quality Alliance, *January 2000 Provider Satisfaction Survey for Medicaid Managed Care: Final Technical Report* (Austin, Tex., July 27, 2000), p.16.

[58] Texas Health and Human Services Commission, *Medicaid Managed Care Report* (online).

[59] Ibid.

[60] Ibid.

[61] Ibid.

[62] Ibid.

[63] Senate Bill 1299 Workgroup, *Border Rate Workgroup on Medicaid and SCHIP Final Report* (Austin, Tex., 2001), Appendix C, p.1.

[64] FFS costs in an SDA are currently not what they would be had there been no managed care. Therefore the FFS data used must be from 1996, before FFS was affected by the presence of a new delivery system. FFS costs for inpatient hospital, outpatient hospital, and physician services are taken into account, but not prescription drug services.

[65] Texas Department of Health, *HMO Rate Setting Methodology FY 2002* (Austin, Tex., 2001), p. 19.

[66] Presentation by Olga Garcia, Texas Health and Human Services Commission, Presentation to the Senate Bill1053/1299 Workgroup, Austin, Texas, November 15, 2001.

[67] Texas Department of Health, *HMO Rate Setting Methodology FY 2002*, p. 7.

[68] Texas Health and Human Services Commission, *Medicaid Managed Care Rate Setting*, p. 1.

[69] Texas Department of Health, *January 2000 Provider Satisfaction for Medicaid Managed Care: Final Executive Summary* (Austin, Tex., July 27, 2001), p. 3.

[70] Ibid.

[71] Texas Health and Human Services Commission, *Medicaid Managed Care Report* (online).

[72] Texas Health and Human Services Commission, presentation to SB 1053 Workgroup, Austin, Texas, November 15, 2001.

[73] John Holahan, Suresh Rangarajan, and Matthew Schirmer, "Medicaid Managed Care Payment Methods and Capitation Rates: Results of a National Survey," (Washington, D.C.: Urban Institute, 1999), pp. 20-35. Online. Available: http://newfederalism.urban.org/html/occa26.html. Accessed: October 29, 2001.

[74] Ibid.

[75] Ibid.

[76] Texas Health and Human Services Commission, *Cumulative Application, Enrollment, and Eligibility Determination Activity for 1-14-02.* Online. Available: http://www.hhsc.texas.gov/SCHIP/ weeklysumrpt.htm. Accessed: January 31, 2002.

[77] Elizabeth Shenkman and Jana Col, *Children's Health Insurance Program in Texas: The New Enrollee Survey Report* (Gainesville, Florida: Institute for Child Health Policy, January 2001), pp. 17-18.

[78] American Academy of Pediatrics, *Pediatricians Participation in Medicaid/SCHIP*, p.2.

[79] Texas Department of Human Services. *Budget and Statistics: SCHIP Program* (2001). Online. Available: http://www.bms.dhs.state.tx.us/SCHIP.htm. Accessed: December 13, 2001.

[80] Presentation by David Wilkes, SCHIP Actuary, Birch and Davis, to the SB1053/1299 Task Force, Austin, Texas, November 15, 2001.

[81] Paul Thomas and Lynne Hudson, "The Texas Children's Health Insurance Program (CHIP) One Year Later—Where Do We Go From Here?" *Texas Journal of Rural Health,* vol. IXI (2001), p. 44.

[82] Texas Health and Human Services Commission, *Budget Brief: October 2001* (Austin, Tex., October 2001), pp. 2-4.

[83] Wilkes presentation.

[84] Allison Wollam, "Financial Aches Dog Houston HMOs," *The Houston Business Journal* (April 6, 2001). Online. Available: http://houston.bcentral.com/jouston/stories/2001/04/09/story1.html. Accessed: November 25, 2001.

[85] Senate Bill 1299 Workgroup, *Border Rate Workgroup on Medicaid and SCHIP Final Report* (Austin, Tex., May 2000), Attachment B, p. 1.

[86] Senate Bill 1299 Workgroup, *Border Rate Workgroup on Medicaid and SCHIP Final Report*, p. 1.

[87] Senate Bill 1053 Workgroup, *Preliminary Report to the Texas Legislature* (Austin, Tex., 2000), p.4.

[88] Texas Health and Human Services Commission, Advisory Committee for Senate Bill 1053 and Senate Bill 1299, *Percent of Uninsured in Adults Ages 19-65 in 2000* and *Percent of Children under 19 Uninsured in 2000* (Austin, Tex., October 26, 2001), n. p. (draft paper).

[89] Texas Health and Human Services Commission, Advisory Committee for Senate Bill 1053 and Senate Bill 1299, *Population Living in Poverty in 2000* (Austin, Tex., October 26,2001), n. p. (draft paper).

[90] Ibid.

[91] Senate Bill 1299 Workgroup, *Border Rate Workgroup on Medicaid and SCHIP Final Report*, p. 2.

[92] Ibid.

[93] Senate Bill 1053 Workgroup, *Preliminary Report to the Texas Legislature*, p. 3.

[94] Ibid, p. 1.

[95] Senate Bill 1299 Workgroup, *Border Rate Workgroup on Medicaid and SCHIP Final Report*, p. 1.

[96] Ibid., Appendix C, p. 1.

[97] Senate 1053 Workgroup, *Preliminary Report to the Texas Legislature*, p. 3.

[98] Texas Health and Human Services Commission, *Quarterly Medicaid Report: Fiscal Year 2002* (Austin, Tex., 2002), p. 1.

Chapter 7. Expanding Health Insurance Coverage with the Texas Health Insurance Risk Pool

by Jed MacKay Perry

Introduction

As medical costs increase and managed care plans find cost containment more difficult, health insurance carriers have become more aggressive in their underwriting practices, particularly in the individual market. As such, more and more people in Texas are facing either extremely high premiums or are simply denied coverage for individual insurance. The Texas Health Insurance Risk Pool, as Texas's method of complying with federal guaranteed issue provisions, was designed to provide an avenue for these types of people. However, many of those who are eligible fail to participate, in most cases because of the high cost.

This paper will examine how the Texas Health Insurance Risk Pool could be modified to cover more of those who are eligible, but do not participate. The paper will first review the current state of the individual insurance market in Texas. Then, it will discuss the history and key characteristics of the pool. Next, the pool will be compared with high-risk pools from other states to determine improvements that could be applied to the Texas model. Finally, the improvements will be developed into policy options for improving the level of health insurance coverage through the Texas pool.

The Individual Insurance Market in Texas

In 1993, the small employer health insurance market was reformed to ensure access to health insurance coverage. Reforms included guaranteed issue, guaranteed renewal, and a prohibition on the use of pre-existing conditions to deny coverage. While high insurance costs still remain a difficult hurdle for small employers to overcome, all companies with two to 50 employees have access to health insurance coverage.

Reform of the individual insurance market in Texas has been much more limited. Insurance carriers are able to deny coverage to individuals with health conditions, both currently and in the past (five-year look-back period), and can impose limitations on coverage (such as limiting coverage of certain body parts). Standardized plans are not mandatory, allowing carriers to make any plan variation they deem necessary.[1]

The small market reforms of 1993 also placed limitations on carriers' ability to fluctuate premiums. Though underwriting for medical experience was not eliminated, rate bands were put in place. Thereby, the highest rate for a particular plan may not be more than 67 percent higher than the lowest rate. On the individual insurance market, consumers do not have the same guarantee. Carriers are currently allowed to raise rates as high as they wish based on the health status of individuals, and carriers may further increase rates during renewal periods.[2]

In effect, the individual insurance market is designed with many barriers to access for consumers. The direct barriers to the small employer insurance market, such as guaranteed issue, have been eliminated completely and indirectly by preventing unlimited price increases. The individual market has no such protections, with many people having no access to coverage at all.

History of the Texas Health Insurance Risk Pool

In 1989, the Texas State Legislature passed SB 832, sponsored by Representative John Gavin, enacting the Texas Health Insurance Risk Pool (THIRP). The plan was originally designed to provide health insurance access to uninsured individuals who were denied insurance coverage because of preexisting conditions. At that time, the program was funded by state general revenue. However, the legislature failed to appropriate funding for the program to operate, leaving THIRP dormant.[3]

In 1996, the U.S. Congress passed the Health Insurance Portability and Accountability Act in part to address the issue of preexisting conditions. According to the Act, individual coverage is guaranteed to those who meet all of the following criteria (those who meet the criteria are referred to as "HIPAA-eligible"):

1. at least 18 months of continuous creditable coverage without any significant breaks;
2. recent coverage was under a group health plan;
3. ineligible for coverage under another group health plan;
4. recent health coverage was not cancelled for committing fraud or not paying premiums;
5. ineligible for Medicare or Medicaid;
6. not offered COBRA, Temporary Continuation of Coverage (TCC), or State continuation coverage, you purchased and exhausted the coverage; and
7. did not accept a conversion policy or a short-term limited duration policy.[4]

Coverage for eligibles is guaranteed regardless of medical history and preexisting condition exemptions cannot be applied.[5]

To meet these federal requirements, states have three options, including making guaranteed issue mandatory for the individual insurance market (e.g., New York), requiring HIPAA-eligibles to purchase specific policies identified by the insurance issuer, or offering coverage through the state's high-risk pool (29 states).[6] Texas chose the third option, to use a high-risk pool model. Accordingly, the Texas Legislature passed HB 710, sponsored by Senator David Sibley and Representative Kip Averitt, during the 75th Texas Legislature (1997). In addition to statutorily identifying THIRP as the method to attain HIPAA compliance, the bill also made improvements to the existing pool, including a dedicated funding mechanism and $500,000 in start-up funds.[7]

THIRP is funded by two sources: premiums paid by program participants and an assessment on health insurance carriers. Table 7.1 shows the amount of funds obtained through both sources over the past four years.

Table 7.1
THIRP Funding Sources

Year	Assessments	Premiums
2001	$26,783,863	$61,881,679
2000	$66,378,938	$38,497,568
1999	$13,830,078	$16,365,666
1998	$10,056,940	$ 4,902,391

Adapted from: Email from Steve Browning, Executive Director, Texas Health Insurance Risk Pool, "RE: One last piece of information," to Jed Perry, April 8, 2002.

Although THIRP was reinvigorated to comply with HIPAA, the pool covers more than just HIPAA-eligibles. The pool provides eligibility to all Texas residents under age 65 who meet one of the following criteria:

1. Notice of rejection or refusal by an insurance company to issue substantially similar individual health insurance due to health reasons;
2. A certification from an agent or salaried representative of an insurance company that states the representative is unable to obtain substantially similar individual health insurance for the person with any state-licensed insurance company, because the person will be declined for a medical condition due to standard underwriting practices;
3. Either an offer (by an insurer or HMO) to issue or an in-force substantially similar individual health insurance policy that excludes a medical condition or conditions;
4. Either an offer (by an insurer or HMO) to issue or an in-force substantially similar individual health insurance policy at a premium rate greater than the current health pool rate;
5. The individual has been diagnosed with one of a number of "Qualifying Medical/Health Conditions;"[8]
6. The individual is not eligible for group insurance either as an employee or as a dependent of an employee.[9]

Under these eligibility requirements there are no restrictions due to ability to pay. All of those who can afford the premium are allowed to purchase a policy from THIRP. With these guidelines, the scope of who is eligible seems to be fairly large.

The first THIRP policies were activated on February 1, 1998.[10] Since that point, the program has seen a steady increase in the number of enrollees, which can be seen in Figure 7.1. In December of 2000, THIRP had 11,783 members, increasing at a rate of approximately 400 members per month.[11] In January 2001, THIRP's enrollment stood at 12,179 and grew to 16,391 by the end of the year. Enrollment was 16,610 as of early January 2002.[12]

Figure 7.1
THIRP Enrollment (1999-2002)

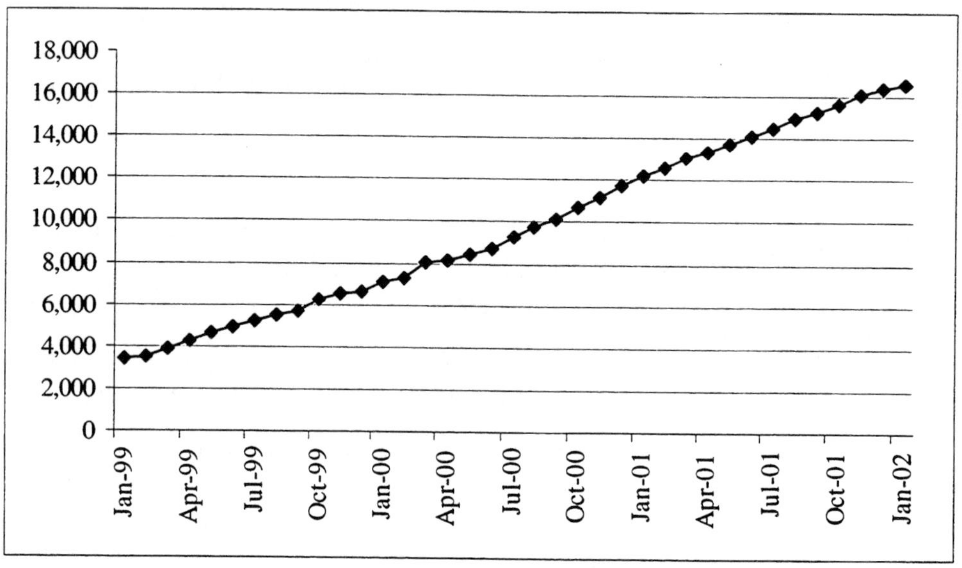

Adapted from: Blue Cross Blue Shield of Texas, "Total Enrollment by Month," *Board of Directors and Committee Meetings—Briefing Book* (Austin, Tex.: Texas Health Insurance Risk Pool, January 2002), p. 2; and Blue Cross Blue Shield of Texas, "Total Enrollment by Month," *Board of Directors and Committee Meetings—Briefing Book* (Austin, Tex.: Texas Health Insurance Risk Pool, January 2001), p. 2.

Unfortunately, not everyone who is eligible is able to participate in THIRP. Though no data is available to indicate specifically how many people are eligible but are not using THIRP, there seems to be an indication that the pool is only serving a fraction of its potential base. Figure 7.2 shows the breakdown of THIRP enrollment by age.

Figure 7.2
THIRP Enrollment by Age

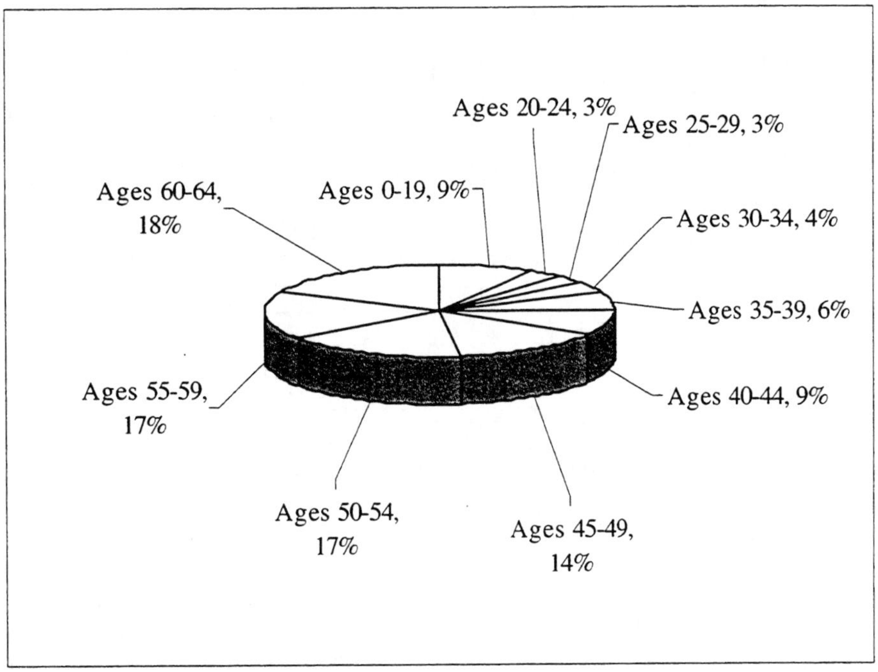

Adapted from: Email from Steve Browning, Executive Director, Texas Health Insurance Risk Pool, "RE: Pool Project," to Jed Perry, January 25, 2002.

Note: Data as of December 12, 2001.

Figure 7.2 indicates that 52 percent of those covered in the pool are over age 50.[13] Generally, it is believed that these older Texans can better afford higher premiums but cannot obtain market insurance because of a preexisting condition. On the other hand, it is believed that many lower-income eligibles do not seek coverage from THIRP due to the above-market premium rates required by statute.[14] Table 7.2 shows the rates for a typical geographic region in Texas under THIRP.[15]

Table 7.2
THIRP Monthly Premiums

	Plan I Monthly Rates ($500 Deductible)		Plan II Monthly Rates ($1000 Deductible)		Plan III Monthly Rates ($2500 Deductible)	
	User Rates		User Rates		User Rates	
Age	**Male**	**Female**	**Male**	**Female**	**Male**	**Female**
0-18	$173	$173	$135	$135	$93	$93
19-24	$200	$263	$153	$199	$106	$138
25-29	$240	$363	$181	$273	$125	$189
30-34	$261	$379	$198	$288	$137	$198
35-39	$295	$404	$224	$307	$154	$212
40-44	$341	$438	$260	$333	$179	$230
45-49	$406	$481	$308	$366	$214	$251
50-54	$502	$546	$381	$416	$262	$287
55-59	$668	$662	$510	$504	$351	$346
60-64	$855	$814	$650	$621	$448	$427

Adapted from: Texas Health Insurance Risk Pool, *Premium Rate Table* (January 1, 2002). Online. Available: http://www.txhealthpool.com/010102%20Rate%20table.pdf. Accessed: March 3, 2002.

Despite creating a method to guarantee access to health insurance to those with preexisting conditions, the state did not guarantee that the prices would necessarily be affordable to all who are eligible. The *statutory* cap on THIRP premiums limit is 200 percent of the "standard" rate. The rate increase in effect for 2002, beginning January 1, took premiums to 180 percent. According to officials at THIRP, the rate table is expected to increase to 200 percent in 2003.[16] Table 7.2 clearly displays the impact of such a high limit on rates for THIRP participants. With rates as high as they are, few lower-income eligible people choose to participate.

According to Table 7.3, premiums have increased as a percentage of the standard insurance rate since the programs inception in 1998. The premium increases have been made to offset the growing cost of providing coverage for risk pool participants.

Table 7.3
THIRP Premium Rate History Summary

Date	Percent of Standard Rate	Rate Change Mechanism
January 1, 1998	137.5%	Pool begins
August 1, 1999	150%	20% flat increase
January 1, 2001	165%	20% average increase to raise standard multiplier to 165%
July 1, 2001	165%	3% average increase to maintain standard multiplier at 165%
January 1, 2002	180%	15% average increase to raise standard multiplier to 180%
January 1, 2003	200%	Anticipated rate increase

Adapted from: Texas Health Insurance Risk Pool, *Board of Directors Summary* (Austin, Tex., January 18, 2002), p. 1.

State-by-State Analysis

If it is going to reach more eligibles through THIRP, the state could consider looking at how other states operate their high-risk pools and apply certain best practices to the program in Texas. The following highlights certain characteristics of THIRP and compares them with high-risk pools in other states. Then, specific best practices are considered for possible application in Texas.

Cost Sharing

Insurance carriers are under increasing pressure to lower their own risk and outlay of funds for medical care. In some states, this requires broad reduction of certain services or more cost sharing. Texas carriers face the same challenges as well, but have more latitude in underwriting to manage their risk. As such, carriers in Texas are increasingly denying individual coverage for preexisting conditions. In some cases, these individuals may be relatively healthy, but have a minor blemish on their medical record and are deemed high-risk. Consequently, they may turn to THIRP for coverage. Unfortunately, many find the premiums offered by THIRP to be far too high and therefore remain uninsured. In these cases, individuals may only be seeking catastrophic coverage and do not necessarily want preventative care. Providing flexibility in deductible and coinsurance rates might reach more of these individuals and persuade them to participate in THIRP.

Texas

THIRP currently offers three coverage plans to participants. The cost-sharing requirements are shown in Table 7.4.[17]

Table 7.4
THIRP Cost Sharing Requirements

Plan Type	Deductible	Coinsurance for PPO Providers	Coinsurance for Non-PPO Providers	Coinsurance Maximum for PPO Providers*
Plan I	$500	20%	40%	$2,000
Plant II	$1,000	20%	40%	$3,000
Plan III	$2,500	20%	40%	$7,500

Adapted from: Texas Health Insurance Risk Pool, *Health Pool Benefits* (January 1, 2002). Online. Available: http://www.txhealthpool.com/benefits.html. Accessed: March 4, 2002.

* There is no coinsurance maximum for non-PPO providers.

Despite the cost-sharing shown above, premiums remain high for THIRP participants.

Other States

Though many states have similar cost-sharing levels as Texas, some have at least one level higher for deductibles (between $5,000 and $10,000). This necessarily reduces premiums for the additional plans. The Louisiana Health Insurance Association reduces premiums by 50 percent for older participants when deductibles are increased from $1,000 to $5,000.[18] In the CoverColorado high-risk pool, a woman age 50-54 years old would face a $565 premium per month with a $500 deductible, but only a $187 premium per month with a $5,000 deductible.[19] Those states that do not have a higher deductible tend to have premiums similar to Texas.

Policy Options and Implications

One of the primary differences for in-network coverage between Plans I, II, and III is the deductible. As the deductible increases, the rates go down, as shown in Table 7.2. Table 7.5 expresses the percent reduction in premiums as the deductibles are increased.

Table 7.5
Percent Reduction in Cost with Higher Deductible

	Percent Cost Reduction (Non-Tobacco User)			
	Plan I to Plan II ($500 to $1,000 Deductible)		Plan II to Plan III ($1,000 to $2,500Deductible)	
Age	**Male**	**Female**	**Male**	**Female**
0-18	21.97%	21.97%	31.11%	31.11%
19-24	23.50%	24.33%	30.72%	30.65%
25-29	24.58%	24.79%	30.94%	30.77%
30-34	24.14%	24.01%	30.81%	31.25%
35-39	24.07%	24.01%	31.25%	30.94%
40-44	23.75%	23.97%	31.15%	30.93%
45-49	24.14%	23.91%	30.52%	31.42%
50-54	24.10%	23.81%	31.23%	31.01%
55-59	23.65%	23.87%	31.18%	31.35%
60-64	23.98%	23.71%	31.08%	31.24%
Average	**23.79%**	**23.84%**	**31.00%**	**31.07%**

Adapted from: Texas Health Insurance Risk Pool, *Premium Rate Table* (January 1, 2002). Online. Available: http://www.txhealthpool.com/010102%20Rate%20table.pdf. Accessed: March 3, 2002.

Table 7.5 shows an average reduction in premiums of approximately 24 percent as the deductible is increased from $500 to $1,000. Table 7.5 further shows an average reduction in premiums of approximately 31 percent as the deductible is increased from $1,000 to $2,500. If 25 percent reductions were taken on Plan III, and then taken again on those results, the following rates displayed in Table 7.6 would occur.

Table 7.6
Premium Rates for Higher Deductibles

	Premiums (Non-Tobacco User)			
	Plan IV ($5,000 Deductible)		**Plan V ($10,000 Deductible)**	
Age	**Male**	**Female**	**Male**	**Female**
0-18	$70	$70	$52	$52
19-24	$104	$104	$60	$78
25-29	$142	$142	$70	$106
30-34	$149	$149	$77	$111
35-39	$159	$159	$87	$119
40-44	$173	$173	$101	$129
45-49	$188	$188	$120	$141
50-54	$215	$215	$147	$161
55-59	$260	$260	$197	$195
60-64	$320	$320	$252	$240

Adapted from: Texas Health Insurance Risk Pool, *Premium Rate Table* (January 1, 2002). Online. Available: http://www.txhealthpool.com/010102%20Rate%20table.pdf. Accessed: March 3, 2002.

These reduced rates could be achieved by increasing the deductible. Possible deductible limits could be $5,000 and $10,000, respectively.

Since the inception of Plan III, there has been a steady migration from the lower deductible plans to the higher deductible plans. As show in Table 7.7, over the course of 2000, Plan I enrollment has dropped 9 percent while Plan III enrollment has increased by 9 percent. This trend seems to support the thesis that even higher deductible plans would be purchased if offered.

Table 7.7
Percent of THIRP Participants by Plan Type

Date	Plan I ($500 Deductible)	Plan II ($1,000 Deductible)	Plan III ($2,500 Deductible)
March 1, 2001	45%	32%	23%
June 1, 2001	43%	32%	25%
September 1, 2001	39%	32%	29%
December 1, 2001	36%	32%	32%

Adapted from: Texas Health Insurance Risk Pool, *Report to Board Members* (Austin, Tex., January 2002), p. 6.

Another option for THIRP to consider is modifying the coinsurance maximums. Currently, Plan I not only has a low deductible, but also a low coinsurance maximum. THIRP could allow more flexibility in the plans by varying coinsurance maximums. In other words, Plan I participants could be given three choices for coinsurance maximums ($2,000/$3,000/$7,500), thereby lowering the premium, while retaining a low deductible.

Managed Care

Like most insurance carriers, high-risk pools may offer various forms of managed care, including HMOs and Preferred Provider Organizations (PPOs). By using managed care mechanisms, pools can impose some control over medical expenditures. Most pools around the country use PPO-based plans, reducing participants' costs for obtaining care through a set network. Few pools use the more restrictive HMO model.

Premiums for all high-risk pools are always higher than average market rates. Consequently, many who participate in high-risk pools have higher incomes. These same people may only see the benefit of participating in a high-risk pool, and spending more money, if they have a less restrictive health plan. This group of high-risk pool eligibles is not necessarily looking for cheaper rates, only the ability to obtain coverage at all.

Lower income individuals eligible for high-risk pools are not likely to have the funds necessary to meet the higher premiums available through most PPO plans. In this case, restrictions in how medical care is accessed are less important than simply obtaining coverage at a reasonable cost. In order to provide coverage for lower-income individuals through high-risk pools, a paradigm shift may be necessary, in which more restrictive plans are considered.

Texas

Texas currently uses a PPO model to provide coverage to pool participants. Pool participants may obtain coverage from any willing provider, but have increased cost sharing if they go outside of the PPO network. There are no additional restrictions made on provision of care.[20]

Other States

As mentioned before, most states utilize indemnity or PPO models for their high-risk pools. The few states that do use HMO models show significant reductions in premiums.

Table 7.8
California Managed Risk Medical Insurance Program Premium Rates: Area 3, Subscriber Only

Age	BC	BS HMO	BS PPO	CC	KPNC
<15	$113.75	$185.00	$174.00	$128.75	$166.11
15-29	$146.25	$185.00	$174.00	$128.75	$212.46
30-34	$177.50	$307.00	$322.00	$168.75	$232.79
35-39	$198.75	$307.00	$322.00	$168.75	$262.09
40-44	$260.00	$386.00	$444.00	$206.25	$267.28
45-49	$295.00	$386.00	$444.00	$206.25	$280.86
50-54	$391.25	$502.00	$597.00	$257.50	$318.66
55-59	$456.25	$502.00	$597.00	$257.50	$399.02
60-64	$456.25	$667.00	$780.00	$332.50	$416.69
65-69	$511.25	$822.00	$961.00	$332.50	$489.68
70-74	$538.75	$990.00	$1,156.00	$332.50	$519.45
>74	$570.00	$1,170.00	$1,368.00	$332.50	$549.23

Source: California Major Risk Medical Insurance Program, *Area 3 Rates*. Online. Available: http://www.mrmib.ca.gov/MRMIB/MRMIP.html. Accessed: March 3, 2002.

Table 7.8 shows the premium rates for California's Major Risk Medical Insurance Program (MRMIB) in Area 3 (Alameda, Contra Costa, Marin, San Francisco, San Mateo, and Santa Clara Counties). Blue Shield (BS) offers an HMO and PPO model, both of which allow significant flexibility for plan participants. BS PPO offers an expansive provider network with very few coverage restrictions. BS HMO utilizes a gatekeeper PCP model, but allows patients to obtain specialist care without referrals for an additional copayment. Blue Cross (BC) uses a broad PPO network and requires higher payment for out-of-network coverage. Kaiser Permanente Northern California (KPNC) uses an HMO model that restricts patients to 15 major medical centers and over 14 outpatient medical offices. Contra Costa Health Plan (CC) also uses an HMO model, but adds further restrictions. Members may only obtain coverage in Contra Costa County and are restricted to the network of providers in the plan.[21] The level of restriction in these plans is reflected in the cost for premiums shown above—the higher the level of restriction, the lower the premium.

Policy Options and Implications

From a technical standpoint, adding more restrictive plans to THIRP would not be difficult. There are no restrictions regarding the use of more restrictive managed care in the Texas Insurance Code, so the only difficulty would be with administration of additional plans. The percent reduction between the most expensive PPO model in Table

7.8 (Blue Shield PPO) and the least expensive HMO (Contra Costa) is expressed in the Table 7.9.

Table 7.9
Rate Reduction with Increased Managed Care Restriction, California MRMIB

Age	Blue Shield PPO	Contra Costa	Percent Reduction
<15	$280.00	$115.00	59%
15-29	$208.00	$115.00	45%
30-34	$283.00	$151.25	47%
35-39	$283.00	$151.25	47%
40-44	$393.00	$185.00	53%
45-49	$393.00	$185.00	53%
50-54	$528.00	$231.25	56%
55-59	$528.00	$231.25	56%
60-64	$689.00	$298.75	57%

Adapted from: California Major Risk Medical Insurance Program, *Area 3 Rates*. Online. Available: http://www.mrmib.ca.gov/MRMIB/MRMIP.html. Accessed: March 3, 2002.

Table 7.10 depicts the resulting premiums if similar percent reductions were taken from the rates set in THIRP's Plan I for a non-tobacco using male.

Table 7.10
Effects of Managed Care on THIRP Premiums

Age	THIRP Plan I	THIRP HMO
30-34	$261.00	$139.49
35-39	$295.00	$157.66
40-44	$341.00	$160.52
45-49	$406.00	$191.12
50-54	$502.00	$219.86
55-59	$668.00	$292.57
60-64	$855.00	$370.73

Adapted from: California Major Risk Medical Insurance Program, *Area 3 Rates*. Online. Available: http://www.mrmib.ca.gov/MRMIB/MRMIP.html. Accessed: March 3, 2002; and Texas Health Insurance Risk Pool, *Premium Rate Table* (January 1, 2002). Online. Available: http://www.txhealthpool.com/010102%20Rate%20table.pdf. Accessed: March 3, 2002.

If similar reductions could be made by introducing stricter managed care practices THIRP could reach-out to a much greater percentage of those who are eligible.

Subsidies

For many of those who are eligible to participate in high-risk pools, the premium is simply too high, regardless of any modifications to the benefits structure or cost sharing. In these cases, only direct financial assistance will give these individuals the means to participate. Some high-risk pools around the country have addressed this problem by using subsidies.

Texas

Other than limiting the cost of coverage, Texas does not currently offer further subsidies to THIRP participants, providing no additional funds for those with lower income. Participants must pay the entire premium. The only "subsidy" is the loss covered by the assessment to carriers. However, THIRP premiums are lower for enrollees who do not use tobacco products.

Other States

Seven states currently offer subsidies for low-income high-risk pool participants.

1. Colorado: 20 percent subsidies are offered to pool participants who live outside of the Denver-Boulder area and have annual incomes less than $30,000.
2. Connecticut: The annual deductibles for enrollees below 200 percent FPL are reduced from $500 to $200. After the enrollee reaches the deductible, the plan

pays providers 75 percent of the Medicare reimbursement level, which they must accept as payment in full.

3. Louisiana: Discounted rates are available to persons who have not smoked cigarettes, cigars, pipe, or utilized other tobacco products in the last year.
4. New Mexico: Enrollees below 200 percent FPL are eligible for as much as a 25 percent premium subsidy.
5. Oregon: The state's Family Health Insurance Assistance Program (FHIAP) provides a subsidy to people with incomes of up to 170 percent FPL. The subsidy pays 70-90 percent of premiums for individuals who have been uninsured for six months or who are leaving Medicaid. As of June 1999, FHIAP subsidized one-fourth of the pool's members.
6. Washington: Washington has special discounts to enrollees ages 50-64 below 300 percent FPL and those in the Washington State Health Insurance Program for more than three years.
7. Wisconsin: The Wisconsin Health Insurance Risk Sharing Plan's (HIRSP) Premium and Deductible Plan offers an income-related premium and deductible to enrollees with annual household incomes of less than $25,000. Subsidy recipients receive a 20-35 percent premium reduction and lower deductibles. The subsidy program is financed with a state appropriation, periodic assessments of health insurers, and adjustments to provider payments, but is subject to the availability of HIRSP funds.[22]

Tennessee also offers assistance to high-risk pool participants. However, the state's high-risk pool is embedded within TennCare, a program that collapses multiple sources of funding, including Medicaid and SCHIP. Therefore, it is difficult to determine how and from what revenue source the subsidy is being paid for high-risk pool participants.

The State of New York does not use a high-risk pool because there is guaranteed issue for both the individual and group markets. However, the state has developed a program called Healthy NY to provide reinsurance to small employer and individual policies for coverage between $30,000 and $100,000 (the state pays 90 percent of costs within this range). This has brought down rates by roughly 10-15 percent. In this program, the state pays for the program through general revenue.[23] However, it may be possible to use a high-risk pool as a reinsurer for those who cannot afford normal premiums on the individual market. In effect, carriers would be responsible for expenses up to $30,000 and then the high-risk pool would assume responsibility up to $100,000. In order to work, such a system would have to be necessarily cheaper than simply having the individual use the high-risk pool.

Policy Options and Implications

Because funds are limited, a standard by which to determine how much of a subsidy is necessary could be helpful. One standard would be to limit participant premium contributions to a certain percentage of their income and then subsidize the remaining portion.

Table 7.11 shows the total number of uninsured parents by percent of the federal poverty level. In this case, the income range associated with the percent of the federal poverty level depicted is based on a family of four (used here for purposes of analysis). The table further shows both 5 and 10 percent of the income range, broken down into a monthly figure. The difference between these numbers and the premiums currently offered for THIRP plans indicates the amount of money necessary for a subsidy. This does not necessarily mean that 5 or 10 percent of income should be the basis for subsidy determination; other thresholds could certainly be used.

Table 7.11
Total Number of Uninsured Parents by Income in Texas

Percent of Federal Poverty Level	Income Range	Number of Uninsured	5% of Income (Monthly)	10% of Income (Monthly)
Less than 50%	Less than $9,050	74,299	$37.71	$75.42
50-99%	$9,050-$17,919	211,814	$37.71 - $74.66	$75.42 - $149.33
100-149%	$18,100-$26,969	185,862	$75.42 - $112.37	$150.83 - $224.74
150-199%	$27,150-$36,019	152,252	$113.13 - $150.08	$226.25 - $300.16
200-249%	$36,200-$45,069	120,925	$150.83 - $187.79	$301.67 - $375.58
250% or higher	$45,250 or higher	135,381	$188.54	$377.08

Adapted from: U.S. Department of Labor, Bureau of Labor Statistics, *1999 March Current Population Survey*. Online. Available: http://www.bls.census.gov/cps/cpsmain.htm. Accessed: April 8, 2002; U.S. Department of Labor, Bureau of Labor Statistics, *2000 March Current Population Survey*. Online. Available: http://www.bls.census.gov/cps/cpsmain.htm. Accessed: April 8, 2002; and U.S. Department of Labor, Bureau of Labor Statistics, *2001 March Current Population Survey*. Online. Available: http://www.bls.census.gov/cps/cpsmain.htm. Accessed: April 8, 2002.

Table 7.12 uses the same subsidy methodology for childless adults.

Table 7.12
Total Number of Uninsured Childless Adults by Income in Texas

Percent of Federal Poverty Level	Income Range	Number of Uninsured	5% of Income	10% of Income
Less than 50%	Less than $4,430	243,428	$18.46	$36.92
50-99%	$4,430-$8,771	224,736	$18.46-$ 36.55	$36.92-$73.10
100-149%	$8,860-$13,201	322,016	$36.92-$ 55.01	$73.83-$110.01
150-199%	$13,290-$17,631	268,065	$55.38-$ 73.46	$110.75-$146.93
200-249%	$17,720-$22,061	262,369	$73.83-$ 91.92	$147.67-$183.85
250% or higher	$22,150 or higher	853,707	$92.29	$184.58

Adapted from: U.S. Department of Labor, Bureau of Labor Statistics, *1999 March Current Population Survey*. Online. Available: http://www.bls.census.gov/cps/cpsmain.htm. Accessed: April 8, 2002; U.S. Department of Labor, Bureau of Labor Statistics, *2000 March Current Population Survey*. Online. Available: http://www.bls.census.gov/cps/cpsmain.htm. Accessed: April 8, 2002; and U.S. Department of Labor, Bureau of Labor Statistics, *2001 March Current Population Survey*. Online. Available: http://www.bls.census.gov/cps/cpsmain.htm. Accessed: April 8, 2002.

In light of the fiscal constraints the state currently faces, use of a subsidy could be very difficult to enact. If additional funding was made available, a subsidy might be possible. However, assessing how much the subsidy would be and to whom the subsidy would be given make the option difficult. Texas could simply lower the limit on premiums from the current 200 percent of the base market rate to a lower rate (such as 150 percent). In effect, this would be a universal subsidy for the entire pool. It, too, would require additional funds to make up the increased loss.

Small Employer Buy-In

High-risk pools were designed for the purpose of providing health insurance coverage to those who are unable to obtain coverage because they have been deemed a significant health risk by health insurance carriers. Pools were not intended for use by employers. However, many small employers face significant premium increases when only one employee develops a serious medical condition or a new employee with a preexisting condition is hired. These increases can often mean the end of the small employer providing health insurance benefits to employees because they cannot legally offer health insurance to some employees and not others. It is these situations that have brought some to suggest that high-risk pools be used to provide some sort of coverage for the high-risk employees of small businesses.

Texas

When small employer health insurance carriers begin providing service in Texas, they must notify the Texas Department of Insurance (TDI) whether they will be a "risk-assuming" carrier or a "reinsured" carrier. If they are risk assuming, they must bear all risk of those they enroll. A carrier that elects to be reinsured typically pays for a reinsurance carrier to assume coverage for high risk individuals or groups. One method of reinsurance available to reinsured carriers is through the Texas Health Reinsurance System.

The Texas Health Reinsurance System is a non-profit entity designed to provide reinsurance for reinsured small market carriers. When insuring a new group, carriers may elect to have individual employees or an entire group covered by the system to mitigate perceived risk. Carriers may also reinsure any new, high risk employees that join the group.

Participating carriers must pay premiums for each life reinsured through the system. Base premium rates are determined by the system's board and then increased based on the risk of the individual or group. Premiums for groups may not exceed 1.5 times the base rate. Premiums for individuals may be as high as five times the base rate. Participating carriers are also assessed a fee to cover the system's annual loss (this assessment is similar to the one used by THIRP).

As of March 2002, the Texas Health Reinsurance System serves approximately 54 small employer health insurance carriers.[24] Reinsurance rates vary based on age, coinsurance amount, gender, and deductible level.[25]

Other States

In its original design (pre-HIPAA), the New Mexico's high-risk pool, the Comprehensive Health Insurance Pool (NMCHIP), allowed employees of companies that offer health insurance benefits to participate. The eligibility criteria for NMCHIP include the following two items: the individual's insurance premium is, or will be, higher than their NMCHIP premium rate for a policy with a $500 deductible; and the individual's coverage is being substantially reduced or limited to exclude or reduce benefits for a specific health condition.[26] Under this scenario, employers could essentially carve-out high risk individuals to NMCHIP as long as they made the same monetary contribution as that provided to employees remaining on the company's plan.[27]

Since implementation of HIPAA, the practice of allowing small employers to "buy into" NMCHIP has been significantly reduced. According to NMCHIP officials, the Centers for Medicare and Medicaid Services (CMS) currently allows companies that have never provided health insurance to carve-out high risk employees to the risk pool. However, the practice is rare.[28]

Policy Options and Implications

At this point, the apparent limitations posed by HIPAA, in which employers must provide equal coverage to all employees if they provide health insurance benefits, make replication of New Mexico's buy-in in Texas highly unlikely. However, if HIPAA was amended at the federal level to allow a carve-out of high risk employees to state high risk pools, Texas might be able to utilize this modification. The main difficulty would be insuring that adverse selection was not occurring and that carriers did not rate more employees as risky to carve them out to THIRP. In addition, it remains to be seen whether the change would encourage more small employers to purchase health insurance or simply encourage employers already offering coverage to carve-out their high risk employees.

If such a change to federal statute were made and Texas allowed the practice of employer buy-in to occur, use of the Texas Health Reinsurance System would likely decrease substantially because the rates in THIRP would be much better than the system. Therefore, it would be necessary to assess small employer carriers for THIRP.

Financing

For the most part, any enhancements to THIRP to encourage and enable more low-income eligibles to join the pool would require an increase in funds. Without additional funds, THIRP will be forced to impose higher assessments on carriers who may feel compelled to leave the Texas insurance market completely as a result.

Texas

THIRP is currently financed through premiums from plan participants. Losses are made up through regular and interim assessments on participating carriers. Each year, actuaries (currently Milliman USA) perform an analysis to predict the net loss for THIRP in the upcoming year. THIRP then assesses carriers a percentage of that net loss based on their relative market share. At the end of the year, THIRP determines the actual net loss for the year and recomputes the assessment to carriers. If the original assessment was too high, the overpayment is credited to the carrier's payment for the following year. If the initial assessment is not enough, the carrier will be assessed further.[29]

Texas currently faces several hurdles when assessing carriers. First, carriers are allowed to make exemptions to their market share from 16 categories, including Medicare, Medicaid, and dental. One of the biggest exemptions is all small employer market insurance. This exemption alone results in a significant loss of funds from which assessments could be based ($2.38 billion for 2001).[30] Appendix H shows the amount of money exempted for each category and the total assessment for 1998-2000.

Other High-Risk Pools

The majority of high-risk pools around the country finance their pools with a similar assessment mechanism as Texas. Determination of the assessment amount does vary from state to state, however. Many assess carriers based on their market share. Other states assess carriers, but use alternative mechanisms for determination of share, including premium value and the number of individuals insured. States also include varying groups of carriers to which assessments can be applied. In some states, all carriers are assessed regardless of whether they participate in the high-risk pool. States may broaden the definition of "carrier" to include HMOs, Multiple Employer Welfare

Associations (MEWAs), and prepaid health clinics. Accident insurance carriers may be assessed in some states as well. Many states that require assessments allow carriers to deduct a portion or all of the assessment from their premium taxes.[31]

High-risk pools may also acquire revenue from sources other than carriers. Some simply receive state general revenue funds from annual appropriations. Generally, these high-risk pools are limited in size and scope. Other states use specific taxes as funding sources, such as hospital and provider taxes. Finally, some states use money derived from tobacco as a source of revenue. In California, the Major Risk Medical Insurance Program receives money from a tax on tobacco and cigarettes. Other states use funds from the recent tobacco settlements.[32] The State of Minnesota recently allotted the Minnesota Comprehensive Health Association $70 million of the state's tobacco settlement.

Policy Options and Implications

Texas could eliminate the exemption for small market carriers to increase the assessment base. For the year 2000, this would add $2.4 billion to the Net Assessable Health Insurance Premiums for THIRP (See Appendix H). However, it remains unclear what sort of financial impact that would have on the small market. Many small employers already face difficulties affording health insurance on the small market. If the small market assessment were passed on to small employers through additional premiums, the result might be a net loss. THIRP might be able to cover a few more individuals, but a larger number of employees may lose coverage in the process as employers drop health insurance benefits.

ERISA and the High-Risk Pool

As mentioned previously, THIRP currently assesses insurance carriers in the state for the pool's annual loss. Exempt from assessment are companies that self-insure – assuming the risk of their employee's health benefits and not purchasing insurance through an outside carrier.

Companies that self-insure are exempt because of the federal Employee Retirement Income Security Act (ERISA). ERISA is the main federal law regarding employee pensions. However, the law also applies to employee welfare benefit programs, including health care. Specifically, the law asserts that states may not directly regulate employer-sponsored health insurance plans. States are able to regulate the insurance carriers and HMOs that provide insurance services to employers, but are limited if the employer continues to bear risk. Therefore, states may not directly impose restrictions, such as an assessment for the high-risk pool, on employers with regard to health benefits.[33]

Initially after passage of ERISA, courts narrowly defined ERISA denying states the ability to even impose indirect action, such as provider taxes, on self-insured plans. However, in 1997 the Supreme Court ruled in the De Buono case that New York State had the authority to tax health care providers, even those serving self-insured health plans.[34]

When ERISA preemption is used to challenge a state law, the courts ask two questions:

1. Does the state law "relate to" an ERISA plan: direct regulation; regulation of the same areas as ERISA; regulation of plan benefits, structure, or administration; or imposition of substantial costs?
2. Is the preemption waived because the law regulates insurance?

As a result, any attempt to impose an assessment on self-insured plans must be able to account of these two questions.[35]

State Case Studies

Several states currently use methods to obtain revenue for their high-risk pool that indirectly capture funds from self-insured, ERISA plans.

Minnesota currently funds its high-risk pool, the Minnesota Comprehensive Health Association (MCHA), through assessments on carriers, similar to Texas. However, in 1997, the Minnesota Legislature began to augment MCHA with funds from the Health Care Access Fund. The fund, primarily used to pay for the state's MinnesotaCare program, derives revenue from the following two sources:

- Provider Tax: The state imposes a 1.5 percent tax on the gross revenues from patient services provided by health care providers and hospitals. The tax also applies to wholesale drug distributors' sales of prescription drugs.
- Gross Premiums Tax: The state imposes a one percent tax on premiums received by nonprofit health plans, HMOs, and ISNs. However, this tax was not collected in 2001 due to surplus in the Health Care Access Fund.

Minnesota also collects taxes on other providers, but uses the revenue for the general fund. These taxes include a hospital surcharge of 1.56 percent on the net patient revenues of each Minnesota hospital and a nursing home surcharge requiring each nursing home in Minnesota to pay an annual tax of $625 per licensed bed.[36]

Louisiana funds its high-risk pool, the Louisiana Health Plan (LHP), primarily with two types of provider taxes: a $2 charge to hospital patients admitted for any other treatment besides psychiatric care or alcohol/substance abuse for every day they are confined to inpatient care, and a $1 charge to patients admitted to an ambulatory surgical center or to a hospital for outpatient ambulatory surgical care for each admission to that facility. Public program participants and those covered by the State Employees Group Benefit Program do not have to pay either tax. Both taxes are passed onto the patient's payor, even if that payor is a self-insured plan.[37] Any additional loss to LHP is made-up with assessments on health insurance carriers.[38]

Other states use taxes to secure revenue from self-insured plans, but use the money for uncompensated care. These states include Connecticut, Massachusetts, and New York.

Some self-insured plans purchase stop-loss insurance to cover losses that exceed a certain threshold. This enables companies to prevent high-end medical costs that could severely impact the pool. Oregon currently assesses stop-loss carriers in addition to regular commercial insurance carriers to pay for the state's high-risk pool (the Oregon Medical Insurance Pool). In effect, Oregon is able to partially assess some self-insured plans with this mechanism.

Oregon's system of assessing insurance carriers for pool revenue is based on the number of insured individuals. Carriers pay a portion of the pool's loss in proportion to the percent of lives covered. Reinsurance companies are assessed on a per person basis, as well. However, reinsurers are allowed to exclude individuals who have already counted for the primary insurer.[39] This would still mean that reinsurers are assessed for employees of self-insured companies trying to supplement risk.

Policy Options and Implications

The following show the impact in Texas of revenue raising options similar to those listed in state analysis detailed above.

- Physician visit fee: In 2000, the total number of physician visits in Texas was 121,842,054.[40] Therefore a $1 fee per visit could generate about $121,842,054.
- Hospital surcharge: In 1999, Texas hospitals generated $45,029,548,352 from inpatient and outpatient care.[41] A 1.5 percent surcharge on those revenues (similar to Minnesota's tax) would result in $675,443,225.
- Outpatient Admit Fee: In 1999, Texas hospitals made 26,957,113 outpatient admissions.[42] If Texas used a $1 admit fee (similar to Louisiana's ambulatory surgery fee), an estimated $26,957,113 could be generated.

This information provides only a small glimpse into the revenue-generating capacity of alternative taxes and assessments. If these or other such mechanisms were used to fund THIRP, the ERISA exemption problem could be circumvented and the program could greatly enhance its ability to serve more enrollees.

Conclusion

The Texas Health Insurance Risk Pool is a valuable mechanism for reaching those who are unable to obtain individual health insurance on the open market. However, the potential of THIRP as a means to reduce the number of uninsured in Texas has yet to be realized. With further innovations the pool could provide coverage to many more people and ensure that the spirit of HIPAA is met.

Notes

[1] Institute for Health Care Research and Policy, Georgetown University, "Chapter 3. Your Protections When Buying Health Insurance." *A Consumer's Guide to Getting and Keeping Health Insurance in Texas.* Online. Available: http://www.healthinsuranceinfo.net/tx03.html. Accessed: March 3, 2002.

[2] Ibid.

[3] Texas Senate Research Center, *HB 710, Bill Analysis*, 75th Legislative Session. Texas State Legislature. March 19, 1997. Online. Available: http://www.capitol.state.tx.us/cgi-bin/tlo/textframe.cmd?LEG=75&SESS=R&CHAMBER=H&BILLTYPE=B&BILLSUFFIX=00710&VERSION=4&TYPE=A. Accessed: April 28, 2002

[4] Health Care Financing Administration, *HIPAA Online: What is guaranteed availability of individual coverage?* Online. Available: http://www.hcfa.gov/medicaid//hipaa/online/230021.asp. Accessed: December 5, 2001.

[5] Ibid.

[6] Ibid .

[7] *Texas House Bill 710, Bill Analysis*, 75th Legislative, regular session (1997).

[8] Texas Health Insurance Risk Pool, *Health Pool Eligibility.* Online. Available: http://www.txhealthpool.com/eligibil.html. Accessed: March 3, 2002.

[9] Texas Insurance Code Annotated, ch. 3, art. 3.77.

[10] Texas Health Insurance Risk Pool, *Frequently Asked Questions.* Online. Available: http://www.txhealthpool.com/faq.html. Accessed: March 3, 2002.

[11] Texas Health Insurance Risk Pool, *The 2000 Annual Report of the Texas Health Insurance Risk Pool* (Austin, Tex., June 1, 2001), p. 3.

[12] E-mail from Steve Browning, Executive Director, Texas Health Insurance Risk Pool, "Texas Health Reinsurance System," to Jed Perry, January 25, 2002.

[13] Texas Health Insurance Risk Pool, *The 2000 Annual Report of the Texas Health Insurance Risk Pool,* p. 5.

[14] Interview by Jed Perry with Steve Browning, Executive Director, Texas Health Insurance Risk Pool, Austin, Texas, November 15, 2001.

[15] Texas Health Insurance Risk Pool, *Premium Rates For Health Pool Coverage.* Online. Available: http://www.txhealthpool.com/rates.html#Tables. Accessed: March 3, 2002.

[16] Browning email, January 25, 2002.

[17] Texas Health Insurance Risk Pool, *Premium Rate Table*, (January 1, 2002). Online. Available: http://www.txhealthpool.com/010102%20Rate%20table.pdf. Accessed: March 3, 2002.

[18] Louisiana Health Plan, *High Risk Health Pool Rates Table.* Online. Available: http://www.lahealthplan.org. Accessed: March 3, 2002.

[19] CoverColorado, *PPO Rate Bulletin.* Online. Available: http://www.cuhip.com/main/index.html. Accessed: March 3, 2002.

[20] Texas Health Insurance Risk Pool, *Health Pool Benefits.* Online. Available: http://www.txhealthpool.com/benefits.html. Accessed: March 3, 2002.

[21] Major Risk Medical Insurance Program, *Description of Plans and Benefit Highlights.* Online. Available: http://www.mrmib.ca.gov/MRMIB/MRMIP.html. Accessed: March 3, 2002.

[22] Lori Achman and Deborah Chollet, "Insuring the Uninsurable: An Overview of State High-Risk Health Insurance Pools" (New York, NY: The Commonwealth Fund, August 2001), pp. 11-12. Online. Available: http://www.cmwf.org/programs/insurance/achman_uninsurable_472.pdf. Accessed: March 3, 2002.

[23] Interview by Jed Perry with Terri Marchon, Public Affairs Associate, New York Department of Insurance, New York, NY, October 9, 2001.

[24] E-mail from Archie Clayton, Texas Department of Insurance, "Texas Health Reinsurance System," to Jed Perry, March 8, 2002.

[25] Memoranda from Pool Administrators Inc., "Reinsurance Rates Effective August 1, 2001," to All Reinsuring Carriers in Texas, *Texas Health Reinsurance System*, July 27, 2001.

[26] New Mexico Comprehensive Health Insurance Pool, *New Mexico Comprehensive Health Insurance Pool.* Online. Available: http://www.aidsinfonet.org/322-chip.html#anchor21641. Accessed: March 3, 2002.

[27] Ibid.

[28] Telephone interview by Jed Perry with Patty Jennings, Chair, New Mexico Comprehensive Health Insurance Pool, Roswell, New Mexico, March 1, 2002.

[29] Browning interview.

[30] Steven Browning, "Health Insurance Premiums Reporting Form: Amounts Reported for Health Insurance Premiums for Texas Residents," *Board of Director and Committee Meetings—Briefing Book* (Austin, Tex.: Texas Health Insurance Risk Pool, July 2001), p. 89

[31] State Coverage Initiatives, *State-Only High-Risk Pool.* Online. Available: http://www.statecoverage.net/highrisk.htm. Accessed: March 3, 2002.

[32] Ibid.

[33] Patricia A. Butler, *ERISA and State Health Care Access Initiatives Opportunities and Obstacles* (New York, N.Y.: The Commonwealth Fund, October 2000), p. 2. Online. Available: http://www.cmwf.org/programs/insurance/butler_erisa_411.pdf. Accessed: March 3, 2002.

[34] Ibid.

[35] Ibid.

[36] Minnesota Department of Revenue, *Tax Reform Assessment Phase Health Care Tax Background.* Online. Available: http://www.taxes.state.mn.us/reform/stdygr/healbkgnd.html. Accessed: January 27, 2002.

[37] Louisiana Revised Statutes, Title 22. Insurance, Chapter 1. Insurance Code. Part VI-A. Louisiana Health Plan. La. R.S. 22:239 (2001), § 239 "Service charges."

[38] Louisiana Revised Statutes, Title 22. Insurance, Chapter 1. Insurance Code. Part VI-A. Louisiana Health Plan. La. La. R.S. 22:239.1 (2001). 239.1 "Fees assessed to participating health insurers for plan losses attributable to federally defined eligible individuals."

[39] Oregon Revised Statutes. Title 56. Insurance. Chapter 735. Alternative Insurance. Medical Insurance Pool. ORS § 735.614 (1999). "Assessments for expenses of pool."

[40] American Medical Association, *Physician Socioeconomic Statistics* (Chicago, IL, Center for Health Policy Research, 2000-2002), p. 49.; and Texas State Board of Medical Examiners, *Physicians In and Out of State.* Online. Available: http://www.tsbme.state.tx.us/demo/docs/d2002/0102/inout.htm. Accessed: February 22, 2002.

[41] Texas Department of Health, *Hospital Survey Data on Diskette* (Austin, Tex.: Office Of Health Information and Analysis, 1999) (database on disk).

[42] Ibid.

Chapter 8. Education Needs and Health Insurance Options: Critical Gaps and Potential Solutions for Texas

by Scott Atnip, Karla Buitrago, Kristen Lindberg, and Dan Starr

Introduction

In Texas, a large number of individuals lack health insurance, and a considerable number of businesses, many with fewer than 50 employees, do not have a company insurance plan. One key underlying cause is lack of awareness among businesses and consumers of the options available to them, and the costs and benefits of these changes. As the Texas Department of Insurance (TDI) State Planning Grant (SPG) Interim Report states, "many of the uninsured do not understand how health insurance works, how to shop for coverage or how to use it."[1] Participants in recent focus group interviews provided several reasons for the large number of Texans without health insurance, as well as common questions and concerns raised by the uninsured, and potential means by which they can learn more about different health insurance options. Participants represented three uninsured populations: employed individuals, unemployed individuals, and small employers.[2, 3] In the public sector, this population consists of a large number of children from low-income families potentially eligible for Medicaid or SCHIP, but not enrolled. The private insurance market is comprised of three separate groups: self-employed individuals and company employees without an employer-sponsored insurance plan, small business owners and employees, and larger employers. In Texas, small employers are defined as having two to 50 eligible employees and larger employers are defined as having 50 or more eligible employees. A significant percentage of the population in both sectors is Hispanic.

Based on the information gathered from the focus groups, the primary reason for so many individuals being uninsured in Texas is the costs of insurance: premiums, co-pays, deductibles, and other necessities. Other factors are employment and economic conditions, provider issues, limited consumer knowledge about health insurance, and factors unique to Texas, such as the high migrant worker population. There are also factors unique to small employers, such as the composition of groups, individual underwriting requirements, limited knowledge of available options, and the difficulty of purchasing health insurance. Group participants raised questions and concerns over issues such as coverage, policies and procedures, ensuring consumer satisfaction, and options for small employers.[4]

In addition, overcoming language barriers is extremely important. Many consumers who do not speak English are either unaware of their insurance options or have great difficulty applying for and enrolling in insurance programs. Uninsured levels are higher among Hispanics than the overall population, and although English is the primary language for a significant percentage of Hispanics in Texas, most Hispanic firms that market health insurance do so only in Spanish.[5]

In light of these issues, significant efforts to assuage consumer fears and misconceptions about health insurance will be needed in order to insure many within the target populations. Widespread availability of assistance with application, enrollment, and renewal will also be needed given the fact that many consumers struggle with complexities in the insurance system. The focus groups identified several ways to educate consumers on health insurance. These include establishing a central access point, such as an insurance hotline; providing information for small employers, possibly through a training or Ombudsman program; releasing published information such as a glossary of insurance terms and materials in Spanish; involving significant personal contact in outreach efforts; holding public meetings and special events; and mass distribution of program materials.[6]

Methods such as these may help to enroll many Medicaid- or SCHIP-eligible families who are unaware of the low premium, co-pay and deductible costs (if any), or that they actually qualify. Even so, an enrollment cap and waiting list may soon have to be implemented for SCHIP, which will present a potential ceiling on how far public sector education efforts can go in reducing the uninsured. In addition, large employers are most often able to purchase a group insurance plan fairly easily. Education, therefore, is needed most among the individual private insurance market and small businesses. A PPRI telephone survey of non-poor uninsured indicated that most individuals who did not accept insurance coverage from their employer did so because they felt the costs were too high, that they did not need the insurance, or they did not like the offered plan.[7] Small businesses make up the largest portion of the uninsured in the private sector, and 97 percent of the survey respondents agreed with the statement, "health insurance plans for small employers should be revised to make coverage more affordable."[8]

Efforts are already underway in both the public and private sectors to increase the distribution of simpler and bilingual program materials, to increase the opportunities for face-to-face interaction with uninsured consumers, to inform them of program policies and benefits, and to help them with the application process. In addition, several recently enacted laws have facilitated application to public programs and provided for more thorough family education upon enrollment, and have also improved coverage opportunities and availability for small businesses.

This report focuses on means of educating uninsured consumers and businesses on the availability and benefits of health insurance in Texas. The first section begins by describing the current outreach efforts for the Medicaid and SCHIP programs from the perspectives of key state agencies and community-based organizations (CBOs), the TexCare Partnership (TCP) strategic plan for the 2002-2003 biennium, and public insurance program outreach in other states that could serve as models for enhancing education in Texas. The second section provides an overview of the private insurance market, and the third section emphasizes the roles played by the Texas Department of Insurance, the Office of Public Insurance Counsel (OPIC), and the Texas Health Care

Information Council (THCIC), as well as past and current education efforts by these agencies. The fourth section provides comparisons with commercial insurance markets and education programs in other states and presents an overview of the national development of ombudsman programs. The final section presents policy options for improving education efforts in both the public and private sectors.

Public Sector Research and Findings

Current Outreach and Education Efforts: SCHIP and Medicaid

State Activity

Since the implementation of SCHIP in April 2000 in Texas, much has been done to make uninsured Texans aware of the benefits, and to assist them in the application and enrollment process. The primary focus of outreach efforts to date has been getting more eligible children enrolled and assisting families with the renewal. The passage of Senate Bill 43 of the 77th Texas Legislature simplified the Medicaid application (integrating it more closely with SCHIP) and mandated education to Medicaid families to increase their understanding of the program and help address the problem of losing coverage due to missed renewal deadlines.

At the state level, the TexCare Partnership has coordinated numerous initiatives and media campaigns through state agencies, community organizations, radio and television stations, and printed advertisements to promote SCHIP since September 2000. Current ongoing efforts include distribution of TexCare Partnership (TCP) informational inserts through mailings and staff networking at the Attorney General's Office and the Department of Public Safety, and through corporate sponsorship alliances and endorsements. Sponsors, which have included HEB, Randall's, Diamond Shamrock, and Reliant Energy, have significantly increased awareness by providing added campaign visibility.[9] TCP posters and brochures, printed in English and Spanish, emphasize the message that health insurance is available to families for $18 per month or less. The TCP telephone number and website address are clearly visible, as is a listing of the key services covered. Photos of children usually include at least one in a wheelchair or using special equipment, to illustrate that services for children with special needs are very much a part of both Medicaid and SCHIP. This strategy has proved highly successful, as indicated by SCHIP enrollment exceeding the TexCare Partnership's established goal for 2001 by 17 percent.

The TexCare Partnership has made a special effort to reach out to schools. Since 1999, TexCare Partnership flyers have been included in Free and Reduced School Lunch Program packets in all school districts in Texas. In 2001, the flyers included one parent's story of a positive experience with TCP. The Texas Education Agency (TEA) collected information on school districts to determine which areas had the greatest proportion of students eligible for free and subsidized lunches, and passed this information to CBOs, which used it to target schools with high numbers of potentially Medicaid- or SCHIP-eligible children. TEA also encouraged every school superintendent to distribute TCP information.[10]

The TexCare Partnership has been heavily advertised by the Health and Human Services Commission (HHSC) through multiple media avenues, including television, radio and transit billboards during the four-week back-to-school campaign in each of the last two years. The 12 major media markets in Texas cover 147 of the 254 counties. Back-to-School campaigns integrating statewide media marketing with local grassroots outreach are planned for August and September 2002. In addition, information and applications were mailed to school nurses and health coordinators. A cover poster urges them to contact the nearest CBO to help them provide information and assistance to families.[11] One standing objective for school outreach is that school health personnel become TCP community partners.

The TexCare Partnership has made extensive use of the media in promoting Medicaid and SCHIP. In addition to purchasing radio and television ads, TexCare Partnership information has been displayed on transit ads, billboards, ethnic community print, and media tours in which state staff speak to newspaper staff about their positive experience with the TexCare Partnership. The goal behind all media marketing is to increase the name recognition of TCP; to promote the message that through TCP, families can afford to keep their children healthy and protected in the event of illness. This is particularly emphasized in the Children's Health Minute, a series of one-minute radio spots covering issues of illness and safe activities, taped in both English and Spanish. The message of the Children's Health Minute is specifically associated with TCP. Community grassroots efforts are centered around a trusted member of the local community carrying the TCP message, in an effort to win the trust of other community members.[12]

Statewide Medicaid outreach efforts have been carried out through Project Alberto, the Texas state program under the national Covering Kids Initiative, a market advertising campaign for children's health insurance which targets eligible uninsured families, with special emphasis on Hispanics and African-Americans. Project Alberto, which began in 1999 with a $1 million federal grant, developed community-based outreach programs to increase knowledge and understanding of the Medicaid programs, and to provide assistance with the application process.[13] The Texas Association of Community Health Centers coordinates these programs, and has also held application workshops and outreach conferences to provide information on public insurance programs throughout the state. Materials provided include a Medicaid brochure, general contact information, and verification checklists, and are available in both English and Spanish.[14] The TexCare Partnership has also posted similar outreach materials on its website.

Senate Bill 43, approved by the 77th Texas Legislature in 2001, was implemented into Texas Department of Health (TDH) policy on January 20, 2002. It provides for the simplification of Medicaid by creating a joint TCP application for Medicaid or SCHIP, adding new DHS rules to help prevent lapses in coverage due to missed renewal or for families transitioning from one program to the other, and requiring parents of Medicaid-enrolled children to complete a Health Care Orientation to educate them on Medicaid benefits and procedures.[15] The TexCare Partnership now uses a uniform application, printed in both English and Spanish, to enroll applicants in either Medicaid or SCHIP, depending on eligibility. The front pages of the application booklet carry the same information as TCP posters and brochures. Assets questions are now included and no longer represent an additional step in the application process. In addition, TCP offers assistance in applying for Social Security numbers as needed. Almost a quarter of all TexCare Partnership applicants to date failed to provide a Social Security number, a crucial means of identification.[16] New Department of Human Services (DHS) policies increase "seamlessness" between Medicaid and SCHIP, and facilitate enrollment and re-enrollment by allowing processing of applications to occur by mail or telephone, provide six months of continuous eligibility to applicants age 19 and under, regardless of income changes, and adjust the administrative system to minimize the chance of families in transition from Medicaid to SCHIP or vice versa suffering a temporary loss of coverage by allowing for one- to two-month manual extensions of the renewal period.[17] Renewal packets are now mailed to families after four months of coverage.

Families enrolled in Medicaid in 2001 are now required to complete the Health Care Orientation, which can be done over the phone or in person, usually during an office visit or checkup, or at a CBO event. During the Health Care Orientation, the TCP or CBO worker/volunteer will explain how Medicaid works; provide educational information on basic preventive services, managed care, Texas Health Steps and case management; walk parents through the process of choosing a doctor and dentist; and hand out important contact information.[18]

The Texas Health Education Assistance Resources and Training organization (Texas HEART) operates a statewide toll-free helpline to assist families enrolled in STAR, the Texas Medicaid managed care system. The helpline, called the Medicaid STARLink, was mandated by the Texas Legislature in 1995 in anticipation of family difficulties in navigating the complex managed care system, and became operational in January 2001. Service is available weekdays from 8 AM to 6 PM. STARLink provides information on STAR health plans and where to go for other benefits (such as mental health services), consumer rights, complaint and appeal procedures, and important phone numbers. Helpline staff also coordinate with providers and appropriate state entities to connect families with urgently needed medical services. In addition, STARLink gathers statistical data on the nature of calls received in every public health region, and presents these in quarterly reports to Medicaid agencies in order to help them evaluate their performance and identify any problems.[19]

CBO Activity

In addition to the state efforts, the TexCare Partnership contracts with CBOs in each of the state's 11 public health regions to provide outreach at the local level. These organizations develop educational kits on health insurance programs, which are distributed through community events (often faith-based), networking through employers, and health center presentations. Activities conducted by CBOs focus on promoting health insurance availability, assistance with applications, and developing future outreach strategies, while working with other organizations in their area to minimize duplication of efforts.[20] Many CBOs also perform "inreach" activities through which they provide training within other organizations to help craft health insurance messages relevant to their communities. An example is training Head Start workers to help families with applications.[21]

Among the noted CBO best practices is the West Texas SCHIP Coalition in Lubbock, which provides town hall meeting presentations on insurance programs and inserts TCP messages into Halloween and carnival treat bags. Also included are the Insure-a-Kid initiative through Austin/Travis County Health and Human Services, which provides health insurance information through kindergarten or early childhood registration and follows up by offering application assistance, and the United Way of San Antonio and Bexar County, which works with neighborhood associations to provide TCP information and application assistance in their neighborhoods.

In Houston, Families Under Urban and Social Attack has collaborated with the Harris County Department of Health and Environmental Services, HOPE for Kids, and Episcopal Health Charities to establish training partnerships with hospital district and school nurses, Head Start counselors, and ministry staff on TexCare Partnership information and application assistance, as well as sponsor volunteer-driven "enrollment days" at local Fiesta supermarkets.[22] CBOs in Harris County work closely together and stay involved with what the others are doing through regular interaction, including conference calls. They also share resources and staff with one another to help with outreach events. Finally, they each played a major role in helping to organize recent statewide collaborative outreach events, including the State Health Care Conference and the County Judge Challenge, a contest to see which CBO could get the most children enrolled in Medicaid or SCHIP within a given period of time.[23]

Gaps in Education/Outreach Efforts: SCHIP and Medicaid

Estimated enrollment in SCHIP as of December 31, 2001, is 500,169, which is 117percent of the TCP projected goal.[24] Nonetheless, there are an estimated 83,482 uninsured children in Texas. Of these, 49,192 are potentially Medicaid-eligible, and 1,412 are potentially eligible for SCHIP.[25] A high percentage of the families deemed potentially Medicaid- or SCHIP-eligible but not enrolled are Hispanic or African American.[26]

The main barrier to enrolling uninsured children near the poverty level is difficulty in motivating parents to apply. Low-income families may be unsettled by the prospect of a monthly premium. Timely re-enrollment into both programs, in order to avoid lapses in coverage, is also still a major problem. Many families lose coverage for at least 30 days because they miss the renewal application deadline, which is every six months for Medicaid and 12 months for SCHIP. In addition, delays can occur in transferring a family's application from one program if they are deemed or become eligible for the other.[27]

Current Plans to Fill Existing Gaps

State Activity

TCP has established an outreach work plan for the 2002-2003 biennium. Between January 23 and February 6, 2002, regional stakeholder wants-assessment meetings were held in Houston, Dallas/Ft. Worth, Abilene, McAllen, El Paso and Austin. These meetings brought TCP officials together with contracted CBO representatives, health plan officials, Texas Health Steps contractors and employees, project grantees, Regional Advisory Committee members, and advocates to review recent literature and studies on SCHIP and Medicaid, and develop future outreach strategies and identify key messages to reach families who are potentially eligible.[28]

Key concerns raised by the stakeholders regarding barriers to enrollment included:

- Parents do not understand how Medicaid and SCHIP work, and there is a lack of educational efforts.
- Parents assume they are ineligible.
- Some children seldom get sick, and their parents tend to wait until medical care is absolutely necessary before seeking help.
- Families cannot afford to wait during the 90-day wait period before coverage begins.

Among the barriers to coverage renewal, the most critical to the stakeholders were the following:

- Some families are "lost" to program staff after they move.
- A negative Medicaid stigma discourages families from renewing coverage.
- Families either do not understand the renewal process, or they fail to complete it.
- Renewal information is sometimes lost in the mail.

Finally, stakeholders identified the following as the most important barriers to utilizing health insurance:

- HMOs are not available past the working hours of some parents.
- There is a general lack of providers.
- Families do not know how to access all of the services within their health plans.[29]

The key provider concern is that 40 percent of patients (on average) do not keep their appointments. In addition, CBO representatives in Harris County emphasized the need to develop more formalized relationships between families and HMOs, as well as the importance of keeping families informed of program changes before they are implemented.[30]

Personal interviews with parents of Medicaid children are currently being conducted to determine their emotional needs and identify any missing motivational factors (constraints on parents' awareness of the programs and on parents' decision-making) from TCP's outreach strategy. CBOs will launch new outreach and inreach programs based on identified community needs, and will continue providing ongoing assistance with application and renewal to families. Effectiveness of the new messages and programs will be tested through focus group meetings with consumers in ten regions during March and April 2002. A statewide quantitative baseline study on family attitudes and awareness levels on Medicaid and SCHIP will also be conducted in April. The results of this study and analysis of the wants assessment and focus group meetings will be used to identify additional barriers and develop a new strategic framework by May. Program materials will be modified as needed and creative concepts developed for integration into a new strategic plan for reaching potentially eligible families and application and renewal assistance. This new plan is scheduled to be developed by June 2002.[31]

CBO Activity

TCP has also laid out objectives and strategies to be carried out by contracted CBOs during the 2002-2003 biennium. First and foremost, the CBOs will represent TCP in their communities, devoting roughly 40 percent of their activities on assisting with TCP outreach and inreach. A critical strategy for this objective will be the establishment of an account system of all community partners assisting with TCP activities, and giving each a classification used to determine the frequency of contact. Providers, businesses and organizations that serve or interact with Medicaid and SCHIP-eligible families will be classified as "high priority impact" and will be contacted in person at least monthly. Independent providers of outreach and inreach will be contacted at least quarterly, and new community partners or organizations that have received training from TCP will be contacted as time allows.[32] Another 30 percent of CBO efforts will go into application and renewal assistance. CBOs will also be expected to participate in workgroup meetings, trainings and conference calls, and perform any special projects requested by HHSC. Finally, CBOs will work with HHSC to organize and sponsor marketing outreach and media events, and will regularly conduct evaluation reports of all outreach and inreach activities using data they collect, including the number of applications received by TCP referencing the CBO, as well as levels of program enrollment.[33]

Key performance measures that will determine the success of CBO efforts include the number of new or existing community partners performing TCP outreach and inreach in a given quarter, the renewal response rate in each area, and the level of reduction in the uninsured population in each area as a result of application drives. The standards for evaluation reports are an 85 percent renewal response rate, and 50 percent reduction in uninsured.[34]

State Program Comparison: Washington

Some other states have achieved a considerable enrollment increase in public health insurance programs due to highly successful outreach efforts. These have included many of the activities laid out by TCP in the 2002-2003 plan in Texas. Of particular interest is the Healthy Kids Now! program in the state of Washington.

Healthy Kids Now! is a statewide campaign to promote the availability of health care to uninsured children in Washington state. The program, managed by the Washington Department of Social and Health Services (DSHS), won the 2001 Silver Anvil Award for best practice in public relations.[35]

DSHS contracted with Desautel Hege Communications and the Health Improvement Partnership in Spokane to conduct an extensive grassroots and media outreach campaign. Community stakeholder meetings were held around the state to assess the needs of each area in Washington and determine how each of these could be addressed. The information gathered was used to develop a template for community outreach, which is used by CBOs throughout Washington. It also helped DSHS develop a simplified application for both Medicaid and Washington's SCHIP program, a four by 12 inch handout card with useful program information to be distributed in communities, and training programs for CBO workers on assisting families with understanding their eligibility rights, applying for insurance, and renewal.[36] Training manuals and videos were prepared for all contracted CBOs. The handout and front cover of the application booklet both advertise the availability of free or low-cost health insurance to children and teenagers in Washington, and clearly display the toll-free DSHS number. The handout also shows the number of the nearest CBO. The flip side of the handout and second page of the application booklet both contain an income eligibility table for both Medicaid and SCHIP, and a simple worksheet to determine family income. The common application is in English, but services are available in seven different languages. Questions on whether the enrollee has difficulty understanding English, requires materials in another language, or requires an interpreter appear early in the application.

The ongoing success of Healthy Kids Now! is determined through regular meetings of focus groups around the state. During the program's first two years, an additional 50,000 children were enrolled in Medicaid and SCHIP combined. To date, over 1 million Healthy Kids Now! handouts have been distributed. Currently, less than 10 percent of children from families with incomes below 200 percent of the federal poverty level are uninsured. Key to the campaign's success has been the state's connecting with communities, which now includes regular electronic communication, interconnection and binding among communities, and the emphasis on health insurance being free or low-cost.[37]

Need for Greater Focus on Private Sector

Although material improvements and outreach efforts by TCP with CBO participation have led to enrollment in Medicaid and SCHIP exceeding TCP goals for 2001, there are limitations that will inhibit continuing enrollment in SCHIP. Between 35,000 and 38,000 new children are enrolled in SCHIP each month on average, and the current total enrollment is almost 30,000 over the estimated program capacity.[38] Although Texas is not currently taking steps to limit the total enrollment, it may need to establish an enrollment cap and/or a waiting list for SCHIP in the near future, as state statutes require if program funds are insufficient to cover all enrollees. Further strain will be put on the SCHIP program with increasing Medicaid enrollment (estimated to increase by 8.6 percent during 2002 and 10.2 percent during 2003), and a projected Medicaid budget shortfall of $205 million for the 2002-2003 biennium.[39] Further Medicaid growth is anticipated with the application simplification of SB 43. Because of these potential constraints, planned outreach efforts in the public sector may prove only marginally effective in reducing the number of uninsured.

For this reason, greater attention must be paid to educating consumers about opportunities in the private sector. This is especially important in light of a number of facts drawn from past research on outreach efforts. The population that has proven hardest to reach is families between 185 and 200 percent of the FPL.[40] These families are eligible for SCHIP, but enrollment may no longer be certain in a matter of months. Another population with high needs is individuals between the ages of 55 and 65 without private insurance.[41] In addition, there are still difficulties connecting with some Hispanic communities because Hispanic firms marketing health insurance have done so only in Spanish, yet English is the primary language for a good portion of the Hispanic population in Texas.[42] Finally, a key factor in getting individuals and families to enroll in insurance programs is establishing their trust in the provider. More direct outreach by private sector firms could go a long way toward accomplishing this endeavor.

Overview of Private Insurance Market

Survey of Outreach and Education Efforts: Private Insurance Subgroups

Private Insurance Consumers

Private insurance consumers can be broken down into three subgroups based on their resources for obtaining health care for themselves and their families: individuals, small businesses and their employees, and employees of large businesses. The individual health insurance market includes employees who work for a company without a group health plan, the self-employed, and people who do not work. Individuals who are not covered through an employer and do not qualify for public health insurance must purchase coverage in the individual market, which provides coverage for about 1 million Texans.[43] These individual health plans, offered by some insurance companies and HMOS, are typically the most expensive health plans and are offered primarily on a fee-for-service basis.

Small business owners and employees are a second subgroup of the private health insurance market. Small employers are defined in Texas as having two to 50 eligible employees. Both nationwide and in Texas, much of the uninsured problem lies with small businesses. Recent interview data show that 43.5 percent of workers in small companies were not offered insurance coverage.[44] While many believe that those without health insurance are unemployed, data show that this is not the case. In fact, of all uninsured Texans ages 18 and older, studies indicate that 68.7 percent actually have jobs.[45] Of the 43 million Americans without health insurance, 62 percent are accounted for by small business owners or employees.[46] In Texas, about 60.2 percent of the

2,089,800 uninsured workers over age 18 were employed by companies with fewer than 100 employees in 2000. Forty-six percent of these uninsured workers worked for companies with fewer than 25 employees.[47]

Because small employers do not usually have the purchasing clout of large businesses, their health insurance costs are much higher and are rising quickly. According to focus groups on the uninsured, "The cost of obtaining health insurance cannot be underestimated as a barrier to access… Health insurance is becoming increasingly more expensive and the medical inflation rate continues to outpace the core rate of inflation."[48] According to the NFIB, small employers pay about 18 percent more for a given benefit than do large employers.[49] Even if a small business does manage to offer health coverage to its employees, the cost of extending that coverage to family members is often prohibitive. Thus a large group of the uninsured is children of small business employees.[50]

Large employers are the third subgroup of private insurance purchasers. Defined in Texas as employers with over 50 employees, large employers offer insurance to employees at a far greater rate than do small employers. Nationwide, for instance, virtually all businesses (99 percent) with 200 or more workers offered coverage in 2000.[51] In Texas in 2000, only 12.9 percent of uninsured workers over age 18 worked for companies with 100 to 1000 employees.[52] Because large employers find it easier to offer employees health insurance, and often have benefits counselors to educate employees about health insurance options, education efforts should focus on small businesses owners, small business employees, and individuals.

Political Context: Legislation and Regulation

Health Insurance Portability and Accountability Act

The Health Insurance Portability and Accountability Act of 1996 (HIPAA) was an attempt by the federal government to enable small employers to access affordable health coverage. This statute mandates that if an insurer in a given state offers insurance to any single small group, it must offer insurance to all small groups in that state. HIPAA even guarantees coverage to groups that have members with pre-existing major medical problems.[53]

Structure of Small Employer Health Insurance Market

Small employers make up more than 40 percent of the market for private group health insurance in Texas.[54] As mentioned above, insuring small groups in Texas has proven to be a difficult task, as a majority of uninsured workers are associated with small employers.[55] According to TDI, the number of small employers offering health coverage to their employees has more than doubled as a result of recent reforms (guarantee issue, stricter rating restrictions, and standard benefit plans) implemented by the Texas Legislature.[56,57] For instance, the number of small employers with insurance rose from 36,952 in 1993 to 97,793 in 2000, representing an increase from 10.6 percent to 25.6 percent of all small firms.[58] Still, TDI's State Planning Grant SPG) Interim Report states that Texas' small employer reforms have had "limited success" in increasing affordability and availability.[59] The State Planning Grant's small employer survey final results indicate that 62 percent of respondents have either tried to purchase small group insurance and found it to be too expensive (35 percent), or simply assumed that the coverage will be unaffordable (27 percent).[60] In order to explore ways to improve upon progress to date and address continuing problems, the structure of the small group health insurance market must be examined.

The year 1993 brought guaranteed issue in health insurance markets to Texas. HB 2055 provided that carriers who choose to insure one small group within a certain market cannot refuse coverage to any other group within the same market. Health conditions, type of industry, size of the group, and other factors that may influence risk to the carrier may not be considered in the decision of whether to insure a given group. The state Insurance Code states: "Each small employer carrier shall provide the small employer health benefit plans without regard to health status related factors."[61] HB 2055 gave guaranteed issue to small groups, defined as 3 to 50 eligible full-time employees. Eligible employees are those who work 30 hours per week or more, are not classified as temporary, part-time or seasonal and do not have coverage through another health insurance plan.[62] In 1997, guaranteed issue was extended to groups of two employees, bringing Texas into compliance with the federal HIPAA regulations.[63] In addition, small employer plans are "guaranteed renewable" and may not be canceled unless the terms of the contract are not met by the purchaser.[64]

While small employers are not mandated to provide health insurance to their employees, if an employer offers coverage to any one employee, coverage must be offered to all eligible employees as well as their dependents. Carriers are allowed to require as many as 75 percent of eligible employees to be covered, though insurers are permitted to offer lower participation levels as long as they apply the same lower participation level to all small employers.

Chapter 26 of the Texas Insurance Code specifies that small employer carriers have to offer two small group plans: the catastrophic plan and the basic coverage plan. The current plans were introduced in 1996. The two standard plans, intended to simplify the information-gathering and enrollment processes for small businesses represent only 0.4 percent (398 plans) of total plans.[65] Both the basic and the catastrophic plan cover the following services: physician or other health care provider services, hospital and outpatient services, anesthesia, x-ray and lab services, and maternity benefits. In addition, carriers may offer riders at additional cost (for prescription drugs, alcohol and drug abuse, and mental health services) to either of these plans as well as additional plans that comply with the code.[66] By law, agents and insurers must provide small employers with a summary of the Basic Coverage Benefit Plan and the Catastrophic Benefit Plan when soliciting their business.[67]

Devised as a low-cost option for small businesses, there appear to be two problems with the standard plans. The first is that the plans do not provide small employers with a desired benefits package at an acceptable cost. The second is that small employers, whether because of lack of education or reluctance on the part of agents/carriers to advertise the plans, are not aware that the plans are available to them. The second problem was one that was discovered in TDI's State Planning Grant activities and also in the conference breakout sessions.[68,69]

The lack of enrollment presents strong evidence for revision of these plans. It would be helpful if different stakeholder groups could be involved in revising these plans. These stakeholders could include groups such as TDI, small group carriers, small employers, and small business associations. More extensive information and recommendations on this topic can be found in the SPG conference paper, "Options for Expanding Health Insurance in Texas—Small Employer Market."[70]

Small employers often have trouble insuring even their healthiest employees under HB 2055. The bill does not allow employers to insure only a portion of their employees. In addition, since full-time workers are defined as working at least 30 hours per week, small businesses have an incentive to employ many of their staff members for less than 30 hours per week. It is entirely possible that these two provisions together have increased, rather than decreased, the number of uninsured in the state.[71] Although HB 369 eliminated some of the initial problems with HB 2055 in 1997, some insurers had already abandoned the market. The remaining carriers found that because there is no way to control their risk in the small group market, they had to raise their small group rates to three or four times the normal rates in order to stay in the market.[72]

The Texas small group market is not a community-rated market. This means that carriers may take into account group or individual characteristics such as age, sex, and family coverage when insuring small employers. For this reason, health insurance rates vary tremendously among small businesses. Instead of employing community rating, the market employs a rate band, which is dependent upon the risk levels of individual groups. In a rate band setting, carriers must file a minimum index rate with TDI that serves as a basis for applying the rate band. They also must file measures of the variability in rates as determined by health risk. These rates are determined through competition with other insurers and do not vary much from carrier to carrier. By statute, "The index rate for a rating period for any class of business may not exceed the index rate for any other class of business by more than 20 percent."[73] The "underwritten rate," or the actual rate charged to the small business, is allowed by law to vary by 25 percent on either side of the index rate. This variation is dependent upon health, risk, age, gender, and certain demographic characteristics.[74,75] Because the code does not allow rates for small group plans to exceed those for large groups by more than 20 percent, it appears that the fundamentally larger premium costs charged to small groups must arise in the adjustments to the small group premiums within the rate band.

The process of obtaining health insurance for small employers is difficult. As it is currently structured, small employers must overcome significant obstacles in obtaining health coverage quickly and cost-effectively. A small employer is generally quoted an initial rate that is based only on a few basic group characteristics. This rate, though, is not necessarily the premium the group will be charged. In order for the agent to get a "real" premium quote from the insurer, the insurer requires not only significant amounts of paperwork from each employee but payment of a month's estimated premium. For small employers, who often suffer from constrained cash flows, this premium charge makes it virtually impossible for the company to obtain more than one premium quote at a given time. Therefore, the search for health coverage may extend for months, or even years, while the employer goes through this process several times. These practices are unduly hard on small employers and discourage these employers from pursuing the best policy for their workers.[76]

Small Employer Rate Guide

SPG focus groups and conference participants demonstrated support for a small employer rate guide, although differences on the potential usefulness and feasibility of a rate guide remain.[77] Because search costs, as well as the actual insurance costs, are much higher for small businesses than for large businesses, TDI should focus first on obtaining and publishing average rates (perhaps for several small groups with different characteristics) for the two standard benefits plans offered by carriers to small employers as well as several additional benefits packages that are deemed to be representative of plans purchased by small employers.

Currently, the employer receives an initial quote through the agent based only on a few initial characteristics such as group size and location. In order to obtain a final price quote, the carrier requires detailed health information (from which it makes its final rate determination) and at least a month's premium. Because small employers are often short on cash flow, most cannot afford to even obtain final quotes from more than one carrier at a time, stretching the length of time their employees go without health insurance for months or even years.

While the benefits of a rate guide have been relatively well defined, it is still unclear exactly how a rate guide would work. According to TDI staff, the development and publication of a rate guide does not require specific enabling legislation. TDI currently produces rate guides in other areas of insurance provision without such legislation.[78] However, legislation requiring carriers to release their rates for the "standard" plans to TDI would have to be enacted to guarantee one hundred percent participation.[79] This will engender strong opposition on the part of insurance carriers as they see this information as proprietary. Filing numerous rates with TDI on a regular basis, whether monthly or weekly, also imposes further costs on carriers, a notion that may be resisted. In addition, according to insurance company representatives at an SPG conference focus group, insurance rates change quite quickly.[80] Thus even updating a rate guide weekly (which would probably necessitate some sort of automatic rate-reporting system) may not provide consumers with an accurate picture of the market at any given point in time. Obstacles to creating a rate guide cited by TDI are the large number of companies offering health insurance in Texas, the lack of standardization of insurance plans, and the large array of benefits packages.[81]

Several remaining obstacles to publishing a rate guide were mentioned at the TDI conference breakout sessions and relate to more profound questions of what the rates published in a rate guide actually represent. The point was made that, even provided with spreadsheet of rates published by all small carriers for various plans, a small employer may not necessarily be able to tell the types of benefits included in each plan.[82] The solution to this problem might be to establish not only the standard rating plans for a given group of employees with various characteristics, but also a standard benefits package for each group of employees. While more exploration of the logistics of a rate guide is necessary, it might be possible to establish only a few (three to five) different hypothetical small employers, requiring carriers to publish three rates for each small employer based on differing sets of benefits. The SPG conference papers describe TDI's initial ideas on rate guide templates.[83]

Other states have published rate guides for their small employer markets, including New Jersey, Colorado, Vermont, and North Dakota. Online locations of rate guides are included in Appendix I. These guides illustrate how these states have handled the problem of informing consumers of insurance rates.

During the 77th Texas Legislature, legislation was proposed that would have mandated the development, printing, and distribution of a health insurance rate guide for Texas employers. Under Senate Bill (SB) 771, the Texas Department of Insurance would have been required on an annual basis to "prepare a consumers' guide on health plans so that employers may compare different plans, premium rates, and the coverage and benefits available under each plan."

In addition, the bill included a provision allowing the commissioner to determine any other information that may "assist employers in assessing employer health benefit plans." The Commissioner would also have been allowed to "adopt rules as necessary" to satisfy the requirements of the proposed legislation. In the engrossed version of the bill, the role of the commissioner is further clarified: "The Commissioner would receive broad rule-making authority to implement these requirements." SB 771 stipulated that TDI would have carried out this legal mandate in conjunction with the Office of Public Insurance Counsel.

TDI provided estimates of the staff positions and levels that would have been required to meet the legal mandate of SB 771. A full-time attorney and a full-time program administrator would have been the initial staff for the first year of operation. After FY 2002 (which would have been the start-up year of the program), TDI concluded that the initiative would have only required a part-time attorney and full-time program administrator. In order to develop the rate guide, the attorney hired for the program "would have to work with other TDI programs to propose and adopt a rule enabling the TDI to gather the information necessary to publish the guide." More specifically, TDI noted that the staff "would need to gather information from over 100 carriers offering health benefit plans to small and large employers in Texas." The information gathered would have been entered and stored in a database. TDI expected to make that database available for Texas employers on the Internet. Online visitors would have been able to search the database for the information they were seeking. At the time of the bill's review, TDI estimated that the new proposed database would receive approximately 7,000 hits per year.[84]

SB 771 was introduced by a sponsor in the Senate and passed through review of the Senate Business and Commerce Committee. In the House of Representatives, however, SB 771 did not emerge from the Insurance Committee. Therefore, SB 771 did not become law in Texas.[85]

Past Reform Efforts

Proposed Consumer Assistance Program: HB 2430

In 1999, the 76th Texas Legislature passed HB 3021, a law that officially recognized the needs of HMO customers in Texas by creating an office of the Health Care Ombudsman. Under this statute, "Texas HMO consumers will now have someone to look out for their interests and help make their health insurance work for them."[86] The Ombudsman's Office was to be run by a nonprofit agency hired by TDI. Its purpose was to assist HMO consumers with HMO complaints or appeals, Medicaid and Medicare hearings, and other appeals outside of HMOs.[87]

Texas House Bill 2430, proposed during the 77th Legislature (2001), was designed to replace the Health Care Ombudsman program with a more comprehensive service for all health insurance consumers, and to supplement the current information services offered by TDI and STARlink.[88] Although the Ombudsman program provides an important service, it is estimated that about half of Texans with private insurance are covered by health plans not regulated by TDI and therefore are not covered by the existing services.[89] Another estimate by TDI states that about 3.5 million Texans were covered by self-insured employer group plans not subject to state regulation in 1998.[90] HB 2430 provided for the creation of a consumer assistance program "to provide information to *all* health insurance consumers who have questions about insurance options and assist persons who are experiencing problems with their insurance coverage" [emphasis added].[91] This bill would have amended the Insurance Code to establish the Health Benefit Plan Consumers Assistance Program in the Office of Public Insurance Council (OPIC). The program would have been operated by a non-profit organization possessing the necessary expertise and would have been available to virtually any consumer with health insurance coverage, including both individual and group plans. Eligible consumers would include those covered by insurers and Health Maintenance Organizations (HMOs), as well as those enrolled in public health insurance programs such as SCHIP, Medicare, and Medicaid.[92]

The estimated costs of this proposed program, referred to as an ombudsman program by various publications, were $1,271,531 in FY 2002 and $1,623,316 during fiscal years 2003-2006. These funds would have paid for an eventual 30 full-time positions, as well as the creation and maintenance of a toll-free consumer hotline, a clearinghouse for objective consumer information, and an interactive Internet site.[93] Operators staffing the hotline would provide information about private health coverage plans available in Texas, as well as public health insurance programs. They would also take information from consumers who wish to appeal denials, terminations, or reductions in coverage. Health insurance counselors in the Research and Resolution unit would then conduct in-depth interviews with these consumers, researching and providing assistance in resolving their health insurance issues. By one OPIC estimate, thousands of Texas residents might have been helped through this new program.[94]

HB 2430 mandated that the new consumer assistance program supplement, rather than duplicate, existing services. The bill would have required issuers of health insurance plans to notify their consumers of the existence of the program, providing the toll-free hotline number in their initial program enrollment materials. Further, the bill mandated that this information be provided to any consumer who decides to file either an oral or a written complaint about health insurance coverage. TDI would be required to inform consumers about the assistance program if their complaints did not involve plans regulated by TDI.[95]

As a means of investigating the political attitude towards health insurance reform in the state, the reasons for the failure of HB 2430 must be taken into account. The proposed Health Benefit Plan Consumers Assistance Program was vetoed by Texas Governor Rick Perry. In his veto proclamation, Governor Perry stated that HB 2430 was insufficiently funded in the General Appropriations Act.

Advocates believe that the consumer assistance program has the potential to provide a necessary service that will benefit all Texas state residents and will not require enormous fiscal resources to implement. A small allotment of funds, either from the state or from a private organization, could be used to start a small consumer assistance office, which would offer only basic services at the outset. As residents become aware of the importance of the services offered, political support for the office could potentially grow.

The consumer assistance program, or ombudsman program, would incorporate many and various aspects of health insurance education and outreach that are currently not provided in Texas. The primary suggestion of consumer advocates around the state in terms of insurance education was the creation of a central place for assembly and dissemination of educational materials, as would have been created by HB 2430.[96] Additional recommendations arising from TDI's grant-funded focus groups in the area of education include:

- Establishing a public information program about health insurance
- Providing one-on-one contact with people who could help to educate others about insurance
- Advertising more about available insurance options
- Establishing a central toll-free number people could call for information about health insurance
- Having a help-line with trained staff who could answer questions about insurance
- Educating people about all the health care options available to them."[97]

A majority of the above recommendations were incorporated in HB 2430 as proposed in the 77th Legislature. In addition, the proposal incorporated many of the program design recommendations of Families USA, a national consumer health advocacy organization. For instance, the program was designed to be broad in scope, covering all health insurance plans in Texas regardless of type of plan, means by which the consumer obtained health insurance, and whether the plan is regulated by TDI. The implementation of HB 2430 by a nonprofit agency also concurs with one of the program recommendations made by Families USA.

The ombudsman program appears to be one of the few health insurance reform proposals that could potentially find support from many types of stakeholder groups. The concept of a general health insurance ombudsman's office was mentioned repeatedly during TDI's State Planning Grant conference and in the conference papers. State Planning Grant focus group participants, as well as conference participants, seem to support it.[98] As demonstrated by the passage of HB2430 through the Texas Legislature, ombudsman programs might find political support in the future.[99,100]

The interest groups that supported HB 2430 are expected to lobby for a similar version of HB 2430 in the next legislative session. Should public funding for an ombudsman program not become available through the legislative process, interest groups are also seeking private funding for the development and implementation of such a program.[101]

Current Reform Efforts

State Planning Grant

The Texas State Planning Grant was implemented in March 2001 to build upon the work begun by the Blue Ribbon Task Force. Its mission is to develop a comprehensive statewide plan to eliminate "the disparity in health care coverage amongst members of the population of Texas" by increasing access to, as well as augmenting, current public and private insurance coverage.[102] This project is overseen by the Texas Department of Insurance and many stakeholders were invited to participate in grant efforts through inclusion in the Project Oversight and Implementation Working Group.

A preliminary survey of Planning Grant Working Group members indicated that there is a high level of interest in the proposals at the end of this section. The policy option entitled "Inform Public of Recent Insurance Reforms" garnered the most support from these members. "Group/Individual Health Insurance Rate Guide" was the third most popular potential policy option, and a "Standardized Insurance Plan for Individual Policies, With Rate Guide" ranked in fifth out of 20 options.[103]

State Planning Grant efforts have been particularly focused on the small group market for health insurance. The results of these efforts were publicized at the Texas State Planning Grant Conference on January 31 and Feburary 1, 2002. The Small Employer Health Insurance Survey results show that, although some progress has been made recently, almost 50 percent of Texans without insurance are employed by firms with fewer than 25 employees and 75 percent of firms with fewer than 50 employees do not offer any health insurance.[104]

The need for improved or new education and outreach programs in the small employer market is strikingly demonstrated by the recent Small Employer Health Insurance Survey by TDI. The survey asked whether the small employer was aware of three recent reforms in Texas small employer coverage regulations. These reforms are listed below:

- Small employers cannot be denied insurance due to pre-existing conditions or poor health status;
- Small employers can purchase standard plans with limited benefits at a lower cost;
- Small employers can join together to form a purchasing alliance.

Survey results indicate that only 28 percent, 18 percent, and 26 percent of small employers, respectively, know about these three reforms. These figures affirm the strong need for increases in educational efforts for small employers.[105]

House Bill 3038

House Bill 3038, enacted by the 77th Texas Legislature, mandates development of means for small employers to offer SCHIP coverage to children of their employees through the company insurance plans.

Health Insurance Education in Texas

Information on individual and small group health insurance in the state of Texas is scattered and not comprehensive, similar to the situation on the national level. Unless an individual has a significant amount of time and the use of an Internet connection, it would be seemingly very difficult to obtain an optimal health insurance plan without access to a benefits counselor in the state of Texas. Several national agencies provide general information on private health insurance. In addition, three primary state agencies/associations provide educational materials regarding private health insurance for these consumer subgroups: the Texas Department of Insurance (TDI), the Office of Public Insurance Council (OPIC), and the Texas Health Care Information Council (THCIC).

Those eligible for public insurance have benefited from coordinated advertising, outreach and education efforts (especially for the SCHIP program) over the past few years, but there has been no corresponding coordinated effort to educate potential consumers of private insurance. Information sources are offered by various agencies, but a consumer looking to purchase health insurance as an individual or a small employer would be forced to spend huge amounts of time and effort investigating his or her options.

Internet resources on private health insurance information are the most readily accessible for those looking to research private insurance options. Several federal agencies offer online consumer brochures that outline insurance options for individuals and small employers. The best of these information sources are the following:

- "Looking for Value: An Employer's Guide to Evaluating Quality Health Plans," by the Employer Quality Partnership. This brochure, recommended and distributed by the National Federation of Independent Businesses (NFIB), offers summaries of the types of insurance plans and factors to consider when evaluating health plans.[106] In addition, this brochure provides additional resources that can be used by employers to evaluate health care plans.

- The mission of the national Consumer Health Education Council, under the Employee Benefits Research Institute, is "to reduce the number of uninsured Americans and improve the health of the general public through information and research that helps individuals and plan sponsors understand the value and uses of private and public health insurance."[107] The Council provides both a "Consumer Gateway" and an "Employer Gateway" online. A document called "Getting and Keeping Coverage" provides "Getting Insurance Links."[108] Some of these links are specific to certain states, although there are no Texas links provided. There are also links to other national agencies, as well as websites that provide free insurance quotes (insure.com, simplyhealth.com, and ehealthinsurance.com).

- Insure.com, recommended by the American Association of Health Plans (AAHP), states that the individual health insurance market is a "wild frontier." This website provides a good summary guide to purchasing individual health insurance called "Tips for Buying Individual Health Coverage." It gives tips on how to reduce individual policy costs and warns that premiums for individual plans can vary by as much as 50 percent for the same product from different companies.[109] The website also provides a "Health Plan Comparison Worksheet" for keeping track of various costs and services as one investigates insurance coverage options.[110]

- The Health Insurance Association of America (HIAA) website provides consumer information in the form of health insurance guides. Two that are especially useful are "Guide To Health Insurance," which helps consumers understand the different types of plans offered, and "The Insurance Guide for Business Owners," which describes the small group insurance market and provides guidance in comparing policies.[111,112] The latter guide is a good source of information for small business owners in terms of learning the basic policies. The "Guide To Health Insurance" warns that purchasing individual insurance requires careful shopping because costs and covered services vary radically between insurers. HIAA also produces guides on disability insurance and long-term care, which can be ordered from its 800 number. HIAA offers a selection of books on health insurance that could be helpful. These include: *Health Insurance Nuts and Bolts: An Introduction to Health Insurance Operations; Health Insurance Terminology: A Glossary Developed by HIAA Insurance Education; The Health Insurance Primer: An Introduction to How Health Insurance Works; and Employment Based Health*

Insurance Coverage. Finally, HIAA offers self-study courses in health insurance and managed care.

Texas Department of Insurance

The Texas Department of Insurance (TDI) is the agency required to provide consumer information and consumer protection in the state. According to its mission, TDI is to regulate the insurance industry "firmly, fairly effectively and efficiently."[113] Among others, TDI lists the following duties as part of its mission:

- to support an industry "dedicated to the long term concept of insurance and its contributions to society"
- to insure the availability of "quality insurance products for all Texans at reasonable prices and under reasonable terms…"
- to enforce "solvency standards and promote competition in the industry while protecting consumers from fraud, misrepresentation and unfair practices"
- to educate the public "about insurance so that Texans can make more informed choices, and TDI insists that the industry be responsive to its customers"
- to ensure that Texas is a "place where industry will want to do business."[114]

There are 13 divisions under the commissioner's jurisdiction, many of which have several subdivisions. The organizational structure of TDI can be seen in Figure 8.1. Following the organizational chart is a brief discussion of some of the divisions related to health care and health education.

Figure 8.1
Texas Department of Insurance Organizational Structure

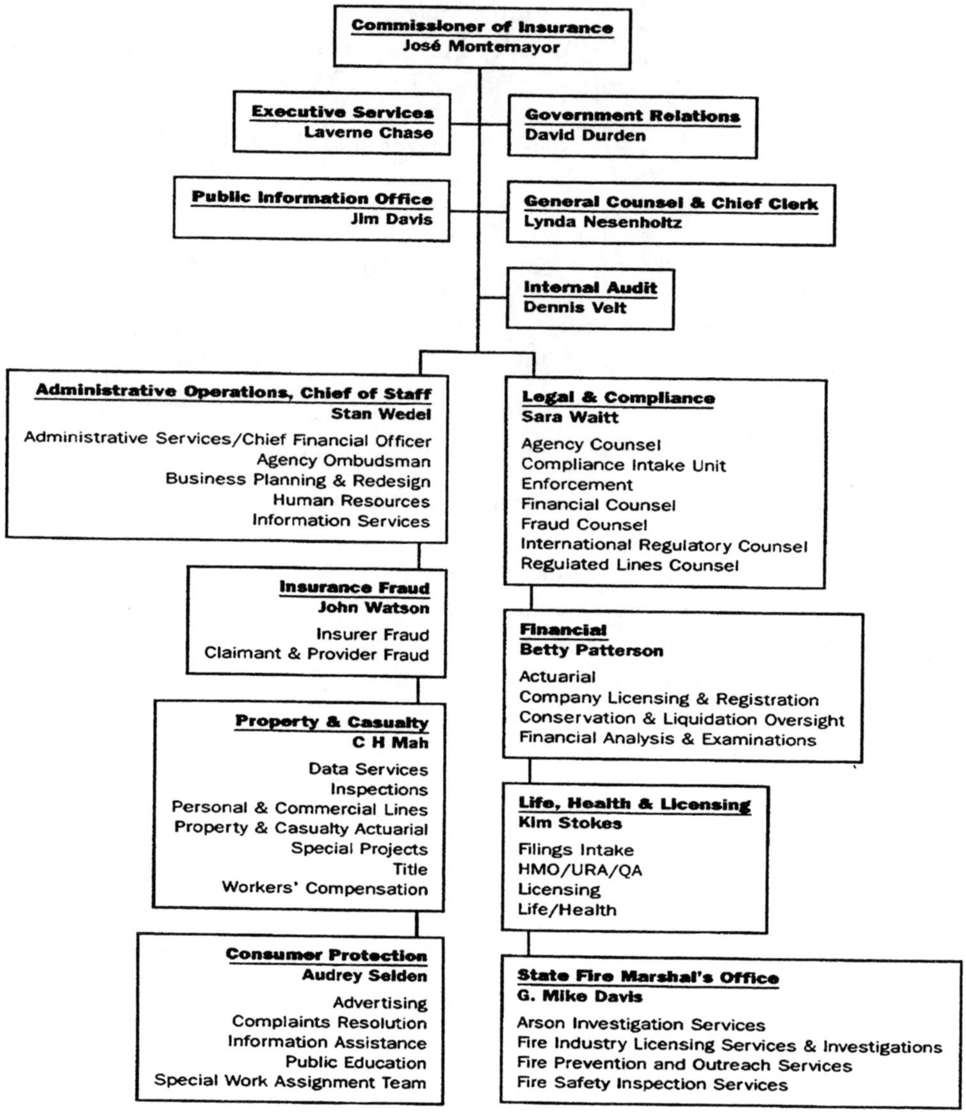

Adapted from: Texas Department of Insurance, *2001 Annual Report* (Austin, Tex., November 2001), p. vii. Online. Available: http://www.tdi.state.tx.us/commish/annual01.html. Accessed: January 2, 2002.

The Commissioner of Insurance

The commissioner is appointed by the governor of Texas and confirmed by the Senate. The commissioner is the agency's chief executive officer as well as the administrative officer in charge of developing operating procedures, overseeing regulatory functions, enforcing the laws under the agency's jurisdiction, and appointing individuals to advisory boards and committees.[115] As of this writing, the Texas Commissioner of Insurance is Jose Montemayor, who was originally appointed by then Governor George Bush and reappointed by Governor Perry to a two-year term, effective February 1, 2001.[116]

Public Information Office

The public information office helps with the education efforts by providing a service called NEWSline, a toll-free information line that provides radio stations with prerecorded insurance information. This office is the agency's contact with the media, consumers, the insurance industry, regulators, and other government agencies, and responds to information requests from these groups.[117]

Insurance Fraud Unit

This unit prepares and refers fraud related criminal cases for prosecution. According to a study by a Connecticut research firm, fraud cost the insurance industry $120 billion in 1995, a 33 percent increase from 1990. These costs are passed on to the consumer in the form of higher premiums.[118] This unit has doubled in size since FY 1995 with the addition of criminal analysts and investigators, and now has law enforcement agency status, which allows it to have peace officers, access to criminal intelligence, make arrests, and execute warrants.[119]

Life, Health, and Licensing Program

This Office regulates HMOs and many different types of life, health, and related coverage. It also is responsible for licensing the following groups: insurance agents, third party administrators, viatical and life settlement providers, provider representatives and brokers, premium finance companies, utilization review agents, and independent review organizations. This office also handles and resolves HMO grievances and performs quality of care examinations of HMOs.

Some of the primary responsibilities of the Life, Health, and Licensing Program include regulating policy forms and reviewing rate filings for credit, life, accident, and health, as well as for Medicare supplement, Medicare select, long-term care, and HMO coverage. This division is also responsible for implementing legislation and monitoring federal government activities related to life insurance, health coverage, and licensing issues. This is the office that is responsible for the State Planning Grant, which is studying the expansion of health coverage to uninsured Texans.[120]

Licensing Division

The licensing division is a section of the Life, Health, and Licensing Program, and is led by a Deputy Commissioner overseeing the processes of licensing and regulating insurance agents, adjusters, risk managers, life insurance counselors, reinsurance intermediaries, TPAs, premium finance companies, and people involved in selling insurance products in the following settings: travel agencies, self storage facilities, retail establishments, and rental car companies.

The Licensing Division includes subsections on Applications, Customer Assistance, Renewals, Appointments and Continuing Education, an Administrative Review and Data Management Section, and a Third Party Administrator and Premium Finance Section. The Continuing Education Section responds to inquiries and telephone calls from agents, companies, and the public including questions regarding licenses, appointment status, and general inquiries about the licensing process.[121]

Life/Health Division

This section is also led by a Deputy Commissioner, and is responsible for reviewing virtually all life and health policies to ensure compliance with both state and federal statutes and regulations. The Division also registers life, settlement and viatical providers, provider representatives and brokers, and reviews contracts related to life and viatical settlements. Life/Health reviewed and processed 26,228 forms during FY 2001, including settlement forms, certifications, reports, calculations, and rates.[122]

Health Maintenance Organization Division

The HMO Division is also under the umbrella of Life, Health, and Licensing, and is responsible for regulating HMOs, certifying and regulating URAs, certifying IROs, and investigating complaints against licensed groups. These responsibilities can lead to enforcement actions based on issues of availability, accessibility, or quality of care provided by HMOs. There is a Quality Assurance Staff that is responsible for providing direct responses to consumer or provider complaints over the complaint line. This staff was kept busy with 7,131 complaints solely against HMOs, along with 457 IRO case reviews, during FY01. The Division is also responsible for conducting quality of care examinations and reviewing form filings to ensure that they are in compliance with state and federal statutes.[123]

Finally, and most importantly for education and outreach within the HMO Division, is the role of educating "industry, provider and consumer groups through bulletins, compliance workshops, manuals, checklists, and speaking engagements." The Division also provides technical assistance to several groups and state agencies.[124]

Consumer Protection

This division is the most important for the purposes of this section, as it is responsible for assisting consumers with resolving complaints and maintaining the toll free Customer Help Line (1-800-252 3239), as well as maintaining consumer publications on the

Internet website and reviewing insurance advertising.[125,126] In FY01, Consumer Protection responded to over 338,000 inquiries.[127]

The Consumer Protection Division has recently been recognized for its accomplishments through several awards. The division was given an "A" for its website and publications by the Consumer Federation of America. It received two additional awards; one from the Health Care Financing Administration (HCFA) for "Outstanding Services to the National Medicare Education Program," and another for its outreach activities.[128] The division has five different subsections as described below.

Complaints Resolution

The Complaints Resolution section involves reviewing disputes between consumers and either companies, agents or other regulated insurance businesses. In FY01, this staff processed almost 29,000 written complaints.[129] It is important to note that this only applies to insurance businesses that TDI regulates, which do not include health insurance plans provided by governments, churches, some school districts, ERISA, out-of-state Blue Cross organizations, and self-insured companies.[130,131] Self-funded insurance plans often go through an HMO or Third Party Administrator to coordinate providers and administer claims and paperwork while the employer still assumes the insurance risk. Self-insured companies cannot be regulated by the states due to federal law, and are instead regulated by the U.S. Department of Labor.[132] TDI's hotline cannot help with any of the insurance plans that are out of its jurisdiction. These plans would have been addressed by the consumer ombudsman legislation in the vetoed HB 2430.[133]

Complaints Resolution also looks at possible violations of the Texas Insurance Code and the Texas Administrative Code and will request enforcement action as warranted. There are four different areas to which complaints can be directed, including Auto/Home, Life, Accident and Health, Real Estate/Title Insurance, and Physician/Provider. Complaints can be made online as well as over the telephone.

Information Assistance

Information Assistance responds to calls to the agency's Consumer Help Line, which is open Monday-Friday from 8 a.m. to 5 p.m. Central Standard Time. There are 16 paid hotline employees who do not generally specialize in specific areas of insurance.[134] During these hours, the operators are able to answer questions about most insurance types, the license status of companies and agents, and other company information such as complaint records and financial ratings. In addition, operators can advise consumers about filing complaints. There are also operators available to speak to consumers in Spanish, or to those that are hearing or speech impaired.[135] The employees are equipped with a keyword Infobase to access information. The long-range plan at present is to eventually open these databases up to the public.[136] The help line accepted 337,134 phone calls during Fiscal Year 2001, which were broken down as follows:

- 17 percent for life, accident, and health issues;
- 21 percent for Property/Casualty;

- 6 percent for agent inquiries;
- 30 percent for company information;
- 21 percent for miscellaneous information such as complaints and referrals;
- 3 percent for Spanish speakers; and
- 2 percent for Medicare.

The 17 percent of phone calls for life, accident, and health care issues in FY 2001 is an increase from the 14 percent of calls going to these topics in both FY 1999 and 2000.[137]

While TDI does not have jurisdiction over certain plans, such as self-funded plans and other governmental plans mentioned above, the hotline employees will attempt to help these groups if they can, and if not, they will refer them to the Department of Labor.

Once a complaint is received, it is filed in writing. The hotline staff employee will inform the consumer what information is required to file a formal complaint with TDI, and in some cases, the hotline staff will take the complaint over the phone. After receiving a complaint, the staff member will submit the complaint to the appropriate Complaint Resolution staff for handling.

As far as advertising the hotline, TDI advertises the telephone number by printing it on insurance policies and in TDI publications, as well as in press releases and Public Service Announcements.[138]

Public Education

The mission of the Public Education Office is to provide information to the public in order to increase consumers' understanding of insurance products, to encourage wise insurance shopping, and to promote TDI consumer services. This department includes both the publications and Speakers Bureau groups. There are nine people on the staff, all of whom are responsible for both Speakers Bureau and Publications duties. One person serves as the Health Information, Counseling and Advocacy Program (HICAP) coordinator, one is capable of speaking to bilingual audiences, and one is responsible primarily for responding to open records requests.[139]

There are four performance measures set by the legislature that the Public Education office tries to meet, as follows:

1. There is an annual goal of 500 for number of presentations made. These informational presentations are often made based on the "hot topic" of the year, which in 2001, for example, was the mold problem in the Houston area.

2. There is an annual goal of 2 million for the number of publications distributed.

3. There is an annual goal is 600,000 for the number of rate guides distributed (there is no rate guide for health insurance in the state of Texas).

4. To produce and distribute rate guides at an average unit cost of 60 cents or less (again, keeping in mind that there currently is no rate guide for health care in the state of Texas).[140]

In fiscal year 2001, the office met all four performance goals. The Speakers Bureau was coordinated or gave 566 presentations, more than 2.188 million publications and more than 662,000 rate guides were distributed, and the rate guides were produced at an average of 37 cents per guide.[141]

The Consumer Protection page on the TDI website recorded almost 333,000 hits in FY 2001. The publications on this site are also accessible by calling 1-800-599-7467, and some are provided in Spanish and Vietnamese.[142] These publications are contracted out for translation, with the ones that are accessed most often being the ones that are translated. If a publication is not translated, and someone asks for one in a specific language, then TDI will have the document translated. Not all of the materials have been translated into Spanish due to relatively few requests for these materials.[143] There is a statutory requirement to translate materials into Spanish for an automobile insurance glossary. There is no such requirement for health insurance materials. However, according to TDI staff, no new legal requirement would be needed to translate all health insurance-related materials into Spanish or other foreign languages.[144]

The publications are chosen for production based on what consumers want or need, as well as on the recommendations of advocacy groups such as the AARP.[145] However, there is no marketing plan for Public Education, as TDI looks at the performance targets as guides at the beginning of each fiscal year. They also plan to ensure that services are spread out throughout the state.

Once TDI decides what to produce, the products are tested for readability by conducting "Flesch-Kincaid" tests and they are tested to see if they can be understood by conducting focus groups. Generally, the publications have a seventh- to eighth-grade reading level. The Office of Public Insurance Counsel is an advocate for insurance consumers, and is required to view publications before their release to the public.[146]

Public Education is also responsible for operating a Speakers Bureau, which delivers public presentations, prepares exhibits and workshops, and makes appearances on talk shows or for various types of groups such as community organizations, consumer groups, business and industry associations.[147,148] There is a calendar of events for the Speakers Bureau on the TDI website.[149] In addition to the Speakers Bureau, Public Education runs the federally funded Health Information, Counseling, and Advocacy Program (HICAP), which trains volunteers statewide to help elderly individuals resolve their insurance concerns by providing one on one assistance in their local communities.[150, 151] HICAP provides extensive information on both public and private options and can make referrals for eligible seniors to help them work through the legal process.[152]

This section offers information on different companies that could be useful to consumers. One list Public Information offers is the List of Companies Offering Small Employer Accident and Health Insurance, which includes all of the companies offering this type of coverage with contact information.[153] They also have a list called Major Texas Insurers, which contains the NAIC Number, the rank by size, the written premium, and the percent of the market share covered by the particular company.[154] Similarly, there is also an annual list of Accident and Health companies including the total number of policies they have with the number of justified complaints. TDI has also created a complaint index so that a consumer can see where a company rates in comparison with other companies when comparing number of justified complaints to the total number of accident and health policies.[155]

Advertising

This is where the review of the industry marketing materials takes place to guard against misrepresentation and to ensure that the material is in compliance with rules and regulations overseeing solicitation and trade practices.[156,157] Important violations are directed to the Legal and Compliance Program to determine if enforcement action is necessary.[158]

Current Enforcement/Regulatory Efforts

TDI must license insurance-related businesses if they are to be allowed to sell their products or services in the state. TDI licenses the following groups:

- Insurance companies
- Agents (discussed below)
- Third party administrators
- Health maintenance organizations
- Premium finance companies
- Consulting care retirement communities
- Insurance adjusters.[159]

TDI also enforces the Texas Insurance Code (available online at http://www.capitol.state.tx.us/statutes/intoc.html). TDI investigates complaints after they have been made through the appropriate channels, and takes enforcement actions against the company or agent who has committed the misconduct.[160] Examples of the type of laws and statutes that TDI regulates can be seen in the following paragraphs.

In Texas and many other states, health insurance options are partially dependent on health status, but the following laws protect an individual even if they are sick. There is a nondiscrimination law which says that companies have to offer all employees of the same status in a company, such as all full-time employees, the same type of plan. The company cannot discriminate based on the health of the individual.

HMOs cannot exclude preexisting conditions, although they can impose a waiting period before coverage begins. Other group health plans must use a look back period, meaning that a preexisting condition is determined if an individual received or was recommended to receive a diagnosis or treatment, or even medical advice during the six months prior to obtaining the plan or beginning the waiting period for the plan. Group health plans cannot exclude a person with a preexisting condition for pregnancy, newborns, newly adopted children, or genetic information.

Most individual health coverage is "guaranteed renewable," meaning that health care coverage cannot be cancelled if an individual becomes sick as long as the individual continues to pay the premium, is not guilty of committing fraud and, if it is an HMO plan, continues to live in the plan service area. Coverage may also be terminated if the HMO withdraws from the individual market. Guaranteed renewal is not applicable if the health plan is a short-term plan, where the length of the contract is limited to a certain time frame.

Guaranteed renewal also applies to all group plans. Coverage to a group cannot be cancelled if someone in the group becomes sick. HMOs, however, can impose other conditions such as requiring the group to meet minimum participation or contribution rates. They can also refuse to continue coverage if the individuals do not pay premiums or commit fraudulent activities. Additionally, they can withdraw the health plan altogether, or withdraw from the small employer market. If they discontinue the plan, they must give the individuals a chance to buy other plans that they sell to other groups of the same size.[161]

Besides the enforcement of the Texas Insurance Code and the licensing of different entities, TDI is also responsible for setting price ranges for auto and homeowner insurance plans sold by the companies in the fields regulated by TDI. These companies are responsible for about 75 percent of auto and 20 percent of homeowner policies in the state.[162]

TDI also monitors the financial condition of the licensed companies in the state to ensure that the companies have the funds available to pay claims and other expenses. Consumers can access this information and look at the company's financial strength by looking at the website or calling the TDI help line.[163] TDI also wants to maintain the financial success of the industry, with a goal to "encourage the financial health of the insurance industry through monitoring and regulation." TDI also attempts to ensure that the industry does not suffer heavy losses through a goal of decreasing "insurance industry loss costs."[164]

TDI also investigates fraud and reports abuses of fraud to the Texas Attorney General, local district attorneys, or United States attorneys.[165] The TDI mission statement lists fraud as an area in which TDI is to protect consumers.[166]

Advertising by the insurance companies is also monitored by TDI, as they ensure that the services of the company are not misrepresented. They also guard against deceptive advertising and unfair trade practices. Companies can be fined for violations in these regards.[167]

TDI also has the right to fine companies for the following reasons: delaying payment of claims, misrepresenting policies, failing to provide the required discounts to consumers, or engaging in other unlawful practices. TDI obtains millions of dollars per year in additional claims and refunds for consumers. Help for this is also available online or by calling the hotline.[168]

Regulation of Agents

For an agent to become licensed, the first step is to find an insurance company that will sponsor the individual. The prospective agent then takes the appropriate classes, after which he or she is required to take an extensive examination to earn an agent license.[169]

The requirements for renewing a license for Life, Accident, and Health (which allows an individual to sell all types of health insurance, including HMO plans, and all types of adjusters) include generally 15 hours of class work with special requirements depending on the type of license each year of the two-year period, or 30 hours every biennium.[170,171,172] Once agents reaches 20 years of service, they are no longer required take the continuing education classes, although they must still renew their license. Agents are required to have hours in Insurance Regulation and Ethics, and adjusters must have hours in consumer protection.[173] There is no exam required to renew a license.[174] In addition to the required continuing education courses, several different associations and groups that represent agents (such as the Texas Association of Health Underwriters) offer educational classes and opportunities throughout the year. There are numerous opportunities and requirements for agent education, so if agents are not sufficiently educated, it is not because of a systematic problem, but rather due to a lack of effort.[175]

When it comes to setting commissions, agents do not have control over the prices they charge; rather, the insurance company that carries the agent is responsible for setting their commission rates. However, some occasional negotiation takes place within larger groups.[176] The Texas Insurance Code regulates the rates that an agent may charge a small group when renewing the group's plan, but not the rates charged for the initial purchase of the plan.[177] Because insuring small groups requires proportionally more time and paperwork than insuring large groups, agents are often given very small commissions for very small groups as a disincentive to sell to these groups. "An obstacle many small businesses have to face when trying to find health insurance for their employees is searching for an agent to market insurance to their group."[178] In addition, some insurance companies, in order to avoid the risk levels of very small groups, provide disincentives to insure small groups, including paying extremely low commissions to agents insuring small groups, setting high premiums, and not renewing the licenses of these agents.[179] House Bill 471, passed during the 77th legislative session, attempted to address this problem, but only in part. The bill "generally prohibits small employer carriers from varying the level of agent commissions according to the size of the group or otherwise reducing access to small employer health benefit plans."[180] Carriers may still charge variable commissions calculated inversely to the size of the small group. In addition, small group carriers may calculate commissions as a percentage of the total premium paid by a small employer.[181] Agent commissions are proportionately higher for small businesses than large businesses. Therefore, prohibitive agent costs as a part of the high cost of health care in general still may remain one of the many obstacles to insuring small businesses.

One possible role for TDI is to regulate all initial rates charged to small employers, in terms of restrictions on agents as well as carriers. As the Blue Ribbon Task force puts it, the state should: "Preclude insurance agent commissions from being calculated in such a way as to preclude Texas small employers from having full access to the small employer health insurance market."[182] This type of regulation seems to have at least some measure of political acceptance, as indicated by the passage of House Bill 471 during the previous legislative session.

In relation to dealings with consumers, the agent acts as the advocate for the client. In the case of very small businesses, the agent acts almost like a human resource employee for health insurance and employee benefits. One way that they will often try to educate consumers or clients is to use publications from TDI. If there is a consumer group that an agent feels could use the publication, the agent will bring several of them to distribute to the group, so these TDI publications take on added importance.[183]

There were two major bills passed in the 77th Legislative Session addressing agents, one of which was HB 949. Agents have nothing to do with the setting of rates for groups with between two and 50 employees; the insurance companies set these. Prior to this bill, the highest rate factor for a small employer plan was prohibited from exceeding the lowest rate factor by more than 20 percent.[184] This rule was very difficult to enforce and was not statutorily required through the insurance code. Some carriers had been charging higher rates by using risk characteristics as a justification for raising the rates. This bill codifies the 20 percent rating rule and requires that the risk load of the small group reflect the risk characteristic of the group.[185]

Another bill that was influential in this area was HB 471, which addresses the issue of undercutting commissions on the smallest groups. Insurance companies determine commission rates for agents. For individual health insurance, as well as small group health insurance for groups of two to 100 employees, the commission is based on the premium paid by the client. This premium can be as low as 1 to 7 percent and as high as 8 to 10 percent of the collected premium. HB 471 tightens the rules pertaining to agent commissions to make them more enforceable and to ensure that small employers have better access to health insurance by prohibiting some commission practices used by insurance companies that keep agents from providing services to small employers.[186,187]

Current Consumer Education Efforts

Comments made during the TDI conference indicate a very low level of knowledge of individual and small employer rights regarding health care coverage, illustrating the need for consumer education. Health care is a difficult subject matter, and consumers need information in order to make informed decisions. The TDI State Planning Grant made some suggestions aimed at educating small businesses on the recent reform efforts. These issues were said to be important when looking at responses from the SPG focus groups and small employer surveys. Suggestions included in the SPG policy options are the following:

- Work with media throughout state to publicize reforms.
- Develop more small employer information on TDI website and coordinate links with trade associations, employer organizations, and other state agencies who provide services to small businesses.
- Develop printed pamphlets and brochures and distribute to local organizations/business groups throughout the state.
- Distribute information to small employers as part of a mail-out of quarterly tax statements by the Texas Workforce Commission.
- Organize local "insurance fairs" for small employers to provide a forum for TDI to provide information and assistance to small employers with health insurance questions.[188]

All of the above recommendations represent relatively low-cost means of improving the situation of the small employer in the health insurance market. The ignorance of small employers of recent reforms despite TDI publications on the subject indicates not only a lack of knowledge of the reforms but a lack of knowledge of where to find information. Purely educational reforms have the advantage of not needing the approval of the legislature in some cases, and in most cases, not needing vast appropriations. The project could be jointly funded by the state and the insurance industry. TDI has the infrastructure in place to implement these reforms, although the optimal situation would be for these reforms to be included in the aforementioned health assistance program.

Despite the need for more educational materials and outreach materials, there are still several sources of information available at this time. Of the state organizations charged with either consumer protection or consumer education, TDI offers consumers the most comprehensive resources on private health insurance-related issues in Texas. TDI develops, updates, and provides a series of general educational materials to Texans on insurance coverage. The majority of the educational materials produced by TDI are in the form of fact sheets and booklets. Many of these fact sheets focus exclusively on topics related to health coverage.

"Your Health Care Coverage," a 35-page document, covers health plan basics, laws regarding different types of plans and conditions, tips on where to look for a health plan, factors to consider when evaluating a health plan, how to file a complaint, and more.[189] This guide provides useful information specific to both individual health insurance and small group insurance. TDI also provides guides specific to small employer insurance, such as "Insurance Resource for Small Businesses" and "Small Employers Health Insurance: Questions and Answers."[190,191] The latter provides information on all facets of small business insurance, from the legal to the financial to the practical. In addition, this document provides a list of the plans that small employer insurance carriers must offer, including deductibles, amount of co-insurance, and maximum out-of-pocket expenses for each type of plan.

Another comprehensive TDI publication, called "Health Care Coverage for Texas Children," provides parents with information on every means of obtaining health insurance for children in Texas, including Medicaid, SCHIP, private coverage, and the risk pool. [192] Descriptions of programs and ways to obtain additional information are included, as well as a list of private health insurers that offer health care coverage for children.

The following is a complete list of the remainder of TDI's health insurance-related publications followed by other relevant general insurance-related publications.

- *Summary of Health Care Coverage Options for Texas Children* is a document discussing the qualifications for a child to be eligible for Medicaid, SCHIP, and the Texas Health Insurance Risk Pool. It contains a very brief statement that says that if a child does not qualify for these plans, TCP can send the consumer a guide listing companies that offer private health plans for children.[193]

- *Health Maintenance Organizations* describes the makeup of HMOs, how they work, their limitations, information about the doctor/patient relationship in an HMO, how to file a complaint, and protections for HMOs with the state laws that they must abide by. There is also a brief glossary of HMO-related terms.[194]

- *HMO Resource* gives the consumer a list of questions to ask an HMO upon considering a plan, with links and contact information on how to learn about the complaints filed against different HMOs and links to various different sources of information regarding HMOs, regulations, and requirements governing the behavior of HMOs.[195]

- *Medicare+Choice Options for Medicare Beneficiaries* provides information on Medicaid+Choice programs, the advantages and disadvantages of the program, and how to determine if a Medicare+Choice program is right for a consumer. It then gives suggestions on how to select a plan and how to get the most out of the plan.[196]

- *HICAP Highlights—Private Fee-for-Service Plans* discusses different options available to the elderly individuals whom HICAP is set up to assist.[197]

- *Long-Term Care Insurance* gives the basics of long term care, some questions that would help an individual decide if long term care is right for them, and what type of policies are available. The document discusses Tax Qualified Long-Term Care Plans and Non-Tax Qualified Long Term Care Plans. This document also states what would be covered in a plan, how to fit a plan to meet one's needs and budget, and how to qualify. Finally, it talks about premiums and shopping tips before giving helpful phone numbers and other links.[198]

- *Insurance for Texans with Disabilities* is a document that discusses central issues involving people with disabilities looking for insurance, including the rights afforded to persons with disabilities, a discussion of pre-existing conditions, and health benefit options. There is also information on how to use the rights, how to get help, how to seek legal advice, and finally, there is contact information and links to get further information.[199]

- *Glossary—Common Insurance Terms* is a fairly comprehensive list of the definitions of health terminology.[200]

- *Insurance Fraud* provides examples of different types of fraud and ways to defend oneself against various different types of fraudulent practices and scams.[201]

- *Helping You With Your Insurance Complaint* gives the consumer tips to understanding a policy and her/his rights, tips to working with both Auto and Homeowner and Accident and Health claims, and information regarding deadlines for the payment of claims. It also walks a consumer through the steps of making a claim, discusses what claims are accepted, and what to do if one is not satisfied with the results from TDI.[202]

- *If My Insurance Company Fails* walks a consumer through the problems involved when an insurer fails, what his/her options are at that point, who will pay his/her claims, and other frequently asked questions. There is also a brief glossary with HMO-related terms.[203]

- *Independent Review Organizations* focuses on consumers with a complaint. If a consumer has a complaint, they can go to an Independent Review Organization to review the decision. This document lays out when the use of an Independent Review Organization would be appropriate and when the use of one would not be available.[204]

- *Insurance on the Internet: Shopping Tips and Dangers* is a publication containing tips on how to shop smart online and confirming company and agent information. It also has tips for identifying fraud and addresses privacy concerns and security tips.[205]

- *Assistance for Providers* is aimed at providers and attempts to help them with issues such as prompt payment, quality of care, common types of complaints against HMOs and insurance companies, claim filing, and the authority of TDI. There is also a section about getting help from TDI as well as other frequently asked questions. Finally, there is contact information for various other sources that might be of interest to providers.[206]

Of the publications mentioned above, *Your Health Care Coverage, Health Care Coverage for Texas Children, Summary of Health Care Coverage Options for Texas Children, Medicare+Choice Options for Medicare Beneficiaries, Glossary-Common Insurance Terms, Helping You With Your Insurance Complaint, Long-Term Care Insurance,* and *HICAP Highlights—Private Fee-for-Service Plans* have been translated into Spanish.

Beyond those listed above, TDI has also translated a consumer-focused section of their website titled *Texas Department of Insurance Working for You* (translated title: *Trabajando para Usted un Guía para el Consumidor*).[207, 208] This section provides highlights of the mandated role of TDI including regulation of the insurance industry, protecting the public via enforcement actions, and consumer assistance programs and services.[209]

In addition to the materials posted on its website, TDI offers free copies of consumer publications through its toll-free publications hotline (800-599-SHOP) and provides answers to general insurance questions via its toll-free consumer help line (800-252-3439). TDI's Information Assistance operators answered about 126,000 accident- and health-related phone calls in FY 2000. Of these calls, about 19,700 were complaints, including complaints resolved by TDI and those initiated by providers.[210]

As another resource for consumer shopping for insurance coverage, TDI publishes rate guides for the following types of coverage: long-term care insurance, automobile insurance, homeowners insurance, Medicare Supplemental insurance, and workers' compensation insurance. The titles for those five guides are, respectively: *2001-2002 Texas Long-Term Care Guide, 2001-2002 Automobile Insurance Rate Guide, 2001-2002 Homeowners Insurance Rate Guide, Medicare Supplement Insurance Handbook and Rate Guide,* and *Texas Workers' Compensation Rate Guide.*[211,212, 213,214,215] Of these rate guides, the only one translated into Spanish and available on the Internet is the guide on Medicare Supplement Insurance. Notably, TDI does not currently provide a rate guide for consumers on health insurance.

Office of Public Insurance Counsel

Organizational Structure

The Texas Office of Public Insurance Council (OPIC) is an independent agency responsible for representing health insurance consumers in hearings before TDI, the State Office of Administrative Hearings, other state agencies, and the courts on issues involving insurance rates, rules and policy forms, among others.[216] The purpose of creating OPIC was to have a counterpart to the legal advocacy provided by the attorneys that work for the insurance industry in the state. OPIC has a staff of 19, including an executive director known as the public counsel, attorneys, an economist, researchers, and support staff. All of the staff members are located in the OPIC office in Austin, as there are no field OPIC offices located elsewhere in the state. The public counsel is appointed by the governor and confirmed by the senate to a two-year term. The public counsel is responsible for all administrative and legal decisions and has authority over the day-to-day operations of the agency. Appointed by then-governor Bush in 1995, Rod Bordelon is currently serving as public counsel.[217]

Current Enforcement/Regulatory Efforts

The statutory authority of OPIC can be found in the Texas Insurance Code (Article 1.35A). In Article 1.35B, OPIC is given the authority to collect funds on behalf of the state's consumers. The agency's enforcement and regulatory efforts are directed at "administrative rulemaking, ratemaking, and policy form approval, primarily before TDI." In other words, the functions of OPIC are mainly dependent on the scope of authority of TDI. [218]

In Texas, for example, the rating system for personal property and automobile insurance is called the "flexband rating system." Once a benchmark rate is set, insurance providers are allowed to deviate from that rate up to 30 percent (above or below the benchmark rate). To deviate any further than that percentage, insurance companies must file a request for approval with TDI. As part of Texas' rating system, annual hearings are held to determine the current benchmark rate. At the State Office of Administrative Hearings (SOAH), an administrative law judge precedes over these benchmark-setting hearings. According to its statutory mandate, OPIC acts as the representative and advocate for the state's insurance consumers. In turn, other attorneys represent the insurance industry and any other interested or relevant parties. As a result of these hearings, SOAH provides recommendations regarding rates to TDI. The Insurance Commissioner acts as "the final arbiter" and makes the decision regarding any change to the existing benchmark rate.[219,220]

In issues related to property and casualty, title, and credit insurance, OPIC has represented Texas consumers regarding "rates, rules, and forms."[221] With regard to life, accident, and health insurance, OPIC has represented consumers of the state only regarding "rulemaking." In rulemaking hearings (which specifically impact life, accident, and health insurance), the Insurance Commissioner listens to presentations from OPIC (as the main representative of consumers) and then from those representing the industry entities. The Commissioner may also seek out the advice of his/her staff. As with changes to the rating system for personal property and automobile insurance, the Insurance Commissioner will make the final decision regarding any proposals or changes to existing rules.[222]

According to the agency description on the OPIC website, "OPIC advocates for lower insurance rates rules that are advantageous to consumers." However, OPIC does not represent consumers as individuals, but rather as a class. Further, OPIC will not "act on individual complaints," but may become involved when the sum of individual complaints "suggest a widespread pattern of practices…" by insurance companies in the state.[223] Individual consumers can file specific complaints through TDI. On the TDI website, consumers can use online forms to file complaints regarding life/health insurance, automobile/homeowners insurance, real estate/title insurance, and physician/providers.[224]

Beyond specific duties at administrative hearings and proceedings, OPIC works generally with members of the state legislature and the Office of the Governor to research insurance matters, as requested. As a result of these requests or research on timely and significant insurance topics, OPIC may publish special reports or other publications. [Currently, the three special insurance interest publications posted on or linked to from the OPIC website are: *A Review of Health Insurance Underwriting Guidelines Used in Texas* (posted),[225] *Health Insurance Coverage in Texas: Context and Demographics*, a

1998 OPIC report submitted to the Senate Interim Committee on Children's Health Insurance (posted),[226] and *Current Population Reports* by the U.S. Census Bureau focusing on health insurance coverage in the United States published in 1997 (link).[227]] Further, as part of its more general role of protecting Texas consumers, OPIC works with TDI, insurance companies, consumer advocacy groups, and interested parties to "resolve problems for consumers as a class." OPIC is also responsible for making recommendations to the Insurance Commissioner regarding candidates for positions on insurance-related boards and committees.[228]

OPIC has developed and produced a Consumer Bills of Rights for the following types of insurance coverage: automobile, homeowners, and credit. The purpose of these publications is to summarize "the rights under Texas statues and rules that apply to consumers of personal lines of insurance." OPIC has not produced a Consumer Bill of Rights for health insurance.[229]

Current Consumer Education Efforts

Over the past several years, OPIC has had to dramatically limit the number of consumer publications to maximize funds. It now sends out material to media sources to allow for a reduction in the number of publications.[230] One publication that OPIC still makes available is the annual HMO report card. The report card can be viewed on the OPIC website or, alternatively, OPIC will send a hard copy upon request.[231] Information on health insurance provided by OPIC is limited, consisting mainly of yearly HMO report cards for seven regions across the state (e.g, "Comparing Texas HMOs, 2000, Central Texas"), in both English and Spanish.[232] Report cards provide standardized measures of quality across all Texas HMOs based on survey data but do not include rates. The report card measures are based on the results of a survey that shows the level of satisfaction of consumers. The publication is designed to help consumers make informed decisions regarding the different HMOs when they are making health care decisions.[233] The agency makes an effort to publicize the existence of these annual HMO report cards by issuing press releases to the media. The media is then expected to inform the public about the report cards.[234]

Texas Health Care Information Council

Organizational Structure

The Texas Health Care Information Council (THCIC) was formed in 1995 and is responsible for providing data on the quality and performance of HMOs in order to help Texas consumers make informed health care decisions.[235] In essence, THCIC is in charge of collecting and maintaining a database of information on different HMOs and hospitals. THCIC is governed by a 19-member board of directors; with 15 of the members are stakeholders of the Texas health care delivery system and the remaining four members are representatives of the four agencies dealing with health or health insurance.[236]

Current Consumer Education Efforts

THCIC offers similar HMO ratings to those offered by OPIC. Called "Straight Talk on Texas HMOs: A Purchaser's Guide, 2001," this guide reports on quality of care for 25 basic service HMOs in Texas.[237] Its intended audience is employer benefits specialists who advise employees on health insurance purchasing decisions. A more consumer-oriented guide published by THCIC is called "Your HMO Quality Check-up: A Consumer's Guide to Texas Commercial HMOs."[238] This guide, published by region, provides fewer measures than does the Purchaser's Guide, and focuses more on preventive services offered by Texas HMOs.

Additional Education Resources

The Institute for Health Care Research and Policy at Georgetown University, funded by a grant from the Robert Wood Johnson Foundation, produced consumers' guides to health insurance for all 50 states. The guide for Texas is entitled "A Consumer's Guide to Getting and Keeping Health Insurance in Texas" and is intended to help consumers understand their rights under Texas state and federal law. [239] It includes separate sections for protections under group health plans, individual health plans, and small group plans. An updated version of this primarily legal guide would be an important component of any centralized information center for private health insurance consumers.

Lastly, the Health Law and Policy Institute at the University of Houston Law Center provides a guide for small employers on purchasing health insurance for employees. The "Small Employers Guide to Health Care Plans" outlines types of small group insurance plans, rights of small business owners in obtaining and keeping health insurance, how to evaluate plans, how to apply for coverage, and additional resources to consult for more answers. [240] Although it is unclear when this guide was written, it could potentially provide a template for similar guides for different audiences.

Education Efforts in Other States

Consumer Health Assistance Programs: A National Trend

Many consumers, for a variety of reasons, have become overwhelmed by the sheer complexity of the health care systems and health insurance markets in the U.S. In response to this consumer need, there has been a nationwide trend of developing and establishing consumer health assistance programs, otherwise known as ombudsman programs. The purposes and scope of outreach of these programs—operating at the national, state, and even local levels—are very diverse. For example, in terms of scope of outreach, some programs focus on serving consumers with particular health problems such as physical disabilities while others are based in certain health care settings, such as long-term care facilities. Across the country, the purposes of the programs also differ widely. Some programs specifically help consumers to find resolutions to problems with their private health insurance providers. Other programs assist consumers with coverage in certain publicly sponsored programs such as Medicare or Medicaid. Still other programs work to address general insurance problems and help consumers who have either public or private coverage, or to help individuals who do not have any type of insurance coverage negotiate with health care providers.[241]

Background on Federally-Mandated Consumer Health Assistance Programs

Federal law mandates that all 50 states have consumer health assistance programs to meet at least certain types of needs of various segments of the health care consumer population. States must provide three types of programs: Long-Term Care Ombudsman Programs, Protection and Advocacy (PandA) Programs, and State Health Insurance Assistance Programs (SHIPs).

Started in 1972 as demonstration projects in five states, the first type of consumer assistance programs, Long-Term Care Programs, "investigate and resolve complaints involving care in nursing homes (and, in some states, other residential settings), represent the interests of nursing home residents before government agencies, and work to protect residents' rights."[242] In 1978, Congress passed the Older Americans Act and each state was mandated to either establish its own long-term care ombudsman program or to contract with a nonprofit organization or a public agency to provide ombudsman services. The U.S. Administration on Aging supports the National Long Term Care Ombudsman Resource Center, which is operated by the National Citizens' Coalition on Nursing Home Reform and generally provides technical assistance, research, and cooperation among long-term assistance programs across the country. Some states include programs both at the state level and at the local level. In FY 1998, the majority of programs (including 35 states and Puerto Rico) were part of the state agency focusing on the aging population. The programs in 15 other states and the District of Columbia were operated as part of other government ombudsman programs, as a separate entity (outside of the state agency focusing on the aging population), or under state contracts by private non-profit agencies.[243]

Begun in 1975 as part of the passage of the Developmental Disabilities Assistance and Bill of Rights by Congress, the second type of consumer assistance programs, PandA Programs, are "authorized under five federal laws to pursue legal, administrative, and other remedies to protect and advocate for the rights of individuals with disabilities." According to federal law, the governors of all 50 states must assign this ombudsman function to a state agency. Like long-term care ombudsman programs, these consumer health assistance programs also receive significant technical support at a national level. The Advocacy Training Technical Assistance Center (ATTC) provides support to these programs in many forms including: developing and distributing publications, providing trainings and conferences, acting as a clearinghouse by distributing model policies, and supplying technical assistance. However, unlike long-term care ombudsman programs, PandA programs "are not required to analyze data on consumer problems or recommend ways to address those problems."[244]

Finally, the third type of consumer assistance programs, SHIPs, focus exclusively on helping those eligible and/or enrolled in Medicare. The focus of SHIPs is to "educate consumers about benefits and claims procedures for Medicare (and Medicaid as well, when necessary), provide information about other types of insurance to supplement

Medicare (so-called "Medigap" policies), and refer consumers to government agencies that can help resolve problems related to health insurance."[245]

Started in 1990, SHIPs were begun as a response to a Congressional mandate to the U.S. Department of Health and Human Services (DHHS), to offer a "health insurance advisory service" for beneficiaries of Medicare. States are able to apply for DHHS grants through the Centers for Medicare and Medicaid Services (CMS) to set up a SHIP for their populations. All 50 states, the Virgin Islands, and Puerto Rico are eligible for this funding through CMS. At the state level, SHIPs are also referred to as SHINE, SHIBA, HICAP, and other names. States and local communities also provide additional funding for these consumer assistance programs. In 36 states, SHIPs were operated through the agencies serving the aging. The rest of the states and U.S. territories have established SHIPs through their departments of insurance or through insurance commissions. In addition to the scope of outreach offered through the operating center of the SHIP (through the aging services agency for example), outreach and counseling on Medicare is offered through local sponsoring organizations. These local sponsoring organizations include social service entities that serve the aging, hospitals, and other general community-based organizations.

Initially, SHIPs focused only on the Medicare populations answering consumer questions regarding Medicare supplemental insurance, also known as Medigap insurance. SHIPs, though, have expanded their services to provide consumers with assistance (counseling and information) on issues related to Medigap, Medicaid, and Medicare. In particular, SHIPs have worked with consumers on resolving problems they encountered with managed care. By law, SHIPs can and are expected to make policy recommendations regarding issues impacting the populations they serve. Recommendations from SHIPs are made to "the appropriate state and federal agencies" that presumably can then take any appropriate further action, if necessary.[246]

Background on State-Sponsored Consumer Health Assistance Programs

In addition to the federally mandated programs mentioned above, there are consumer health assistance programs that have not been mandated by federal law. Instead, these additional programs have been initiated at the state level. Generally speaking, these state-sponsored programs are in two categories: (1) programs that focus on serving Medicaid populations, and (2) programs that focus more broadly on "general health care."[247]

<u>Medicaid-Focused Programs at the State and Local Levels</u>

The programs in the first category, those that focus on serving Medicaid beneficiaries, have varying purposes. Many of the states that began these programs wanted to deliver education to consumers on the following issues: managed care, enrollment, and access in relation to the Medicaid program. These programs can count as "administrative expenses" under the state-federal matching arrangement; therefore, states can use federal matching funds to maintain this consumer education effort. Some programs function in the advocacy role and can "represent them [consumers] through the grievance and appeals process" if necessary. Other programs act as a mediator for Medicaid beneficiaries but do not play a role in grievance and appeals processes.

These programs are structured quite differently from state to state and city to city. Sometimes government agencies (at either the state or local level) administering the state's Medicaid program will contract with nonprofit organizations to handle the education services for Medicaid beneficiaries. In other states, nonprofit organizations are privately funded (no state or municipal funding is provided) to help individuals and families covered by Medicaid, the State Children's Health Insurance Program (SCHIP), and/or private insurance. Some states will provide ombudsman services, including education and counseling, as part of a separate government agency (not within the Medicaid-administering agency itself). In contrast, other states have added ombudsman services within the Medicaid agency. Some of the states and cities with these Medicaid ombudsman programs include: Colorado, Connecticut, Rhode Island, Maryland, District of Columbia, California, Utah, Maine, Missouri, North Carolina, Indiana, Louisiana, New Mexico, Tennessee, Vermont, Kentucky, Mississippi, and New York City.[248]

General Health Care-Focused Programs at the State and Local Levels

The programs in the second category, those that focus on assisting a range of segments of the health consumer population rather than only Medicaid beneficiaries, also have a broad array of purposes and functions. Certain states only serve those with private coverage through the ombudsman program. Still others may simultaneously help consumers with private insurance, consumers with public insurance, and the uninsured. Some states have passed laws to establish new and separate consumer assistance programs. In others, ombudsman services are provided out of the state attorney general's office, the governor's office, or the insurance department. At the municipal level, some of the larger cities such as New York City have established program through city-wide agencies or by contracting out ombudsman services through a local community-based nonprofit organization. In the case of states with no specific legislation creating a mandate for a consumer assistance program, some have found ways of using laws already in place to set up their programs. For example, states may have broad consumer protection statutes and/or insurance regulations that allow for the addition of a consumer assistance unit, characteristically as part of the work of the state attorney general or the state insurance department or commission. Some of the states and cities with these general health care-focused ombudsman programs include California, Illinois, Pennsylvania, Connecticut, Florida, Georgia, Maryland, Maine, Nevada, Texas, Vermont, Chicago, and New York City.[249]

A New Nationwide Study: Measuring the Impact of Consumer Health Assistance Programs

In June of 2001, Families USA, a not-for-profit advocacy organization based in Washington, D.C. that represents the interests of health care consumers, surveyed programs throughout the country. Because of the wide range of diversity in form and function of programs, Families USA developed the following definition for programs to be included in this national survey: "a program independent of health facilities and/or health plans whose primary purposes are (1) to educate consumers about their health care rights and responsibilities and (2) to identify, investigate, and resolve consumers' complaints about health care services."[250]

Beyond finding out the specific services that these programs provide for consumers, the authors of final report on the study, *Consumer Health Assistance Programs: Report on a National Survey*, point out that these programs "...not only provide crucial services to people who encounter problems with the health care system, they serve as the eyes and ears of policymakers, health care providers, and government agencies seeking to improve the management and delivery of health care services to diverse populations."[251]

The methodology of the survey consisted of a written questionnaire mailed out to a wide range of the consumer assistance programs (with a postage-paid reply envelope) and in-depth telephone interviews with 69 programs of varying types. Highlights of the research findings of this study reveal successful outcomes on a number of levels:

- Over two-thirds of cases handled by consumer assistance programs are resolved in the favor of the consumers involved.
- Almost 100 percent of cases are handled without a need for litigation.
- One-fourth to one-third of consumer assistance programs use the data gathered to report to policymakers and other interested parties and to make policy recommendations, as needed.
- In FY 1998, 201,053 complaints were filed with long-term care ombudsman programs and, of those complaints, 121,686 cases were closed.
- PandA programs were able to assist 274,542 consumers through information and referrals and also represented 66,962 consumers in appeals and grievances processes.
- From the fall of 1999 to fall of 2000, SHIPs had 343,405 in-person contacts with consumers and 878,320 over-the-phone contacts with consumers.
- The majority of consumer assistance programs provide help to somewhere between 800 and 2,000 consumers a year.
- SHIPs that operate at a state level provide assistance to approximately 33,500 consumers per year.
- In general, programs report that, according to the date collected, the consumers served approximately reflect the ethnic and racial make-up of the U.S. population.
- Of the statewide SHIPs, PandA programs, Medicaid, and general consumer health assistance programs surveyed in this study, half reported having a member of their staff who was bilingual.
- Long-term care programs and local SHIPs did not have as high a percentage of bilingual staff members (used interpreters and resources from local community-based organizations to reach out and help multi-lingual and multi-cultural populations).[252]

Unfortunately, currently there is no comprehensive national statistical information on how many people are assisted by programs initiated and provided at the state and/or municipal level.

Taking the results of the survey, Families USA concluded that the services provided by various types of consumer assistance programs can be categorized as the following: (1) direct assistance to consumers, (2) community outreach and education, and (3) data collection used to give policymakers and other health policy stakeholders feedback and recommendations. Table 8.1 shows the percentage breakdown of the activities and services provided by the responding consumer assistance programs.

Table 8.1
Program Activities of Consumer Health Assistance Programs

	Percent of programs, by program type, performing these activities						
	State SHIP	Local SHIP	State Long-Term Care	Local Long-Term Care	Protection and Advocacy	Medicaid	General
ASSIST INDIVIDUAL CONSUMERS	100%	98.4%	100%	98.9%	100%	100%	100%
Investigate complaint	85%	78.2%	95.5%	96.6%	92.9%	85.7%	89.3%
Empower consumers to resolve own issues by providing technical assistance	95%	84.7%	100%	93.1%	100%	78.6%	92.9%
Write letters/make calls on consumers' behalf	90%	90.3%	100%	88.5%	100%	78.6%	92.9%
Represent consumers in formal grievance reviews	50%	60.3%	66.7%	65.1%	100%	46.2%	40.7%
Follow case through to complaint resolution	70%	73.4%	95.5%	95.4%	92.9%	85.7%	82.1%
ASSIST GROUPS OF CONSUMERS	55%	37.1%	77.3%	79.3%	85.7%	35.7%	42.9%
OUTREACH AND EDUCATION	100%	96.0%	95.5%	100%	100%	93.3%	89.3%
Provide outreach	100%	96.0%	95.5%	97.7%	92.9%	92.9%	89.3%
Develop educational materials	100%	60.5%	90.9%	74.7%	92.9%	71.4%	85.7%
Train community org./providers	90%	52.4%	90.9%	87.4%	71.4%	57.1%	50.0%
OTHER ACTIVITIES (collect data, prepare/distribute reports, other)	75%	64.0%	90.9%	96.6%	71.4%	86.7%	89.3%

Adapted from: Families USA, "Program Activities of Consumer Health Assistance Programs," table in *Consumer Health Assistance Programs: Report on a National Survey* (Washington, D.C., June 2001), p. 9.

As part of the third category, community outreach and education, many programs develop educational materials and use other methods to explain their rights to the consumer public. Table 8.2 shows the percentage breakdown of the methods used by the responding consumer assistance programs to educate the public.

Table 8.2
How Consumer Assistance Programs Inform the Public of their Rights

	Percent of programs, by type, using each method to inform the public of their rights					
	State SHIP	Local SHIP	State long-term care	Local long-term care	Protection and advocacy	General
Speaking Engagements	95.0%	82.8%	95.5%	94.3%	85.7%	85.7%
Media	70.0%	63.3%	77.3%	59.8%	42.9%	67.9%
Written Materials	90.0%	76.6%	77.3%	78.2%	92.9%	71.4%
Materials in other languages	55.0%	22.7%	45.5%	27.6%	57.1%	32.1%
Low-literacy materials	25.0%	23.4%	13.6%	11.5%	42.9%	28.6%
Website	55.0%	21.1%	59.1%	37.9%	64.3%	78.6%
Audiotapes/recorded messages	5.0%	6.3%	13.6%	12.6%	42.9%	7.1%
Train community organizations' staff	50.0%	26.6%	22.7%	32.2%	35.7%	32.1%
Other	0.0%	9.4%	9.1%	5.7%	7.1%	10.7%

Adapted from: Families USA, "How Programs Inform the Public of Their Rights," table in *Consumer Health Assistance Programs: Report on a National Survey* (Washington, D.C., June 2001), p. 14.

Most importantly, programs must educate the public about the resource of the consumer assistance programs themselves. There are a variety of methods that programs use, from yellow page listings to distributing brochures and flyers and from going through insurers/providers to speaking at community events. The table below shows the percentage breakdown of the methods used by the responding consumer assistance programs to inform the public about their existence and services available to them as consumers.

Table 8.3
Methods Used by Consumer Assistance Programs to Publicize their Programs to the Public

Method	Percent of program using each method to publicize program, by program type						
	State SHIP	Local SHIP	State long-term care	Local long-term care	Protection and advocacy	Medicaid	General
Through insurers/ providers	85.0%	50.0%	45.5%	39.1%	21.4%	86.7%	53.6%
Adverse action notices	25.0%	19.5%	40.9%	19.5%	14.3%	53.3%	46.4%
Post in public agencies/providers	80.0%	73.4%	81.8%	74.7%	92.9%	73.3%	64.3%
Purchasers	5.0%	5.5%	0.0%	3.4%	0.0%	6.7%	3.6%
Government agencies	100%	75.8%	90.9%	78.2%	71.4%	60.0%	57.1%
Yellow pages listings	45.0%	32.0%	22.7%	25.3%	28.6%	46.7%	32.1%
Brochures/flyers	100%	90.6%	95.5%	92.0%	92.9%	73.3%	75.0%
Materials in languages other than English	75.0%	35.2%	59.1%	33.3%	64.3%	53.3%	28.6%
PSAs/media	55.0%	58.6%	40.9%	46.0%	21.4%	26.7%	42.9%
Website	75.0%	31.3%	59.1%	42.5%	64.3%	40.0%	71.4%
Speak at community meetings/events	95.0%	86.7%	90.9%	86.2%	78.6%	60.0%	85.7%
Arrangements with neighborhood organizations	25.0%	18.0%	0.0%	8.0%	21.4%	26.7%	14.3%
Ride circuit	20.0%	20.3%	31.8%	29.9%	42.9%	20.0%	3.6%
Other	10.0%	8.6%	13.6%	6.9%	14.3%	20.0%	14.3%

Adapted from: Families USA, "Methods of Publicizing Program," table in *Consumer Health Assistance Programs: Report on a National Survey* (Washington, D.C., June 2001), p. 12.

In addition to sharing information about delivering their prescribed services, a few responding programs in the survey also shared their experiences in making policy recommendations that ultimately impacted the delivery of health care, strengthened consumer protections, and led to stronger insurance regulations. Programs that are allowed to "recommend improvements and advocate policy change have paved the way for numerous changes in health care policies and regulations that benefit consumers."[253] Few of the programs make such recommendations. Consumer assistance programs that gather data and report that data to policymakers "in ways that paint meaningful pictures" are able to make significant policy recommendations.[254] The table below presents the percentage breakdown of the data gathered and reported by the various types of consumer assistance programs.

Table 8.4
Data Reported by Consumer Assistance Programs

	State SHIP	Local SHIP	State long-term care	Local long-term care	Protection and advocacy	Medicaid	General
Number of consumers served	88.9%	89.1%	81.0%	81.0%	100.0%	73.3%	73.1%
Number of complaints received	50.0%	52.9%	90.5%	89.3%	76.9%	73.3%	69.2%
Number of complaints resolved	27.8%	42.9%	90.5%	88.1%	69.2%	60.0%	61.5%
Type of problem	77.8%	75.6%	95.2%	85.7%	92.3%	66.7%	73.1%
Referral source	44.4%	47.9%	47.6%	72.6%	23.1%	46.7%	46.2%
Amount of time required to resolve	33.3%	28.6%	28.6%	54.8%	7.7%	26.7%	26.9%
How complaint resolved	38.9%	42.9%	47.6%	70.2%	76.9%	46.7%	34.6%
Source of complaint	16.7%	26.9%	38.1%	58.3%	7.7%	66.7%	50.0%
Type of service provided	44.4%	62.2%	71.4%	58.3%	100%	60.0%	46.2%
Whether formal grievances filed	11.1%	31.1%	19.0%	34.5%	30.8%	53.3%	26.9%
Consumer's insurance source	16.7%	36.1%	14.3%	16.7%	7.7%	33.3%	38.5%
Consumer's age	27.8%	58.0%	38.1%	38.1%	100%	26.7%	26.9%
Consumer's ethnicity	27.8%	54.6%	33.3%	38.1%	100%	6.7%	23.1%
Consumer's gender	27.8%	58.0%	47.6%	36.9%	100%	20.0%	26.9%

Adapted from: Families USA, "Data Reported by Programs," table in *Consumer Health Assistance Programs: Report on a National Survey* (Washington, D.C., June 2001), p. 30.

In an effort to provide further support to the existing consumer assistance programs, Families USA will launch a new Ombudsman Support Center in 2002 which they state will "provide training, technical assistance, and educational guidance to 2,200 health ombudsman offices around the country."[255]

Examples from Other States

Texas may find potential solutions to fill the education gap among the identified target audiences mentioned previously by examining education and response models developed and implemented by other states in the U.S. The states reviewed are Illinois, Indiana, and New Jersey. In addition, consumer assistance, or ombudsman, programs are reviewed in general and at the state level.

Ombudsman Programs

Consumer health assistance programs become more and more important as our health care systems increase in complexity. As these programs have begun to proliferate, certain national organizations have recognized the trend and are beginning to publish guides on how to design ombudsman offices. One such guide, "Designing a Consumer Health Assistance Program," by Families USA, enumerates nine issues for states to consider when organizing their own program. These issues are: scope, location, funding, staff, training, outreach, complaints, access, and collecting data.[256]

<u>Scope</u>

Factors to be considered when determining the scope of a state's consumer assistance program revolve around what types of health insurance plans will be covered by the program. Families USA recommends that programs be designed as broadly as possible in order to provide consumers with one central point of contact for information on all plans. In order for consumers to get the best information, though, the recommendation is that, within this broad program, specialists be trained in various aspects of the health insurance system.[257]

<u>Location</u>

The location refers not to the program's physical location but to the agency that runs the program. Existing consumer health assistance programs are operated by several types of institutions, including nonprofits, state insurance departments, and state attorney general's offices. The primary consideration in making the decision of which agency should run the program is who best would advocate for consumers without conflicts of interest. Families USA's recommendation, based on research to-date, is to contract the ombudsman program to a nonprofit organization and protect them from political pressure through multi-year contracts.[258]

<u>Funding</u>

Funding needs vary widely among consumer health assistance programs depending on what types of services the program offers. Funding sources include state funding (general revenue, special taxes or fees, tobacco settlement funds), federal matching funds and grants, and private funding. Programs described as "badly underfunded" spend $.01 per eligible consumer while a more adequately funded program spends $1.57 per eligible consumer. According to Families USA, public funding is the most desirable form of funding because it is the most stable source.[259]

<u>Staff</u>

Staff designation, like funding decisions, depends on the design of the individual state's consumer assistance program. Staff should be divided into groups by specialization so that consumers get the highest-quality help. States should consider hiring an attorney to give legal advice and trained medical professionals (doctors, nurses, or nurse practitioners) to address quality-of-care issues. Especially important are multi-lingual staff in areas that have substantial minority populations. Volunteers can be utilized, especially for community outreach activities in their own communities. Standards for volunteer performance, though, should be maintained and enforced.[260]

Training

Staff training needs will be determined by staffing and individual program structure. In addition to initial training, staff members will require continuing education and training in areas such as legal rights of the insured, structure of various health plans, grievance and appeals procedures, and ethical factors. Training budget should be determined only after consulting with other states and with other ombudsman programs within the state.[261]

Outreach

Consumer assistance programs should devote significant resources to outreach activities in two forms: educating consumers about their health care rights and publicizing the programs services to their target audience. Outreach strategies include promoting services through the insurers, advertising services through traditional media outlets, and contracting with CBOs to provide outreach services. Consumer assistance programs also distribute educational materials through hotlines, websites, and various offices. Recommendations by Families USA include requiring insurance companies to distribute information about the hotline in their initial membership materials and tracking how people find out about the program in order to better target efforts.[262]

Complaints

The crucial decision in how to handle appeals is at what point the ombudsman's office should intervene in the complaint process. Consumer assistance programs, in general, should "offer information and referrals to consumers; make calls or write letters on behalf of consumers and/or give advice on how to appeal; and represent consumers in internal grievance and administrative appeals. Although a few programs have the authority to represent consumers in litigation, this authority is not recommended because most states are not inclined to support this aspect of a proposed program.[263]

Access

Access refers to the right of the consumer assistance program to view the records of consumers that request help through the complaint process. In some states, the program can access the consumer's insurance and medical records only after the consumer has provided written consent; in others (those authorized by federal law), access is guaranteed. It is recommended that the consumer assistance program be required to obtain written authorization by the consumer before accessing medical or insurance files. Procedures should be developed to protect consumers' confidentiality.[264]

Collecting Data

Most ombudsman programs collect data on their services and end users. This information may be used in a variety of ways. The program should determine at the outset what information would be most useful to key stakeholders, such as health plans, policymakers, consumers, regulators, and the program itself. Regular means of sharing information with these stakeholders should be set up. A final consideration is that the laws establishing the program should "reflect its important role in providing information about consumers' experiences with the health care system."[265]

Illinois

The State of Illinois Department of Insurance includes a Consumer Market Division which provides oversight for "consumer protection and education programs, licenses and regulates the activities of insurance producers, and monitors the marketplace operations of insurance companies through policy analysis, complaint investigation and periodic onsite examinations."[266] Within the division, the Consumer Services Section is the main connection between the Illinois public and the Department of Insurance. Staff within the Consumer Services Section investigate and respond to consumer complaints against insurance companies. These consumer complaints target companies providing all types of insurance coverage (including health). Of the division's two Compliance Sections, the Life, Accident, and Health Compliance Section specifically focuses on investigating complaints against health maintenance organizations (HMOs) as well as on overseeing marketing materials produced by companies providing life, accident, and health insurance.[267]

Within its broad mandate, the various sections within the Consumer Market Division engage in a range of consumer assistance and education efforts. The division provides consumers a mechanism for filing complaints against insurance companies, either electronically or in hard copy. Filed complaints initiate a process of investigation by the division staff.[268] Complaint statistics are compiled and published by the department for the information of the Illinois public.[269] As an improvement on its existing complaints process, the division launched a pilot electronic complaint project. Consumer complaints submitted through e-mail are, in turn, electronically transmitted to participating insurance companies. As a result, staff reports that the response time for handling complaints has been cut by at least five days. In its *2000 Annual Report to the Governor*, the division reports that "Industry response has been quite favorable..."[270] As a supplement to its handling of consumer complaints, the division develops, updates, and provides a series of general educational materials to the public on insurance coverage. The majority of the Division's educational materials are in the form of fact sheets (available both on the Internet and in hard copy). Many of these fact sheets focus exclusively on topics related to health insurance coverage. The following is a partial list of titles of health insurance-related fact sheets:

- "Acronyms for Life, Accident, and Health Insurance and Managed Care"
- "Facts about HIPAA-Preexisting Conditions"
- "Comprehensive Health Insurance Program (SCHIP) (Coverage for Persons Who Cannot Find Health Insurance)"
- "Health Insurance Continuation Rights: COBRA"
- "Health Insurance Continuation Rights: Illinois Law"
- "Health Insurance Continuation Rights: Illinois Spousal Law"

- "Women's Health Care Issues"
- "Insurance Coverage for Newborn Children"
- "Coordination of Benefits (COB)"
- "Health Maintenance Organization (HMOs)"
- "Health Insurance for Small Employers"
- "The Small Employer Health Insurance Rating Act"
- "Individual Major Medical Insurance"
- "Illinois Insurance Facts: Insurance for College Students"
- "Frequently Asked Questions: Individual Accident and Health Insurance"[271,272]

Lastly, the division has set up a toll-free Consumer Assistance Hotline for consumers to use for general queries regarding insurance coverage. (There are a total of three consumer hotlines, including the division's consumer hotline for general insurance queries, the Senior Health Insurance Program's hotline for queries from Medicare beneficiaries and their caregivers, and a newly launched health-insurance-specific hotline.)

In addition to these existing divisions and sections within the Department of Insurance, in 2000 the state of Illinois established the Office of Consumer Health Insurance (OCHI). OCHI was created as part of a provision of that state's recently passed Managed Care Reform and Patients Rights Act (effective as of January 2, 2000) which expands the rights of consumers under health care plans through tighter requirements of insurance companies and health care providers.[273] The stated mission of OCHI is to "assist consumers with health related issues and to report trends in the health insurance marketplace."[274] Presumably addressing individual consumers who visit online, the department states on its website that the OCHI staff can "explain your rights as a health care consumer; answer your questions about health insurance; help you understand the coverage provisions of your specific health care plan; and assist you when you have a problem or complaint."[275]

As part of the new law, OCHI was required to set up a toll-free consumer hotline, which became operational on the same date as the law's effective date, January 2, 2000. In 2000, OCHI staff received a total of 10,750 calls from consumers seeking help. The consumer calls came from 1,042 different zip codes throughout the state and focused on a range of topics. The most notable topics of these consumer queries were (in order of frequency): specific claims (1,925), coverage continuation (1,270), and concerns about HMOs and Point of Service (POS) health insurance plans. Responding to consumer queries from the hotline, OCHI staff members also distributed educational printed materials and the division's standard Consumer Complaint Form for those consumers who wanted to submit a written complaint, electronically or through the mail.[276] The new OCHI hotline is listed with the other two consumer help lines on the department's website.[277]

New Jersey

The state of New Jersey has been fairly active in regulating its private health insurance markets. The restructuring of New Jersey's individual and small employer private health insurance markets in 1992 has allowed for increases in the number of insured as well as for more user-friendly information-gathering and enrollment processes. In addition, two Boards dedicated specifically to the individual and small employer markets have produced superior educational materials and made the state more responsive to consumer needs. Detailed below are the structure of New Jersey's health insurance regulation apparatus, the 1992 health insurance reform and its effects, and the educational materials offered by New Jersey for individuals and small employers seeking to obtain private health insurance.

<u>New Jersey Health Insurance Regulatory Agencies</u>

The agency that has responsibility for regulating health insurance in New Jersey is the Department of Banking and Insurance (DOBI).[278] Within DOBI are several offices that manage more specific aspects of the insurance industry. The Office of Life and Health Insurance, for example, disseminates information on individual health care and small employer health programs, as well as on NJ Family Care, the state program of insurance for low-income children and families.[279] The Office of Enforcement and Consumer Protection is also part of DOBI and is responsible for handling consumer complaints and questions about life and health insurance.[280] Review and approval of all individual and group health insurance contracts, as well as rates for these contracts, are handled by the Health Insurance Bureau.[281] Finally, the Managed Care Bureau provides information targeted primarily to HMOs, though its website does provide information of interest to consumers such as HMO enrollment data and financial summaries of New Jersey HMOs.[282]

<u>New Jersey Health Insurance Reform</u>

In 1992, the New Jersey Legislature created two programs designed to guarantee access regardless of health, age, insurance claims history, or other risk factors, to private health insurance for small employers and individuals. These two programs, called the Individual Health Coverage Program (IHC) and the Small Employer Health Benefits Program (SEH), were augmented by a third, the New Jersey Health Access Program, which provided subsidies for low-income individuals to purchase health insurance.[283] Both programs are run by Boards of Directors that are charged with implementing health insurance reform and regulating the insurance market.

The IHC Program was implemented in August 1993 and operates as a standardized, open enrollment, community rated market. Any individual who resides in New Jersey and does not have access to health insurance through either their employer or Medicare qualifies for the program. The IHC Program is led by its nine-member Board of Directors, some of whom are appointed by the Governor. They represent consumers, insurers, HMOs, the AFL-CIO, and the Commissioner of Insurance.[284]

There are several aspects of the IHC Program that were designed to guarantee New Jersey residents easier access to individual health insurance coverage in the private market. One of these aspects is the existence of standard plans. These plans, labeled B, C, D, E, and HMO, were designed by the Boards and are the only plans New Jersey HMOs may offer to individuals. Community rating means that carriers must offer the standard plans to all New Jersey individuals regardless of their age, gender, profession, health status, or geographical location. The combination of standard plans and the community rating methodology is what makes it possible for the Board to publish rate guides for these individual plans to guide consumers in their health insurance purchases. Two other regulations affect the individual health plans market. First, the clause regarding portability and preexisting conditions stipulates that all conditions are covered by standard plans immediately if there has been no lapse in coverage, and after up to one year if there was no prior coverage. The minimum loss ratio stipulation states that carriers participating in IHC must pay out at least $.75 in benefits for every $1 received in premiums.[285]

By the end of 1997, the IHC Program had been cited as a success in expanding the market for individual private health coverage. The number of carriers offering guaranteed issue individual coverage expanded from one prior to reform to 22 in 1997, with 154,000 individuals covered. In addition, about 15 percent of those who purchased IHC Program coverage in the fourth quarter of 1997 had been previously uninsured.[286]

The SEH Program went into effect in January 1994, beginning the sale of standardized, open-enrollment plans with modified community rating. SEH is governed by its own 18-member Board of Directors, who serve without compensation and include, among others, insurance agents, representatives of small business, and a doctor. Both the IHC and SEH Boards are State agencies and are funded by assessments of health insurers and HMOs.[287]

The small employer program was designed to be similar to the IHC program in many aspects. Standard plans B, C, D, E, and HMO are offered and small employers may also renew pre-reform plans under specific conditions. All plans must be offered on a basis of guaranteed issue/guaranteed renewal, meaning that an eligible small employer cannot be denied coverage or renewal. The modified community rating of the SEH plans lets insurers take only age, gender, family status of group employees, and location of the business into account in pricing the plan, a difference from the total community rating of the individual plans. The portability and preexisting conditions stipulation in the small employer market stipulates that a waiting period of up to six months may be imposed on the basis of a preexisting condition only on groups of 2-5 employees with no prior coverage. The minimum loss ratio in the small employer market is the same as that in the individual market.[288]

The SEH program has been judged as "highly successful" in increasing enrollment of individuals covered by small group plans.[289] Enrollment under SEH plans increased 22 percent to 847,000 over the three-year period ending in 1997. In addition, approximately 15 percent of small employers purchasing coverage during the last quarter of 1997 had had no prior coverage.[290]

New Jersey Individual and Small Employer Health Insurance Education

The launch site for an individual or small employer looking for private health coverage in New Jersey is the state's website. It is here that consumers can obtain basic information on health coverage, and link to various health programs offered in the state, such as Medicaid and charity care. This website also offers more specific information such as how to find or apply for coverage with an HMO, lists of New Jersey HMOs, and consumer report cards for these HMOs.[291]

For consumers looking specifically for individual and small employer coverage outside of the arena of publicly-subsidized health insurance, the New Jersey agency website to visit is that of the Department of Banking and Insurance and within that, the Office of Life and Health Insurance. Most of the relevant information was obtained from a website entitled "NJ Health Reform Insurance Information," a link from the Office of Life and Health Insurance on the NAIC website.[292]

The "NJ Health Reform Insurance Information" page provides documents regarding both individual and small employer health insurance plans. Listed below are the most useful educational documents on this website.[293]

- *What is NJ Health Insurance Reform?*: Provides a short but very helpful summary of the statutory aspects of the New Jersey small group and individual markets as established by the 1992 reforms.[294]
- *The New Jersey Individual Health Coverage Program, Buyer's Guide*: Includes steps to follow in obtaining coverage, eligibility rules, key features of the program, details of the delivery system, benefits provided, description of the standard plans, and examples of individuals with coverage under these plans. Also includes Frequently Asked Questions regarding most of these topics.[295]
- *New Jersey Individual Health Coverage Program Rates:* Updated monthly, these rate guides provide premium rates, by company, for a single person, an adult with child(ren), a husband and wife, and a family plan for each of the standard plans A/50, B, C, D, and HMO. Rates are given for two levels of deductibles for plans A/50 through D and four levels of co-pay for the HMO plan.[296]
- *Individual Health Care Program Carriers:* Names, addresses, and phone numbers for 17 carriers that carry individual health insurance plans in the state.[297]
- *Basic Health Benefits Plan:* Provided for each of the five standard plans, these documents serve as templates for the plans. The document for plan A/50 states: "This policy has been approved by the New Jersey Individual Health Coverage Program Board as the standard policy form for a BASIC health benefits plans (A/50)." Individuals, through these documents, can learn exactly what benefits are covered under the different standard plans and what their rights are under these plans.[298]
- Various *IHC Program Documents* provide notification of public meetings, amendments to related statutes, carrier filing deadlines, and miscellaneous rules.[299]

- *New Jersey Small Employer Health Benefits Buyer's Guide:* This guide outlines the basic regulations that apply to health plans for small employers in New Jersey. Contains information on eligibility, features/types of reform, commonly asked questions from employees, description of the standard benefits plans and what is covered.[300] From this document, one can link to summaries, or "snapshots," of the small employer standard plans.[301,302,303,304]
- *2001 Small Employer Health Benefits Premium Comparison Survey:* Provides results of an annual premium survey done by the New Jersey Department of Banking and Insurance. This survey publishes monthly premiums for a sample small employer for all standard plans in three counties in New Jersey. Premium comparison worksheets can be obtained through links from this site.[305]
- *Small Employer Carriers*: Names and phone numbers of 23 small employer carriers in the state.[306]
- *SEH Program Documents*: Include links to *Small Group Health Benefits Basic Policy* for all standard small employer plans. These documents enumerate the benefits and statutes governing each plan.[307]
- Various *SEH Program Bulletins:* provide information on amendments to related statutes, carrier filing deadlines, coverage for certain services, and miscellaneous rules.[308]

Taken together, the educational materials published by the New Jersey Individual and Small Employer Boards seem to give a comprehensive overview of the rights and benefits enjoyed by the insured in the state. These documents are included in Appendix I; some could serve as models for Texas educational materials.

Vermont

In designing a health care ombudsman program in Texas, policymakers must look to other states that have instituted similar programs. Vermont is one state that created an ombudsman fairly recently, in 1998. The Office of Health Care Ombudsman (HCO) was created by the Vermont Legislature "to advocate for Vermonters with health care and health insurance problems. In addition to advocating for individual Vermonters, we act as a public voice for Vermonters on these issues with the Vermont Legislature, United States Congress, state and federal agencies, and health insurance companies and plans."[309] More specifically, the Ombudsman is "charged with assisting consumers with selecting health plans and understanding their rights and responsibilities; providing information to the public agencies and the legislature about problems and concerns of consumers; . . . and, promoting the development of consumer organizations."[310]

The Vermont HCO is run, on contract, by Vermont Legal Aid, Inc. (VLA). A statewide organization, VLA has a history of providing advice and legal representation on health care issues, and has accumulated vast expertise in these areas. Because VLA has considerable resources around the state, these resources can be used to support the HCO program if needed.[311] As Families USA recommends, it is best for these programs to be run by a nonprofit organization in order for the organization to be free from conflicts of interest. The experience and success of Vermont's HCO, it seems, has validated this recommendation.

In addition to directly assisting Vermont health care consumers, the HCO acts as an advocate for health care consumers at the state and federal levels on issues such as access to affordable drugs, confidentiality of and access to medical records, and Medicaid coverage. The Ombudsman's office also reviews consumer education materials that were developed by other agencies and advocacy groups.[312] The office advertised its services at each one of Vermont's 14 hospitals and participated in various media outreach activities.[313] Additional outreach and publicity steps taken in the past year, which perhaps could be considered for other states' programs, include:

- Workshop at Vermont Adult Learning Conference
- Windsor County health care panel sponsored by Senator Cheryl Rivers
- Disability Forum sponsored by the Vermont Center for Independent Living
- "Aging Matters" radio show
- WCAX Special Segment
- Department of Transportation meeting regarding accessibility issues for the disabled
- Community Rounds at Fletcher Allen Health Care
- Regular articles for *The Independent*
- Presentation at the Breast Cancer Conference
- Presentation at the annual meeting of the Vermont Association of Mental Health.[314]

The Vermont HCO has now been in existence for two years, with demand for its services increasing 22 percent from the first year of operation (to 2,141 consumers using HCO services). Of all calls received in 2000, 10 percent were from consumers without insurance. In addition to the simple number of consumers helped, demand for more complex services has also increased over the two years of the program. In the year 2000, there was a 55 percent increase in the need for HCO to intervene with insurance companies, state agencies, or federal agencies on a client's behalf.[315]

The total budget for HCO for the year 2000 totaled $274,753. Total personnel costs were $197,764, and included salaries of the Health Care Ombudsman (1), Attorney (1), Health Care Counselors (5), Administrative Support, and Clerical. The remainder of the costs were operating expenses of $76,859. While it is unclear exactly how many staff members this budget supports, the seven primary assistance providers obviously constitute a low-cost program that provides benefits disproportionate to its costs.[316]

Vermont keeps track of several data points, as is recommended by the Families USA *Designing a Consumer Health Assistance Program.* In the HCO's Annual Report, all calls are broken down into categories by type of call.

Table 8.5
HCO Calls by Category

Issue Category	Description of Issue	Percentage of Calls
Access to Care	Caller has not received needed care	35%
Billing/Coverage	Care received, but claim denied or other billing issues	32%
Eligibility	For state health care programs	11%
Miscellaneous Issues	Including termination of coverage, access to medical records	9%
Consumer Education	Education about a particular issue, but not in relation to a specific denial of care or inability to access care	7%
Buying Insurance	--	5%

Adapted from: Vermont Office of Health Care Ombudsman, *Office of Health Care Ombudsman, Annual Report 2000* (Burlington, Vermont, 2000), p. 4.

Both the percentage and number of access to care and billing/coverage calls increased from 1999. The number of consumer education calls fell; this decrease is attributed to the fact that a major insurer (Kaiser Permanente) left the state in 1999, leaving more than 100,000 residents without health coverage.

Table 8.6
HCO Calls by Type of Coverage

Type of Coverage	Description of Coverage	Percentage of Calls
State Health Care Programs	Includes Medicaid, VHAP, VHAP Pharmacy, Vscript	55%
Commercial Insurance	Includes small and large group coverage and individual coverage	28%
Uninsured	--	10%
Medicare	--	7%

Adapted from: Vermont Office of Health Care Ombudsman, *Office of Health Care Ombudsman, Annual Report 2000* (Burlington, Vermont, 2000), p. 4.

The fact that Vermont has included all types of health insurance in one office is very important. As enumerated in the section regarding designing a consumer health assistance program, there are several advantages to creating a single comprehensive information source for state health insurance consumers. A centralized office costs less on the whole as overhead costs do not have to be duplicated. More importantly, it reduces the effort consumers have to make to find the help they need, increasing the likelihood that they will actually receive assistance. In addition, it makes advertising simpler and less costly and reduces the number of calls that must be referred to separate offices.

Table 8.7
Methods of Case Resolution

How Case Was Resolved	Description of Method	Percentage of Calls
Direct Intervention	Made calls/took other action on behalf of client-up to 2 hours work	47%
Brief Analysis: Advice/Referral	Referral or advice after analysis	29%
Inquiry Answered During Initial Call	--	13%
Complex Intervention	Direct intervention that took more than 2 hours work to resolve case	6%
Client Withdrew	--	5%

Adapted from: Vermont Office of Health Care Ombudsman, *Office of Health Care Ombudsman, Annual Report 2000* (Burlington, Vermont, 2000), p. 4.

While the above charts do not necessarily represent the insurance concerns of Texans, they illustrate the variety of issues addressed by any consumer assistance program or health care ombudsman. In addition, the charts can be used to advise other states on how to distribute staffing, and perhaps funding, within the agency. The Vermont agency also keeps track of program quality through a Client Satisfaction Survey, which is sent to all clients on whose behalf the program intervened.[317] This survey method represents an important way of measuring the success of the program, and can be used to justify to the legislature the program's continued existence or increased funding. Any program instituted by Texas should include some sort of comprehensive quality measures.

The HCO works with various agencies and advocacy groups in order to provide the best assistance to health care consumers. A few of the agencies HCO coordinates with are: the Health Insurance, Counseling and Assistance Program; the Banking, Insurance, Securities and Health Care Administration; the Vermont Ombudsman Project; the Governor's Commission on Women; the Community of Vermont Elders; and the Vermont Low Income Advocacy Council. Quarterly HCO reports are required to be sent to the Banking, Insurance, Securities and Health Care Administration, the Office of Vermont Health Access, and the Health Access Oversight Committee, as well as a number of interested parties.[318]

Options for Education and Regulation Reform in Texas

TexCare Partnership

The outreach work plan for 2002-2003 offers great potential for increasing enrollment in Medicaid and SCHIP in Texas. However, the state may want to consider the following suggestions as activities and materials are being developed and modified.

Include eligibility information in brochures and applications

The message that health insurance options are available to families for a maximum monthly premium of $18 has been a powerful influence to counter families' concerns about being unable to afford insurance. The new application booklets and information flyers do not include eligibility information, however. Providing an easy-to-read eligibility table (and corresponding premium rates for SCHIP) in applications and widely distributed advertising in a manner similar to the Washington program may help prevent more families from simply assuming that they do not qualify, thereby further increasing the number of applications.

Extend media campaign to "hard to reach" counties

Using the media is a key tactic to promote positive influence of TCP to families, particularly with respect to emphasizing positive experiences. Although the media campaign has reached a large number of families within the 12 state media markets, these markets do not serve 107 of the state's 254 counties. Additional advertising and TCP story coverage in rural county newspapers could attract more Medicaid and SCHIP-eligible families from these areas.

Options for Education and Regulation in the Private Sector

The following tables present options for the state of Texas to improve education and regulation that could allow more Texans to obtain access to health insurance. The tables are divided among education options for TDI, OPIC, and regulation possibilities.

Table 8.8
Education and Outreach Options for TDI

Option	Advantages	Disadvantages
Develop Marketing Plan within Consumer Protection Division	• Improves advertising and awareness of publications, hotline, and services. • Proactive rather than reactive. • Less costly because utilizes existing services.	• Requires more intense data collection. • Must market services to hard-to-reach groups so users of TDI services represent entire health consumer market.
Publish Health Insurance Rate Guide (emphasis on small group market)	• Provides benchmark rates and a starting place for small employers. • Can reduce search costs for small employers-may eliminate need to pay for multiple quotes. • Can reduce time without insurance for small employers. • Enjoys support from advocacy community. • Recommended by Blue Ribbon Task Force. • Other state models available.	• Requires new legislation. • Insurer objections. • Insurers not held to the rates in the rate guide. • Rates change quickly. • Would have to establish several defined benefits packages for which rates would be published. • Significant number of insurers.
Overcome Language Barriers-Translate All Health Insurance Materials into Spanish (and other languages, if needed)	• Hispanics comprise 58% of uninsured in Texas.[319] • Would eliminate waiting period for translation of documents. • Would present a more culturally-sensitive image of TDI. • Many consumers now may assume that publications cannot be made available in Spanish if they are not on website.	• Would require advertising of new translated materials. • Might be costly.

Option	Advantages	Disadvantages
Open Information Assistance Database to the Public	• Existing consumer assistance hotline database could be made available online to consumers through TDI website. • Database could be included as part of health care ombudsman's office, if implemented. • TDI currently has long-range plans to implement this option. • Not costly.	• Requires that database be made "consumer-friendly."
Centralized Location of Information	• Significantly reduces search time for all consumers. • Should be part of health care ombudsman's office if implemented.	• Requires coordination between all agencies that provide health insurance education.

Table 8.9
Education and Outreach Options for OPIC

Option	Advantages	Disadvantages
Consumer Bill of Rights	• Gives OPIC a more solid basis for consumer protection and advocacy. • Provides all consumers with a comprehensive source of rights related to health insurance. • Equalizes protections provided to consumers with automobile and homeowners insurance.	• Requires coordination between TDI and OPIC in creating the Bill of Rights and following through on consumer protection efforts.

Option	Advantages	Disadvantages
Expand Agency Resources for Publication	• As the voice of "insurance consumers as a class," OPIC is uniquely positioned to educate consumers about their health insurance rights. • Educational materials should be targeted to specific audiences such as small groups, individuals, etc.	• Efforts would have to be coordinated with TDI.
Enhance Consumer Advocacy Activities	• If rate guide option is implemented, OPIC may have greater advocacy powers in relation to setting index rates for health plans (like it does now for personal property insurance). • In absence of health care ombudsman, OPIC could be designated a "special state health insurance advocate ... on behalf of small businesses."[320]	• Additional resources may be needed at OPIC to expand activities. • Any expanded advocacy activities will require advertising to inform consumers. • A special small business advocacy program would necessitate intense training of several employees to serve this target group.
Establish Health Care Consumer Assistance (Ombudsman) Program	• Well-publicized during 77th Legislature; still has strong support among various stakeholders. • Incorporates and consolidates many individual education options at a lesser cost ($1.3 million in year 1; $1.6 million thereafter). • Would serve *all* health care consumers regardless of type of health plan. • Creates central clearinghouse of health insurance information; collects data; represents consumers at hearings. • Would supplement current TDI services.	• Vetoed by Governor in 2001 because of inadequate appropriations. • Services have to be coordinated with TDI and OPIC to avoid duplication. • Confusion among stakeholders about purpose and services.

Table 8.10
Options for Regulation

Option	Advantages	Disadvantages
Revise the Small Employer Standard Plans	• Low current enrollment in Basic and Catastrophic plans evidences need for revision. • Revising and increasing enrollment in standard plans raises effectiveness of rate guide. • Once plans are revised, informing consumers of new plans can be accomplished through options listed above.	• Requires cooperation among all stakeholders in small employer market.

Research and Findings: The Blurring of the Lines Between Public and Private Insurance

A Need for Coordination Between State Agencies Focusing on Both Public and Private Education and Outreach

Thus far, the research and findings have focused strictly on ways to reach out to and educate consumers as a cost effective way to increase enrollment in either private insurance plans or public insurance plans. The options in the following table do not focus entirely on consumers who qualify for public programs or those who qualify for private coverage, but rather these options blur the line between private and public options presented previously. There is a need for greater coordination between state agencies that focus on the private insurance market (TDI, OPIC, etc) and state agencies that focus on the public insurance programs (CHIP, Medicaid, Medicare). Several state agency officials have recognized the need for the coordination of education and outreach efforts.[321,322] Given this acknowledged need, the following options are low-cost, smaller-scale education and outreach efforts that can be undertaken to decrease the number of uninsured in Texas.

Table 8.11
Options for State Agencies that Blur the Line between Public and Private Insurance

Option	Advantages	Disadvantages
Educate Small Businesses about SCHIP Coverage for Employees' Children	• Cost of family coverage through small employer is often prohibitive. • Employees often do not know children are eligible for public insurance. • Links public and private insurance options. • Could be incorporated in mailings of tax statements by the Texas Workforce Commission. • Effort initialized by HB 3038 in 2001.	• Requires new educational materials (pamphlets) to be designed and produced by TDI. • Would have to be coordinated with HB 3038 effort.
One-on-One Assistance Program	• Can emulate HICAP program for elderly. • Training infrastructure already in place. • Would provide needed education/outreach in hard-to-reach communities.	• Requires training and hiring of new employees. • Not clear how much this resource would be utilized.
Educate Small Businesses on Recent Insurance Reforms (see specific options below)	• State Planning Grant efforts indicate the importance of this option. • Understanding rights is critical to obtaining and using health insurance. • Could be implemented as part of health care ombudsman's office.	

Option	Advantages	Disadvantages
Community Health Insurance Fair	• Allows for one-on-one, in-person assistance. • Would bring together small business owners, individuals, agents, state agencies, and insurance companies. • Could be funded through corporate sponsorship. • Could be locally marketed as "Health Insurance 101." • Creates a win-win situation for both the state regulators in reaching out to the community, the industry by bringing in more clients, and the consumers by providing access to education. • Also serves as an opportunity to educate small employers and individual consumers about public programs.	• Targets a single community at a time rather than any statewide initiatives.
Work with Media to Publicize Small Group Reforms	• Consists of advertising resources that currently exist.	• Could be costly.
Distribute Information to Small Employers through Mailings	• Could be incorporated into mailings of tax statements by the Texas Workforce Commission. • Uses already-existing educational materials.	• Requires cooperation with outside agencies. • Requires significant financial resources and staff time (estimated cost: $30,000 per mailing)[323]

Conclusions

Public sector education and outreach strategies have been enormously successful in increasing the enrollment of Texas children in the SCHIP program. Efforts to insure additional Texans through private health plans may benefit from employing some of these same strategies. Education and outreach efforts focusing on the private health insurance market could be improved through a more directed strategic marketing plan (such as the plan utilized in SCHIP). Further, increased collaboration between state agencies that focus on the private insurance market (TDI, OPIC, etc) and those that focus on public insurance programs (CHIP, Medicaid, Medicare) may reduce the number of Texans without health insurance. Such efforts may insure additional Texans through private insurance plans, thereby possibly reducing the costs of public insurance programs at the state level. Finally, increasing the number of insured Texans may potentially decrease the amount of charity care and the amount of unpaid care provided through the hospital systems.

Two state agencies, the Texas Department of Insurance and the Office of Public Insurance Counsel, have the potential to play a greater role in educating consumers about the private health insurance market. As the key agency for providing information on private health plans, TDI might increase its advertising efforts in order to make consumers aware of the costs and benefits of private insurance plans. Options for expanding education and outreach efforts that could be examined include: translating all health insurance materials into Spanish and other languages; creating additional consumer resources such as a central information location and an online interactive database; and, distributing information to small employers regarding recent insurance reforms. TDI's efforts in developing and distributing a health insurance rate guide might prove to be valuable to small employers. The Office of Public Insurance Counsel could also consider strengthening its role in protecting health insurance consumers. In collaboration with TDI, OPIC may consider expanding its ability to provide consumers with a clearer understanding of their health insurance rights. This might be accomplished through the creation of a Consumer Bill of Rights or additional consumer education publications. Lastly, the establishment of an ombudsman program (following the example of other states) could possibly create a cost-effective means of informing all consumers about their health insurance options.

Health insurance ranks as the job benefit of primary importance for employees. Thus it is important for employers, especially small businesses, to be able to offer affordable health insurance in order to attract high-quality employees, both within Texas and from other states.[324] Given its notably high proportion of residents without health insurance, Texas should undertake an examination of the policy options presented in this report. The outlined options may serve as a cost-effective means of reducing the number of uninsured Texans. Moreover, implementing such options might lead to a more desirable job market and the spurring of economic development within the state.

Notes

[1] Texas Department of Insurance, State Planning Grant Division, *Texas State Planning Grant Interim Report* (Austin, Tex., October 2001). Online. Available: http://spg.tdi.state.tx.us/pubs/interim. Accessed: January 26, 2002.

[2] Texas Department of Insurance, *Working Together for a Healthy Texas*. Online. Available: http://spg.tdi.state.tx.us/pubs/final/index.html. Accessed: April 17, 2002.

[3] Ann Lessem, James Dyer, Steve Borders, and Jason Vendel, "Uninsured Texans: Attitudes Toward Coverage" (paper presented at conference on "Working Together for a Healthy Texas: Expanding Health Insurance Coverage for Texans," Texas State Planning Grant Conference, Austin, Tex., January 31-February 1, 2002), pp. 1-227.

[4] Ibid.

[5] Class presentation by Jose Marrero, President, JAM Creative, at the Lyndon B. Johnson School of Public Affairs, Austin, Texas, November 6, 2001.

[6] Lessem, Dyer, Borders, and Vendel, "Uninsured Texans: Attitudes Toward Coverage," pp. 1-22.

[7] Ibid., pp. 54-62.

[8] Ibid.

[9] TexCare Partnership, *TexCare Partnership Statewide Outreach Initiatives, September 2000—August 2001* (June 2001). Online. Available: http://www.hhsc.state.tx.us/CHIP/cnews/TCP_Initiatives.pdf. Accessed: November 17, 2001.

[10] Texas Education Agency, "Building Bridges to Healthy Kids and Better Students: Strengthening School-Based Outreach and Enrollment for Health Insurance" (Austin, Tex., February 2002), n. p.

[11] Interview by Daniel Starr with Kimberly Davis, Director of Medicaid and CHIP Outreach, Texas Health and Human Services Commission, Austin, Texas, January 18, 2002.

[12] Email from Kimberly Davis, Director of Medicaid and SCHIP Outreach, Texas Health and Human Services Commission, "TexCare Partnership Outreach Workplan 2002-2003—Revised," to Daniel Starr, February 26, 2002.

[13] Covering Kids, *Project Alberto: Texas Outreach Initiative*. Online. Available: http://www.coveringkids.org/projects/state.php3?StateID=TX. Accessed: November 5, 2001.

[14] Texas Association of Community Health Centers, *Project Alberto Report* (Austin, Tex., 2000), p. 8.

[15] Texas Health and Human Services Commission, *Children's Medicaid Simplification—Senate Bill 43 Proposed Implementation Outline* (November 2001). Online. Available: http://www.hhsc.state.tx.us/CHIP/sb43/sb43_simplification_intro.html. Accessed: November 13, 2001.

[16] Ibid.

[17] Davis interview.

[18] Texas Health and Human Services Commission, *Medicaid/Texas Health Steps Health Care Orientation* (November 2001). Online. Available: http://www.hhsc.state.tx.us/CHIP/SB43/SB43_script.pdf. Accessed: November 13, 2001.

[19] Texas Health Education Assistance Resources and Training, *Medicaid STARLink* (January 2001). Online. Available: http://www.txheart.org/starlink.html. Accessed: April 3, 2002.

[20] TexCare Partnership, *Children's Health Insurance Program 2000 Annual Report* (Austin, Tex., 2000), p. 11.

[21] Davis interview.

[22] TexCare Partnership, *CBO Best Practices* (2000). Online. Available: http://www.texcarepartnership.com/Documents/CBO Best Practices.doc. Accessed November 8, 2001.

[23] Interview by Daniel Starr and Scott Atnip with Candace Dorsey, CHIP Outreach Program Manager, Harris County Department of Health and Environmental Services, Houston, Texas; Helen Stagg, CHIP/Health Coordinator, Families Under Urban and Social Attack, Houston, Texas; Carolyn Franks, CHIP/TexCare Program Manager, Institute of Religion, Houston, Texas; Heather Kanenberg, Public Policy Analyst, Children At Risk, Houston, Texas; Anita Garvey, CHIP Regional CBO Contract Manager/Health Plan Liaison, Region 6/5, Houston, Texas; and Sheryl Guilbeaux, CHIP Regional CBO Contract Manager/Health Plan Liaison, Region 6/5, Houston, Texas, February 8, 2002.

[24] Texas Health and Human Services Commission, *Cumulative Application, Enrollment and Eligibility Determination Activity for 12/31/01*. Online. Available: http://www.hhsc.state.tx.us/CHIP/WeeklySumRpt.htm. Accessed: January 10, 2002.

[25] Texas Health and Human Services Commission, Research Department, *Baseline Projection of Otherwise Uninsured Texas Children Under 19 by Poverty Income Status: Years 2000-2006* (Austin, Tex., January 2001) (computer printout).

[26] Texas Health and Human Services Commission, *Cumulative Application, Enrollment and Eligibility Determination Activity for 11/5/01*. Online. Available: http://www.hhsc.state.tx.us/CHIP/WeeklySumRpt.htm. Accessed: November 17, 2001.

[27] Interview by Daniel Starr with Lynn Denton, Communications Director, Texas Department of Health, Austin, Texas, November 8, 2001.

[28] TexCare Partnership, *TexCare Partnership Outreach Work Plan: Children's Medicaid and the Children's Health Insurance Program January 2002-August 2003* (Austin, Tex., January 2002), p. 1 (draft).

[29] Focus Group of Multiple Stakeholders, Computerized Feedback at TexCare Partnership Regional Stakeholder Meeting, Austin, Texas, February 6, 2002.

[30] Dorsey, Stagg, Franks, Kanenberg, Garvey, and Guilbeaux interview.

[31] TexCare Partnership, *TexCare Partnership Outreach Work Plan: Children's Medicaid and the Children's Health Insurance Program January 2002-August 2003* , p. 2.

[32] TexCare Partnership, *TexCare Partnership Outreach: Guidance for Community-Based Organizations' Outreach Projects 2002-2003 Strategic Work Plan* (Austin, Tex., January 2002), p. 1.

[33] Ibid.

[34] Ibid.

[35] Washington Department of Social and Health Services, *DSHS Children's Campaign Wins National 'Best of the Best' Award* (June 2001). Online. Available: http://www.wa.gov/dshs/mediareleases/pr01152.shtml. Accessed: January 8, 2002.

[36] Telephone interview by Daniel Starr with Selia Evans, Healthy Kids Now! Program Director, Washington Department of Social and Health Services, Olympia, Washington, January 16, 2002.

[37] Ibid.

[38] Jason Cooke, "CHIP and Medicaid: Status Report" (presentation at conference on "Working Together for a Healthy Texas: Expanding Health Insurance Coverage for Texans," Texas State Planning Grant Conference, Austin, Tex., January 31- February 1, 2002).

[39] Ibid.

[40] Class presentation by Jose Marrero, President, JAM Creative, at the Lyndon B. Johnson School of Public Affairs, Austin, Texas, November 6, 2001.

[41] Class presentation by DeAnn Friedholm, Director, Children's Defense Fund for Texas, at the Lyndon B. Johnson School of Public Affairs, Austin, Texas, November 13, 2001.

[42] Marrero presentation.

[43] Texas Department of Insurance, *Your Health Care Coverage* (Revised June 2001). Online. Available: http://www.tdi.state.tx.us/consumer/cbo05.html. Accessed: November 11, 2001.

[44] Texas Department of Insurance, "Characteristics of Texans With and Without Health Insurance" (paper presented at conference on "Working Together for a Healthy Texas: Expanding Health Insurance Coverage for Texans," Texas State Planning Grant Conference, Austin, Tex., January 31-February 1, 2002), p. 21.

[45] Ibid, p. 9.

[46] National Federation of Independent Business, *The NFIB Small-Business Growth Agenda for the 107th Congress,* Washington, D.C. (pamphlet).

[47] Texas Health and Human Services Commission, Research and Forecasting, *Demographic Profile of the Texas Population Without Health Insurance in 2000* (Austin, Tex., October 2001). Online. Available: http://www.hhsc.state.tx.us/budget/cons_bud/dssi/TXUNIN2000.html. Accessed: May 6, 2002.

[48] Ann Lessem, James Dyer, Steve Borders, and Jason Vendel, "Uninsured Texans: Attitudes Toward Coverage" (paper presented at conference on "Working Together for a Healthy Texas: Expanding Health Insurance Coverage for Texans," Texas State Planning Grant Conference, Austin, Tex., January 31-February 1, 2002), p. 5.

[49] National Federation of Independent Business, *Association Health Plans (AHP), Talking Points,* Washington, D.C. (pamphlet).

[50] Texas Institute for Health Policy Research, *The Uninsured in Texas, Policy Brief* (Austin, Tex., September 29, 2000). Online. Available: http://www.healthpolicyinstitute.org/publications/policy_briefs/uninsured_paper_policy_brief.pdf. Accessed: November 11, 2001.

[51] Jack A. Meyer and Lise S. Rybowski, The Commonwealth Fund, "Business Initiatives to Expand Health Coverage for Workers in Small Firms" (October 2001). Online. Available: http://www.cmwf.org. Accessed: November 4, 2001.

[52] Texas Health and Human Services Commission, Research and Forecasting, *Demographic Profile of the Texas Population Without Health Insurance in 2000* (Online).

[53] Lyndon B. Johnson School of Public Affairs, *Expanding Health Care Coverage for the Uninsured in Texas,* Policy Research Project Report Series, no. 141 (Austin, Tex., 2001), pp. 151-172.

[54] Ibid.

[55] Texas Health and Human Services Commission, Research and Forecasting, *Demographic Profile of the Texas Population Without Health Insurance in 2000* (Online).

[56] Texas Department of Insurance, "Small Employer Health Insurance Survey Results" (paper presented at a conference on "Working Together for a Healthy Texas: Expanding Health Insurance Coverage for Texans," Texas State Planning Grant Conference, Austin, Tex., January 31-February 1, 2002), p. 1.

[57] Texas Department of Insurance, *Texas State Planning Grant.* Online. Available: http://spg.tdi.state.tx.us. Accessed: January 26, 2002.

[58] Texas Department of Insurance, "Small Employer Health Insurance Survey Results" (paper presented at a conference on "Working Together for a Healthy Texas: Expanding Health Insurance Coverage for Texans," Texas State Planning Grant Conference, Austin, Tex., January 31- February 1, 2002), p. 2.

[59] Texas Department of Insurance, State Planning Grant Division, *Texas State Planning Grant Interim Report* (October 2001). Online. Available: http://spg.tdi.state.tx.us/pubs/interim. Accessed: January 26, 2002.

[60] Texas Department of Insurance, "Small Employer Health Insurance Survey Results," p. 6.

[61] Texas Insurance Code, ch. 26, art. 21, *Small Employer Health Benefit Plans; Employer Election.* Online. Available: http://www.capitol.state.tx.us/statutes/intoc.html. Accessed: January 26, 2002.

[62] Texas Department of Insurance, *Small Employers Health Insurance: Questions and Answers* (Revised January 2001). Online. Available: http://www.tdi.state.tx.us/consumer/cbo40.html. Accessed: February 21, 2002.

[63] Lyndon B. Johnson School of Public Affairs, *Expanding Health Care Coverage for the Uninsured in Texas,* pp. 151-172.

[64] Texas Department of Insurance, *Small Employers Health Insurance: Questions and Answers* (Online).

[65] Texas Department of Insurance, "Small Employer Health Insurance Survey Results," p. 2.

[66] Texas Insurance Code, ch. 26, art. 42, *Small Employer Health Benefit Plans.* Online. Available: http://www.capitol.state.tx.us/statutes/intoc.html. Accessed: January 26, 2002.

[67] Texas Department of Insurance, *Small Employers Health Insurance: Questions and Answers* (Online).

[68] Sue Hart and Esther Blount, "Options for Expanding Health Insurance in Texas—Small Employer Market" (paper presented at conference on "Working Together for a Healthy Texas: Expanding Health Insurance Coverage for Texans," Texas State Planning Grant Conference, Austin, Tex., January 31-February 1, 2002), p. 3.

[69] Texas Department of Insurance, "Concurrent Breakout Sessions to Discuss Options for Expanding Health Insurance" (conference on "Working Together for a Healthy Texas: Expanding Health Insurance

Coverage for Texans," Texas State Planning Grant Conference, Austin, Tex., January 31- February 1, 2002).

[70] Sue Hart and Esther Blount, "Options for Expanding Health Insurance in Texas—Small Employer Market," pp. 1-22.

[71] Lyndon B. Johnson School of Public Affairs, *Expanding Health Care Coverage for the Uninsured in Texas,* pp. 151-172.

[72] Ibid.

[73] Texas Insurance Code, ch. 26, art. 32, *Index Rates.* Online. Available: http://www.capitol.state.tx.us/statutes/intoc.html. Accessed: January 26, 2002.

[74] Lyndon B. Johnson School of Public Affairs, *Expanding Health Care Coverage for the Uninsured in Texas,* pp. 151-172.

[75] Georgetown University, Institute for Health Care Research and Policy, *A Consumer's Guide to Getting and Keeping Health Insurance in Texas* (January 1998). Online. Available: http://www.healthinsuranceinfo.net. Accessed: February 2, 2002.

[76] Texas Department of Insurance, "Concurrent Breakout Sessions to Discuss Options for Expanding Health Insurance."

[77] Texas Department of Insurance, "Policy Options Under Review by SPG" (paper presented at conference on "Working Together for a Healthy Texas: Expanding Health Insurance Coverage for Texans," Texas State Planning Grant Conference, Austin, Texas, January 31- February 1, 2002), p. 3.

[78] Email from Jim Davis, Director, Public Information Office, Texas Department of Insurance, "Information Request/Verification," to Scott Atnip, March 25, 2002.

[79] Diane Longley, "Concurrent Breakout Session on Consumer Education and Outreach: Making Private Insurance Work" (conference on "Investing in Texas: Financing Health Coverage Expansion," Austin, Texas, March 22, 2002).

[80] Texas Department of Insurance, "Concurrent Breakout Sessions to Discuss Options for Expanding Health Insurance."

[81] Telephone interview by Jacqueline Angel, Scott Atnip, Karla Buitrago, and Kristen Lindberg with Richard Lee, Director of Public Education, Texas Department of Insurance, Austin, Texas, February 1, 2002.

[82] Texas Department of Insurance, "Concurrent Breakout Sessions to Discuss Options for Expanding Health Insurance."

[83] Texas Department of Insurance, "Sample Texas Small Employer Rate Guide" (paper presented at conference on "Working Together for a Healthy Texas: Expanding Health Insurance Coverage for Texans," Texas State Planning Grant Conference, Austin, Tex., January 31- February 1, 2002), 50-52.

[84] Texas Legislature, *Senate Bill 771: Proposed Version*. Online. Available: http://www.capitol.state.tx.us/tlo/billnbr.htm. Accessed: February 22, 2002.

[85] Texas Legislature, *Bill History: SB 771*. Online. Available: http://www.capitol.state.tx.us/tlo/billnbr.htm. Accessed: February 22, 2002.

[86] Consumers Union, *Consumer Gains Clouded by Long-Term Effect of Industry Subsidies* (June 2, 1999). Online. Available: http://www.consumersunion.org/other/sesstx699.htm. Accessed: January 25, 2002.

[87] Ibid.

[88] Texas Legislative Budget Board, *Texas House Bill 2430: Introduced Version, Bill Analysis.* Online. Available: http://www.capitol.state.tx.us/tlo/billnbr.htm. Accessed: January 24, 2002.

[89] Texas Academy of Family Physicians, *77th Legislative Compendium: Managed Care*. Online. Available: http://www.tafp.org/Departments/Leg/lc-managedcare.htm. Accessed: January 25, 2002.

[90] Texas Department of Insurance, State Planning Grant Division. *Grant Proposal, Project Abstract.* Online. Available: http://spg.tdi.state.tx.us/grant/abstract.htm. Accessed: January 25, 2002.

[91] Texas Legislative Budget Board, *Texas House Bill 2430: Enrolled Version, Bill Analysis* (Online).

[92] Texas House of Representatives, *House Bill 2430: House Committee Report—Fiscal Note*. Online. Available: http://www.capitol.state.tx.us/tlo/billnbr.htm. Accessed: January 24, 2002.

[93] Texas Legislative Budget Board, *Texas House Bill 2430: Enrolled Version, Bill Analysis* (Online).

[94] Texas House of Representatives, *House Bill 2430: House Committee Report—Fiscal Note* (Online).

[95] Texas Legislative Budget Board, *Texas House Bill 2430: Enrolled Version, Bill Analysis* (Online).

[96] Lessem, Dyer, Borders, and Vendel, "Uninsured Texans: Attitudes Toward Coverage," p. 27.

[97] Ibid, pp. 23-24.

[98] Ibid, pp. 19, 28-29.

[99] Texas Legislature, *Bill History: HB 2430*. Online. Available: http://www.capitol.state.tx.us/tlo/billnbr.htm. Accessed: January 26, 2002.

[100] Ibid.

[101] Email from Cynthia Levinson, Vice President, Texas Health Education Assistance Resources and Training (HEART), "Help with Policy Research Project," to Kristen Lindberg, February 5, 2002.

[102] Texas Department of Insurance, State Planning Grant Division, *Grant Proposal, Project Abstract*. Online. Available: http://spg.tdi.state.tx.us/grant/abstract.htm. Accessed: January 25, 2002.

[103] Texas Department of Insurance, State Planning Grant Division, *Texas State Planning Grant Interim Report* (Online).

[104] Texas Department of Insurance, "Small Employers and Health Insurance: Final Results of the Texas Small Employer Survey" (paper presented at conference on "Working Together for a Healthy Texas: Expanding Health Insurance Coverage for Texans," Texas State Planning Grant Conference, Austin, Tex., January 31- February 1, 2002), p. 1.

[105] Texas Department of Insurance, "Small Employer Health Insurance Survey Results," p. 8.

[106] Employer Quality Partnership, *Looking for Value: An Employer's Guide to Evaluating Quality Health Plans*. Online. Available: http://www.eqp.org/page2.html. Accessed: November 4, 2001.

[107] Consumer Health Education Council, *Consumer Health Education Council*. Online. Available: http://www.healthchec.org. Accessed: November 7, 2001.

[108] Consumer Health Education Council, *Getting and Keeping Coverage*. Online. Available: http://www.healthchec.org/consumer/getkeep.html. Accessed: November 7, 2001.

[109] Insure.com, *Tips for Buying Health Coverage* (February 22, 2001). Online. Available: http://www.insure.com/health/individual.html. Accessed: November 18, 2001.

[110] Insure.com, *Health Plan Comparison Worksheet* (November 9, 2001). Online. Available: http://www.insure.com/health/plancomparison.html. Accessed: November 18, 2001.

[111] Health Insurance Association of America, *Guide To Health Insurance*. Online. Available: http://www.hiaa.org/consumer/guidehi.cfm. Accessed: November 8, 2001.

[112] Health Insurance Association of America, *The Insurance Guide for Business Owners*. Online. Available: http://www.hiaa.org/consumer/guidebo.cfm. Accessed: November 8, 2001.

[113] Texas Department of Insurance, *Mission Statement*. Online. Available: http://www.tdi.state.tx.us. Accessed: January 24, 2002.

[114] Ibid.

[10] Texas Department of Insurance, *2001 Annual Report* (Austin, Tex., November 2001), p. 4. Online. Available: http://www.tdi.state.tx.us/commish/annual01.html. Accessed: January 2, 2002.

[116] Texas Department of Insurance, *Jose Montemayor: Texas Commissioner of Insurance*. Online. Available: http://www.tdi.state.tx.us/commish/jose.html. Accessed: January 2, 2002.

[117] Texas Department of Insurance, *2001 Annual Report*, p. 10.

[118] Texas Department of Insurance, *A Word from the Commissioner: Help Us Fight Insurance Fraud*. Online. Available: http://www.tdi.state.tx.us/commish/help.html. Accessed: January 26, 2002.

[119] Texas Department of Insurance, *2001 Annual Report*, p. 17.

[120] Ibid, p. 34.

[121] Ibid, p. 35.

[122] Ibid.

[123] Ibid, pp. 35-39.

[124] Ibid, p. 37.

[125] Ibid, p. 42.

[126] Texas Department of Insurance, *Texas Department of Insurance*. Online. Available: http://www.tdi.state.tx.us. Accessed: January 2, 2002.

[127] Texas Department of Insurance, *2001 Annual Report*, p. 44.

[128] Email from Audrey Selden, Consumer Protection Division, Texas Department of Insurance, "FY 2002-2003 Business Plan," to Jacqueline Angel, February 14, 2002.

[129] Texas Department of Insurance, *2001 Annual Report*, pp. 42-44.

[130] Texas Department of Insurance, *Helping You with Your Insurance Complaint* (Revised April 2000). Online. Available: http://www.tdi.state.tx.us/consumer/consum83.html. Accessed: January 26, 2002.

[131] Telephone interview by Scott Atnip with Nancy Walker, State Legislative Aid, City of Austin, Austin, Texas, January 24, 2002.

[132] Texas Department of Insurance, *Helping You with Your Insurance Complaint* (Online).

[133] Walker interview.

[134] Telephone interview by Jacqueline Angel, Scott Atnip, Karla Buitrago, and Kristen Lindberg with Anita Pogue, Director of Information Assistance, Consumer Protection Division, Texas Department of Insurance, Austin, Texas, February 1, 2002.

[135] Texas Department of Insurance, *2001 Annual Report*, pp. 42-43.

[136] Pogue interview.

[137] Ibid.

[138] Ibid.

[139] Telephone interview by Jacqueline Angel, Scott Atnip, Karla Buitrago, and Kristen Lindberg with Richard Lee, Director of Public Education, Texas Department of Insurance, Austin, Texas, February 1, 2002.

[140] Ibid.

[141] Selden email.

[142] Texas Department of Insurance, *2001 Annual Report*, pp. 43-44.

[143] Lee interview.

[144] Email from Jim Davis, Director, Public Information Office, Texas Department of Insurance, "Information Request/Verification," to Scott Atnip, March 25, 2002.

[145] Ibid.

[146] Ibid.

[147] Texas Department of Insurance, *What is the Speakers Bureau?* Online. Available: http://www.tdi.state.tx.us. Accessed: January 2, 2002.

[148] Texas Department of Insurance, *2001 Annual Report*, p. 43.

[149] Texas Department of Insurance, *Speakers Bureau Calendar of Events*. Online. Available: http://www.tdi.state.tx.us/consumer.speak.html. Accessed: January 26, 2002.

[150] Texas Department of Insurance, *Senior Issues*. Online. Available: http://www.tdi.state.tx.us. Accessed : January 2, 2002.

[151] Texas Department of Insurance, *2001 Annual Report*, p. 43.

[152] Texas Department of Insurance, *Senior Issues* (Online).

[153] Texas Department of Insurance, *Listing of Companies Offering Small Employer Accident and Health Coverage*, Online. Available: http://www.tdi.state.tx.us/company/lhsmallemp.html. Accessed January 25, 2002.

[154] Texas Department of Insurance, *Major Texas Insurers*. Online. Available: http://www.tdi.state.tx.us/company/top40.html. Accessed: January 2, 2002.

[155] Texas Department of Insurance, *2000 Accident and Health Complaint Index*. Online. Available: http://www.tdi.state.tx.us. Accessed: January 2, 2002.

[156] Texas Department of Insurance, *2001 Annual Report*, p. 42.

[157] Texas Department of Insurance, *Texas Department of Insurance Working for You*. Online. Available: http://www.tdi.state.tx.us. Accessed: January 2, 2002.

[158] Texas Department of Insurance, *2001 Annual Report*, p. 43.

[159] Texas Department of Insurance, *Texas Department of Insurance Working for You* (Online).

[160] Texas Department of Insurance, *2001 Annual Report*, p. 42.

[161] Georgetown University, Institute for Health Care Research and Policy, *A Consumer's Guide to Getting and Keeping Health Insurance in Texas* (January 1998). Online. Available: http://www.healthinsuranceinfo.net. Accessed: February 2, 2002.

[162] Texas Department of Insurance, *Texas Department of Insurance Working for You* (Online).

[163] Ibid.

[164] Texas Department of Insurance, *Mission Statement* (Online).

[165] Texas Department of Insurance, *Texas Department of Insurance Working for You* (Online).

[166] Texas Department of Insurance, *Mission Statement* (Online).

[167] Texas Department of Insurance, *Texas Department of Insurance Working for You* (Online).

[168] Ibid.

[169] Telephone interview by Scott Atnip with Shirly Hutzler, Lobbyist, Texas Association of Health Underwriters, Austin, Texas, February 14, 2002.

[170] Email from Shirly Hutzler, Lobbyist, Texas Association of Health Underwriters, "Question," to Scott Atnip, January 26, 2002.

[171] Texas Department of Insurance, *Continuing Education: Agents, Adjusters, Providers*. Online. Available: http://www.tdi.state.tx.us/agent/agcehome.html. Accessed: January 26, 2002.

[172] Hutzler interview.

[173] Texas Department of Insurance, *Continuing Education: Agents, Adjusters, Providers* (Online).

[174] Hutzler email, January 26, 2002.

[175] Hutzle interview.

[176] Ibid.

[177] Texas Insurance Code, ch. 26, art. 73, *Agents*. Online. Available: http://www.capitol.state.tx.us/statutes/intoc.html. Accessed: January 26, 2002.

[178] Lyndon B. Johnson School of Public Affairs, *Expanding Health Care Coverage for the Uninsured in Texas,* Policy Research Project Report Series, no. 141 (Austin, Tex., 2002), pp. 151-172.

[179] Ibid.

[180] Texas Department of Insurance, *77th Legislature Enacts More Than 80 Insurance Bills*. Online. Available: http://www.tdi.state.tx.us/commish/lege80.html. Accessed: January 25, 2002.

[181] Ibid.

[182] Texas Blue Ribbon Task Force on the Uninsured, *Report to the 77th Legislature* (Austin, Texas: February 2001), p. 40.

[183] Hutzler interview.

[184] Hutzler email, March 5, 2002.

[185] Texas Legislative Budget Board. *House Bill 949: Enrolled Version, Bill Analysis*. Online. Available: http://www.capitol.state.tx.us/tlo/billnbr.htm. Accessed March 7, 2002.

[186] Texas Legislative Budget Board. *House Bill 471: Enrolled Version, Bill Analysis*. Online. Available: http://www.capitol.state.tx.us/tlo/billnbr.htm. Accessed March 7, 2002.

[187] Hutzler email, March 5, 2002.

[188] Texas Department of Insurance, "Policy Options Under Review by SPG" (paper presented at a conference on "Working Together for a Healthy Texas: Expanding Health Insurance Coverage for Texans," Texas State Planning Grant Conference, Austin, Tex., January 31- February 1, 2002), p. 1.

[189] Texas Department of Insurance, *Your Health Care Coverage* (revised June 2001). Online. Available: http://www.tdi.state.tx.us/consumer/cbo05.html. Accessed: November 11, 2001.

[190] Texas Department of Insurance, *Insurance Resource for Small Businesses*. Online. Available: http://www.tdi.state.tx.us/commish/smbiz.html. Accessed: November 11, 2001.

[191] Texas Department of Insurance, *Small Employers Health Insurance: Questions and Answers* (revised January 2001). Online. Available: http://www.tdi.state.tx.us/consumer/cbo40.htm. Accessed: November 11, 2001.

[192] Texas Department of Insurance, *Health Care Coverage for Texas Children* (revised May 2001). Online. Available: http://www.tdi.state.tx.us/consumer/cbo72.html. Accessed: November 11, 2001.

[193] Texas Department of Insurance, *Summary of Health Care Coverage Options for Texas Children* (revised September 2001). Online. Available: http://www.tdi.state.tx.us. Accessed: January 2, 2002.

[194] Texas Department of Insurance, *Health Maintenance Organizations* (revised December 2000). Online. Available: http://www.tdi.state.tx.us. Accessed: January 2, 2002.

[195] Texas Department of Insurance, *HMO Resource*. Online. Available: http://www.tdi.state.tx.us. Accessed: January 2, 2002.

[196] Texas Department of Insurance, *Medicare+Choice Options for Medicare Beneficiaries*. Online. Available: http://www.tdi.state.tx.us/consumer/cbo36.html. Accessed: January 26, 2002.

[197] Texas Department of Insurance, *HICAP Highlights—Private Fee-for-Service Plans*. Online. Available: http://www.tdi.state.tx.us/consumer/hicap/hicapnews200.html. Accessed: January 26, 2002.

[198] Texas Department of Insurance, *Long-Term Care Insurance*. Online. Available: http://www.tdi.state.tx.us/consumer/cbo32.html. Accessed: January 26, 2002.

[199] Texas Department of Insurance, *Insurance for Texans with Disabilities*. Online. Available: http://www.tdi.state.tx.us/consumer/cbo39.html. Accessed: January 26, 2002.

[200] Texas Department of Insurance, *Glossary—Common Insurance Terms*. Online. Available: http://www.tdi.state.tx.us/consumer/glossary.html. Accessed: January 26, 2002.

[201] Texas Department of Insurance, *Insurance Fraud* (revised April 2001). Online. Available: http://www.tdi.state.tx.us/consumer/cbo44.html. Accessed: January 26, 2002.

[202] Texas Department of Insurance, *Helping You with Your Insurance Complaint* (Online).

[203] Texas Department of Insurance, *If My Insurance Company Fails* (revised September 2000). Online. Available: http://www.tdi.state.tx.us/consumer/cbo6.html. Accessed: January 2, 2002.

[204] Texas Department of Insurance, *Independent Review Organizations* (revised January 2000). Online. Available: http://www.tdi.state.tx.us/consumer/iro.html. Accessed: January 26, 2002.

[205] Texas Department of Insurance, *Insurance on the Internet: Shopping Tips and Dangers* (revised February 2000). Online. Available: http://www.tdi.state.tx.us. Accessed: January 2, 2002.

[206] Texas Department of Insurance, *Assistance for Providers* (revised April 2001). Online. Available: http://www.tdi.state.tx.us/consumer/cbo52.html. Accessed: January 2, 2002.

[207] Texas Department of Insurance, *Texas Department of Insurance Working for You* (Online).

[208] Texas Department of Insurance, *Trabajando Para Usted Un Guía para el Consumidor* (revised June 2001). Online. Available: http://www.tdi.state.tx.us/consumer/news3s.html. Accessed: January 2, 2002.

[209] Texas Department of Insurance, *Texas Department of Insurance* (Online).

[210] Texas House of Representatives, *House Bill 2430: House Committee Report—Fiscal Note*. Online. Available: http://www.capitol.state.tx.us/tlo/billnbr.htm. Accessed: January 24, 2002.

[211] Texas Department of Insurance, *2001-2002 Texas Long-Term Care Rate Guide* (revised May 2001). Online. Available: http://www.tdi.state.tx.us/consumer/ltcrgintro.html. Accessed: January 2, 2002.

[212] Texas Department of Insurance, *Texas Workers' Compensation Rate Guide* (December 5, 2001). Online. Available: http://www.tdi.state.tx.us/company/rcomp.html. Accessed: January 2, 2002.

[213] Texas Department of Insurance, *2001-2002 Homeowners Insurance Rate Guide* (revised September 2001). Online. Available: http://www.tdi.state.tx.us. Accessed: January 2, 2002.

[214] Texas Department of Insurance, *Medicare Supplement Insurance Handbook and Rate Guide* (revised September 2001). Online. Available: http://www.tdi.state.tx.us. Accessed: January 2, 2002.

[215] Texas Department of Insurance, *2001-2002 Automobile Insurance Rate Guide* (revised September 2001). Online. Available: http://www.tdi.state.tx.us. Accessed: January 2, 2002.

[216] Texas Department of Health, Statewide Health Coordinating Council, *2001-2002 Texas State Health Plan Update: Ensuring a Quality Health Care Workforce for Texas, Appendix H, Ad Hoc Committee on Consumer Information.* Online. Available: http://www.tdh.state.tx.us/stateplan01/default.htm. Accessed: January 24, 2002.

[217] Office of Public Insurance Counsel, *Office of Public Insurance Counsel*. Online. Available: http://www.opic.state.tx.us/whatis.html. Accessed: January 24, 2002.

[218] Ibid.

[219] Ibid.

[220] State Office of Administrative Hearings, *Welcome to SOAH*. Online. Available: http://www.soah.state.tx.us/Backgrnd/SOAH.htm. Accessed: January 26, 2002.

[221] Office of Public Insurance Counsel, *Office of Public Insurance Counsel* (Online).

[222] Ibid.

[223] Ibid.

[224] Texas Department of Insurance, *Helping You with Your Insurance Complaint* (Online).

[225] Office of Public Insurance Counsel, *A Review of Health Insurance Underwriting Guidelines Used in Texas*. Online. Available: http://www.opic.state.tx.us/health1.html. Accessed: January 26, 2002.

[226] Office of Public Insurance Counsel, *Health Insurance Coverage in Texas: Context and Demographics*. Online. Available: http://www.opic.state.tx.us/Healthykids.html. Accessed: January 2, 2002.

[227] Robert L. Bennefield, U.S. Census Bureau, *Current Population Reports, Health Insurance Coverage* (1997). Online. Available: http://www.opic.state.tx.us/Healthinfo.html. Accessed: January 2, 2002.

[228] Office of Public Insurance Counsel, *Office of Public Insurance Counsel* (Online).

[229] Office of Public Insurance Counsel, *Current Bill of Rights*. Online. Available: http://www.opic.state.tx.us/BOR_intro.htm. Accessed: January 2, 2002.

[230] Office of Public Insurance Counsel, *Office of Public Insurance Counsel* (Online).

[231] Office of Public Insurance Council, *Health Insurance Information*. Online. Available: http://www.opic.state.tx.us/Healthinfo.html. Accessed: January 24, 2002.

[232] Office of Public Insurance Counsel, *Comparing Texas HMOs* (2000). Online. Available: http://www.opic.state.tx.us/counties2000.html. Accessed: October 30, 2001.

[233] Texas Department of Health, Statewide Health Coordinating Council, *2001-2002 Texas State Health Plan Update: Ensuring a Quality Health Care Workforce for Texas* (Online).

[234] Office of Public Insurance Counsel, *Annual HMO Reports Now Available*. Online. Available: http://www.opic.state.tx.us/PRHMO2001.htm. Accessed: January 2, 2002.

[235] Texas Health Care Information Council, *About THCIC*. Online. Available: http://www.thcic.state.tx.us/AboutTHCIC.htm. Accessed: January 24, 2002.

[236] Ibid.

[237] Texas Health Care Information Council, *Straight Talk on Texas HMOs: A Purchaser's Guide* (November 2001). Online. Available: http://www.thcic.state.tx.us/Publications.htm. Accessed: November 4, 2001.

[238] Texas Health Care Information Council, *Your HMO Quality Check-up: A Consumer's Guide to Texas Commercial HMOs* (August 2001). Online. Available: http://www.thcic.state.tx.us/Publications.htm. Accessed: November 4, 2001.

[239] Georgetown University, Institute for Health Care Research and Policy, *A Consumer's Guide to Getting and Keeping Health Insurance in Texas* (January 1998). Online. Available: http://www.healthinsuranceinfo.net. Accessed: February 2, 2002.

[240] University of Houston Law Center, Health Law and Policy Institute, *Small Employers Guide to Health Care Plans*. Online. Available: http://www.lawlib.uh.edu/healthlaw/tccempl.html. Accessed: November 18, 2001.

[241] Families USA, *Consumer Health Assistance Programs: Report on a National Survey* (Washington, D.C., June 2001), p. 1. Online. Available: http://www.familiesusa.org/media/pubs/index.htm. Accessed: February 1, 2002.

[242] Ibid, p. 2.

[243] Ibid, p. 3.

[244] Ibid, pp. 3-4.

[245] Ibid, p. 3.

[246] Ibid, p. 4.

[247] Ibid, p. 5.

[248] Ibid, p. 5.

[249] Ibid, p. 6.

[250] Ibid.

[251] Ibid, p.1.

[252] Ibid, p. 8.

[253] Ibid, p. 17.

[254] Ibid, p. 29.

[255] Families USA, *Career Opportunities*. Online. Available: http://www.familiesusa.org/html.jobs/jobs.htm. Accessed: February 2, 2002.

[256] Families USA, *Designing a Consumer Health Assistance Program* (June 2001). Online. Available: http://www.familiesusa.org/index6.htm. Accessed: February 1, 2002.

[257] Ibid.

[258] Ibid.

[259] Ibid.

[260] Ibid.

[261] Ibid.

[262] Ibid.

[263] Ibid.

[264] Ibid.

[265] Ibid.

[266] State of Illinois, Department of Insurance, *Illinois Department of Insurance: 66th Annual Report and Summary of Annual Statements* (2000), p. 20. Online. Available: http://www.state.il.us/ins/AnnualReportLinks.htm. Accessed: November 18, 2001.

[267] State of Illinois, Department of Insurance, *Department Overview*. Online. Available: http://www.state.il.us/ins/overview.htm. Accessed: November 11, 2001.

[268] State of Illinois, Department of Insurance, *I Want to File a Complaint*. Online. Available: http://www.state.il.us/ins/Complaints/file_complaint.htm. Accessed: November 11, 2001.

[269] State of Illinois, Department of Insurance, *Complaints*. Online. Available: http://www.state.il.us/ins/Complaints/Complaints.htm. Accessed: November 11, 2001.

[270] State of Illinois, Department of Insurance, *Illinois Department of Insurance: 66th Annual Report and Summary of Annual Statements*, p. 20.

[271] State of Illinois, Department of Insurance, *Health Insurance*. Online. Available: http://www.state.il.us/ins/healthInsurance/healthInsurance.htm. Accessed: November 11, 2001.

[272] State of Illinois, Department of Insurance, *Illinois Department of Insurance: 66th Annual Report and Summary of Annual Statements*, p. 20.

[273] State of Illinois, Department of Insurance, *Office of Consumer Health Insurance*. Online. Available: http://www.state.il.us/ins/OCHI/office_consumer_health_ins.htm. Accessed: November 11, 2001.

[274] State of Illinois, Department of Insurance, *Illinois Department of Insurance: 66th Annual Report and Summary of Annual Statements*, p. 20.

[275] State of Illinois, Department of Insurance, *Department Overview* (Online).

[276] State of Illinois, Department of Insurance, *Illinois Department of Insurance: 66th Annual Report and* Summary of Annual Statements, p. 20.

[277] State of Illinois, Department of Insurance, *Contact the Illinois Department of Insurance*. Online. Available: http://www.state.il.us/ins/Contact_us.htm. Accessed: November 11, 2001.

[278] New Jersey Department of Banking and Insurance, *New Jersey Department of Banking and Insurance*. Online. Available: http://www.njdobi.org. Accessed: December 17, 2001.

[279] National Association of Insurance Commissioners, *New Jersey Office of Life and Health Insurance* (June 11, 2001). Online. Available: http://www.naic.org. Accessed: December 17, 2001.

[280] New Jersey Department of Banking and Insurance, *Enforcement and Consumer Protection* (August 8, 2000). Online. Available: http://www.njdobi.org/enfcon.htm. Accessed: January 8, 2002.

[281] National Association of Insurance Commissioners, *New Jersey Health Insurance Bureau* (March 8, 2001). Online. Available: http://www.naic.org. Accessed: December 17, 2001.

[282] National Association of Insurance Commissioners, *New Jersey Managed Care Bureau*. Online. Available: http://www.naic.org. Accessed: December 17, 2001.

[283] National Association of Insurance Commissioners, *What Is New Jersey Health Insurance Reform?* Online. Available: http://www.naic.org. Accessed: December 17, 2001.

[284] Ibid.

[285] Ibid.

[286] Ibid.

[287] Ibid.

[288] Ibid.

[289] Ibid.

[290] Ibid.

[291] State of New Jersey, *New Jersey People—Be Healthy*. Online. Available: http://www.state.nj.us/njpeople/healthy.html. Accessed: December 17, 2001.

[292] National Association of Insurance Commissioners, *New Jersey Health Reform Insurance Information* (September 13, 2001). Online. Available: http://www.naic.org. Accessed: December 17, 2001.

[293] Ibid.

[294] National Association of Insurance Commissioners, *What Is New Jersey Health Insurance Reform?* (Online).

[295] National Association of Insurance Commissioners, *The New Jersey Individual Health Coverage Program, Buyer's Guide* (1998). Online. Available: http://www.naic.org. Accessed: December 17, 2001.

[296] National Association of Insurance Commissioners, *New Jersey Individual Health Coverage Program Rates.* Online. Available: http://www.naic.org. Accessed: December 17, 2001.

[297] National Association of Insurance Commissioners, *Individual Health Care Program Carriers.* Online. Available: http://www.naic.org. Accessed: December 17, 2001.

[298] National Association of Insurance Commissioners, *Basic Health Benefits Plan (Plan A/50).* Online. Available: http://www.naic.org. Accessed: December 17, 2001.

[299] National Association of Insurance Commissioners, *New Jersey Health Reform Insurance Information,* (September 13, 2001). Online. Available: http://www.naic.org. Accessed: December 17, 2001.

[300] National Association of Insurance Commissioners, *New Jersey Small Employer Health Benefits Buyer's Guide.* Online. Available: http://www.naic.org. Accessed: December 17, 2001.

[301] National Association of Insurance Commissioners, *Snapshot Of Standard Health Benefits Plans.* Online. Available: http://www.naic.org. Accessed: December 28, 2001.

[302] National Association of Insurance Commissioners, *New Jersey Small Employer Standard Health Benefits Plan Summary.* Online. Available: http://www.naic.org. Accessed: December 28, 2001.

[303] National Association of Insurance Commissioners, *New Jersey Small Employer HMO Chart.* Online. Available: http://www.naic.org. Accessed: December 28, 2001.

[304] National Association of Insurance Commissioners, *New Jersey Small Employer Health Benefits Parity.* Online. Available: http://www.naic.org. Accessed: December 28, 2001.

[305] National Association of Insurance Commissioners, *2001 Small Employer Health Benefits Premium Comparison Survey.* Online. Available: http://www.naic.org. Accessed: December 17, 2001.

[306] National Association of Insurance Commissioners, *Small Employer Carriers.* Online. Available: http://www.naic.org. Accessed: December 17, 2001.

[307] National Association of Insurance Commissioners, *New Jersey Health Reform Insurance Information* (Online).

[308] Ibid.

[309] Donna Sutton Fay, *Office of Health Care Ombudsman, Annual Report 2000* (Burlington, Vermont: Vermont Office of Health Care Ombudsman), p. 1.

[310] Ibid, p. 11.

[311] Vermont Legal Aid, Inc., "Proposal for Health Care Ombudsman" (presentation at "Families USA Health Action 2002" conference, Washington, D.C., January 2002), p. 1.

[312] Donna Sutton Fay, *Office of Health Care Ombudsman, Annual Report 2000,* p. 11.

[313] Ibid, p. 1.

[314] Ibid, p. 12.

[315] Ibid, p. 1.

[316] Ibid, p. 14.

[317] Ibid, p. 10.

[318] Ibid, p. 13.

[319] Texas Department of Insurance, "Characteristics of Texans With and Without Health Insurance" (paper presented at conference on "Working Together for a Healthy Texas: Expanding Health Insurance Coverage for Texans," Texas State Planning Grant Conference, Austin, Tex., January 31- February 1, 2002), p. 12.

[320] Ann Lessem, James Dyer, Steve Borders, and Jason Vendel, "Uninsured Texans: Attitudes Toward Coverage" (paper presented at conference on "Working Together for a Healthy Texas: Expanding Health Insurance Coverage for Texans," Texas State Planning Grant Conference, Austin, Tex., January 31-February 1, 2002), p. 20.

[321] Texas Department of Insurance, State Planning Grant Division, *Texas State Planning Grant Interim Report* (Austin, Tex., October 2001). Online. Available: http://spg.tdi.state.tx.us/pubs/interim. Accessed: January 26, 2002.

[322] Diane Longley, "Concurrent Breakout Session on Consumer Education and Outreach: Making Private Insurance Work" (conference on "Investing in Texas: Financing Health Coverage Expansion," Austin, Tex., March 22, 2002).

[323] Ibid.

[324] Lessem, Dyer, Borders, and Vendel, "Uninsured Texans: Attitudes Toward Coverage," p. 11.

Chapter 9. Investing in Texas: Financing Health Coverage Expansion

by Kate Brodsky, Evan Christman,
Jamie Dudensing, Kristie Kimbell, and Laura Koenig

Introduction

The number of medically uninsured individuals in Texas is significant and growing. The state is spending increasing sums of money to provide safety-net health care for these individuals. Texas has one of the highest per capita rates of uninsurance in the nation, with an average of 24.4 percent of the population without health insurance per year,[1] or about 4.5 million uninsured individuals.[2] The number of uninsured in Texas has risen steadily from 1988 to 1999. It is projected to continue growing and could reach 6.1 million by 2010.[3] The rising number of uninsured in turn leads to higher costs for the state. The cost of health care has increased in the past decade by as much as ten percent within a single year. It is expected to continue growing at the same rate for each of the next several years. Such cost increases will have further implications on the number of uninsured in Texas.[4] Texas is also experiencing rapid growth of low-income and undocumented segments of the population. At the same time, Texas, like many states, is faced with a possible budgetary shortfall as a result of the nation's economic downturn. In fact, Texas is facing a potential $5 billion shortfall for the 2004-2005 biennium, and has already begun to implement cutbacks for the 2002-2003 biennium.

Many states have sought expansions to their existing Medicaid and SCHIP programs as a means of expanding health insurance coverage. The prevailing thought is that states, by obtaining a federal match on health care dollars spent, can cover more people, while effectively exporting one-half to two-thirds of the cost. For many states, including Texas, the main issue is less about whether or not to expand, and more about where to find the additional funds for the match. Indeed many of the people to be covered by an expansion may be being covered by local public funds on a sporadic basis anyway. Another issue confronting planners is whether the money should come from localities, such as counties or hospital districts, or from the state level, and whether or not it should come from new or existing funds. This report will examine the ability of the state to fund an expansion of health insurance coverage to the uninsured through a Medicaid waiver, with specific focus on a combined "hypothetical" Section 1931 and HIFA waiver model. The report includes research regarding funds that are already being spent on health care as well as potential new revenue sources to fund such an expansion.

The first section of this report examines the current structure of health coverage financing in Texas. The second section describes Texas' current fiscal outlook and a discussion of the importance of accessing available federal funds. In the third section, existing funding sources for health care, including county indigent health care funds and hospital district revenue, are explored in terms of a local contribution option that could be used as state matching funds for a waiver expansion. This section includes the results of a survey of all 254 Texas county judges and hospital/program administrators conducted by the authors. Input from telephone and in-person interviews with state agency, elected, and stakeholder experts is also included. The fourth section outlines *new* revenue options to help fund an expansion, including: provider taxes (hospital, physician, pharmaceutical and nursing home taxes); a medical service sale tax; a re-working of the franchise tax; excise taxes (soda, and cigarette taxes); and a state income tax. Each of these sources has the possibility to generate income for a health coverage expansion program in Texas. Amounts generated would depend on how implementation proceeded. In the fifth section other potential sources of revenue are outlined. These primarily include funds that have already been appropriated for the provision of health care in some manner by the Texas Legislature. The section examines the possibility of rerouting funds from state owned teaching hospitals and medical schools, unclaimed lottery funds, as well as the opportunity for cost sharing in the CHIP program. A brief conclusion is presented in the sixth section.

Research for this report includes national and state document and report reviews, related literature reviews, stakeholder document and report reviews, state-by-state email and telephone questionnaires, state website reviews, a state-wide county survey, and numerous expert interviews with experts.

The Current Healthcare Funding Structure in Texas

In 1998, Texans spent more than $70 billion on health care, an average of $3,514 per person, below the national average of $4,261. Of that $70 billion in statewide spending, the local governmental contribution was $1.17 billion and charity spending was estimated to be $1.08 billion.[5]

Texans who have health insurance obtain their coverage in one of several ways. Individuals may be insured privately through an employer-sponsored group plan or through an individual plan. Between 1996 and 1998, on average, about 56 percent of Texans were insured privately. The other method of insurance coverage is through a *public* source. Public sources of coverage include the federal and state funded Medicare, Medicaid, and SCHIP programs. Between 1996 and 1998, on average, about 19 percent of Texans were covered by a public source.[6] The main providers of health care services for indigent individuals, who do not qualify for one of the above-mentioned public programs, are local entities—counties and hospitals. Counties, specifically, are mandated by state law, Chapter 61 of the Texas State Code, or the Indigent Health Care and Treatment Act of 1985, to provide a specific set of health care services to indigent individuals, primarily those who fall below 21 percent of the Federal Poverty Level (FPL), about $1,800 a year. Counties and hospital districts in Texas spend hundreds of millions of local tax dollars a year to provide health care to medically needy individuals. Texas policymakers have made efforts at both the state and local level to provide basic health care services to the indigent, but a review of these current programs suggests that the indigent care "safety-net" may be inadequate.

Understanding the Delivery of Indigent Care and Who Pays for It

The counties and hospital districts are key players in this "safety-net" system of coverage for the indigent. They are allowed to fulfill their mandate to provide indigent services in one of three ways: 1) creating a *hospital district*, 2) running a *public hospital*, or 3) operating a *county indigent health care program* (CIHCP). Several variations of these arrangements, or hybrids, are also permitted. The result is 254 unique county programs.[7]

The indigent health care safety-net essentially fills the gaps in the Texas Medicaid program. In general under current law, most non-disabled, non-TANF eligible low-income adults under the age of 65 are not eligible for Medicaid, nor does Medicaid cover undocumented or recent legal immigrants. State law has placed responsibility for these individuals with the counties.[8] Changes to federal law in the late 1990s has also made legal immigrants who entered the United States after 1996 ineligible for Medicaid, forcing them to rely on the county safety-net health care system as well.

This devolution of safety-net care to the counties relieves the state of some fiscal burden, but it has also meant that county programs, unlike the state, do not receive federal matching funds for expenditures. Counties that operate a public hospital, either as a municipal entity or as a part of a hospital district, can use payments from the federal Medicaid program through the Disproportionate Share Hospital Program to offset some of the costs of uncompensated care. However, counties that reimburse providers through a CIHCP do not receive federal money.

Currently, 138 counties operate CIHCPs, and the remaining counties meet the state requirement through a public hospital or a hospital district. Counties may also operate a hybrid of the three; for instance, some counties may wish to utilize a hospital in a large urban area and use a CIHCP to provide care in rural areas.

Table 9.1
Indigent Care Entities in Texas Counties

Type of System	Number of Counties	Percent of state uninsured population under 65 in these counties
County Indigent Health Care Programs	114	32%
Hospital Districts	87	58%
Public Hospitals	30	3%
Hybrids	24	7%
Total Number of Uninsured below 65: 4.5 million		

Adapted from: Texas Department of Health, *County Directory*. Online. Available: http://www.tdh.state.tx.us/hcf/ihcp. Accessed: April 8,2002.; and U.S. Department of Labor, *2001 March Current Population Survey*. Online. Available: http://www.bls.census.gov/cps/cpsmain.htm. Accessed: April 8, 2002.

In State Fiscal Year (SFY) 2000, the 138 counties that operate CIHCP spent about $60 million to provide care.[9] Hospital districts in SFY 2000 raised over $1 billion dollars in taxes, a portion of which is used to fund care for the indigent population.[10] About 90 percent of these funds come from the nine large urban hospital districts.

The variations in indigent health care delivery reach far beyond the four systems listed above. Even counties with similar systems may operate very differently. Some counties hire providers themselves, some enter into contracts, and others simply reimburse providers on a fee-for-service basis. Although eligibility is mandated as a minimum below 21 percent of the FPL, some counties do not meet this mandate, and yet others cover upwards of 100 percent of the FPL. Some counties are doing well to cover the required basic set of services, while others cover an expanded set of services. Counties with more active programs will have specialized staff to reimburse providers and enroll applicants, while smaller counties may not have any dedicated staff.

County Indigent Health Care Programs (CIHCPs)

CIHCPs, in operation in 138 counties, provide a state-mandated set of basic primary and preventative services for the county's indigent residents who fall below 21 percent of the FPL. One hundred and ten counties, mostly rural, are covered entirely by CIHCPs, and a combination CIHCP and either a hospital district or a public hospital covers the remaining 28 counties. CIHCPs are funded primarily with local tax money. Although, counties have the flexibility to provide services above the required list of services and to use a higher FPL limit if desired, there has been no financial incentive to do so until recently.

Once a county spends a set amount of its budget on approved health care expenditures for the indigent, it becomes eligible to apply for state assistance. To qualify for state funds counties must meet two requirements: (1) a county must spend a threshold amount, 8 percent of the property tax levy, and (2) the county may only count expenditures for services approved by the state on individuals with incomes lower then 50 percent of the FPL. Counties are free to offer other services or assist individuals with higher incomes, but these expenditures do not count against the 8 percent threshold.[11] After the county has met these requirements and until funds run out, the state will pay 90 cents for every dollar spent on approved services, again only matching expenditures for approved services and only for individuals with incomes below 50 percent of the FPL.[12]

The Indigent Health Care Division (IHCD) of the Texas Department of Health (TDH) is responsible for monitoring county spending and disbursing state matching funds. Counties seeking reimbursement must report their annual tax levies, and must also report their monthly spending on indigent care. Once a county has spent 6 percent of their general revenue tax levy (GRTL) on indigent health care, TDH staff review sample cases to ensure the county is following state eligibility and reimbursement policies. After counties have passed the 8 percent threshold, the counties will begin to draw down state funds on a monthly basis.

The state matching funds are intended as an incentive for counties with CIHCPs, but they are of limited help for counties with fiscally strapped programs. Additionally, basing the expenditure threshold for eligibility on property taxes presents some problems. This method of determining need of counties is not considered to be a very accurate reflection of individual county needs because it does not account for the unique circumstances in each county.[13] Requiring all counties to pay up to 8 percent of their GRTL assumes that all counties have an equal fiscal capacity. Some counties have tremendous difficulty covering expenditures up to this threshold and still maintaining other county services. However, tying indigent spending to a level of fiscal effort also creates some problems. There are no explicit links between a county's general revenue and the demand for indigent care. Some counties easily meet the threshold (21 counties had spending over 10 percent of GRTL in SFY 2001), while others find it difficult. Across the state the demand for county indigent services varies, and counties have different factors driving demand.[14] In SFY 2001, 24 counties received state match funds, 102 counties reported indigent spending below the threshold, and 7 counties reported no indigent expenditures. There are significant spending differences between counties that did and did not qualify for the matching funds. For example, counties that received matching funds averaged 12 percent of GRTL, while those that did not receive state funds averaged only 3.5 percent. The method of determining state assistance is currently being re-evaluated.

Hospital Districts

Hospital districts are special taxing districts created for the sole purpose of providing health care to indigent people within the boundaries of the district. Voters must approve a hospital district, and each district can determine eligibility standards and services to be provided. Most hospital district boundaries mirror those of the county, although some counties have multiple hospital districts within them and some districts span multiple counties. In Texas, 130 hospital districts span all or part of 112 counties. Recently, there has begun to be some mention of the possibility of multi-county hospital districts, but it is unclear how feasible this option really is. f the 130 hospital districts, 109 use their tax dollars to operate a hospital. The hospital district has the authority to impose property taxes annually within its boundaries, but the amount may not exceed the limit approved by voters, and in no event can it be in excess of 75 cents on each $100 valuation of taxable property in the district. The district may also choose to levy a sales tax.

Originally, hospital districts were free to set the income limit of the people that could be served. Many served far above the 21 percent FPL level required by CIHCP counties, even up to 100 or 200 percent of the FPL. However, some took advantage of this flexibility and served very few or none. Hospital districts are now mandated to serve at least the state minimum, and districts that served a higher level in 1984 we mandated to maintain that level. Hospital district taxes account for on average one quarter of their operating revenue. The other three quarters comes from payers (the state, out-of-pocket payers, private insurance, and public insurance).[15]

The state provides some funds to hospital districts through the state Tertiary Care Fund, which helps reimburse public and private hospitals for emergency care provided to people from outside counties, especially large urban hospitals like in Harris County, and is funded through unclaimed lottery prizes. There are two federal programs available that also enable states to provide additional funds to hospitals: 1) the Disproportionate Share Hospital (DSH) Program, and 2) the Graduate Medical Education (GME) funding. The DSH program, actually part of Medicaid, provides money to the state, which in turn reimburses public and private acute care and public psychiatric hospitals (about 150 total) that provide a "disproportionate share" of inpatient health care to indigent individuals—Medicaid and low-income. Texas distributed \$1.5 billion in DSH money in 1997. The \$1.5 billion includes both federal and state funds.

Texas uses a series of intergovernmental transfers from the nine urban hospital districts to fund the state portion of DSH that is redistributed to non state-owned hospitals. The hospital districts transfer money to the state, which then uses the funds to draw down matching funds from the federal government. The Balanced Budget Act of 1997 implemented a series of declining caps that have reduced the amount of federal DSH funding a state can receive. Since 1998 the amount of federal funds the state can receive has declined by 22 percent, from \$979 million to \$765 million in 2002. Under the BBA formula, the allowable amount in future years is tied to the level of spending in Texas' Medicaid program and inflation. There are currently no real limitations on how DSH money can be spent by the receiving institution.[16]

GME money is intended to provide funding to teaching hospitals to help reimburse them for some of the costs associated with medical teaching. The GME payments in effect supplement the Medicare and Medicaid payments that the teaching institution gets for treating these recipients (about \$35 million a year through Medicaid, and about \$180 million through Medicare in Texas). This money allows teaching hospitals to increase their staff and serve more people, especially the medically indigent. The belief is that without GME dollars, these teaching hospitals would be less able to support residency positions, thus reducing the number of indigent patients that would be served.[17] These teaching institutions also receive state general revenue funds for a number of purposes.

Public Hospitals

Public hospitals are hospitals "owned, operated, or leased by a county or municipality." Public hospitals are responsible for providing care for individuals within set geographical service areas; some cover entire counties, some cover only part of a county. Thirty-two counties (mostly rural) are served in whole or in part by a public hospital, 29 of which are served exclusively in this manner, and the remaining three are hybrids. For example, Travis County is served by a public hospital and a CIHCP. Like hospital districts, public hospitals must provide services to individuals who fall below 21 percent of the FPL, and may provide services to individuals above that limit as well. They also must provide a certain set of services for example doctor visits and hospital stays, but can provide additional services such as prescriptions, and home health care. As a whole, these hospitals spent \$65 million in free care for indigent individuals in 1997. Public Hospital funding comes from the same sources, as do hospital district funds. However, public hospital local tax support is not always dedicated, unlike hospital districts, and therefore each year it must compete with other county needs for money. This situation is actually leading many of these hospitals to create hospital districts, sell to a private entity, or close altogether.[18]

Tobacco Settlement Funds

Counties also receive payments from the Tobacco Settlement Trust Fund. In 1998 Texas settled with the tobacco companies. The counties, cities, and hospital districts signed an agreement that reserves some settlement funds for "hospital districts, other local political subdivisions owning and maintaining public hospitals, and counties of the State of Texas responsible for providing indigent care to the general public."[19] The funds were granted to compensate political subdivisions for the cost of tobacco-related illnesses in their health care programs. These entities, the same as the entities required to deliver indigent care under Chapter 61 of the Texas State Code, are referred to in the agreement as political subdivisions.

The total settlement amount of $2.8 billion was to be received over a five-year period. The funds were split into two payment methods, a series of lump-sum payments and a trust fund. The lump sum payments paid a total of $450 million dollars over 1999-2001.[20] Another $1.8 billion was deposited in a Permanent Trust Fund. The return on trust fund investments will be paid to the counties in perpetuity, depending on how much un-reimbursed care each provides. In 2001, the first year of interest payments, a total of $13 million was paid.[21] County tobacco money has no spending requirements, except within hospital districts, which must use it for health care.[22] As a whole, in 1999, counties (those who reported) spent at least $940 million of tobacco money on indigent health care.

SFY 2002 was to be the first year in which tobacco payments to counties was solely from the Permanent Trust Fund created with the initial amount of $1.8 billion. However, due to the poor economic circumstances of 2001 and due to heavy investment of the fund in stocks, the fund has not only failed to gain interest, it has lost a net $30 million in principal.[23] This loss has caused great concern on behalf of hospitals and CIHCPs that had counted on the April 2002 disbursement as part of their current year budget.

Other Providers of Indigent Health Care in Texas

Other providers of indigent health care services in the state include non-profit and for-profit private hospitals (322 in Texas) and clinics, state facilities (hospitals run by state agencies TDMHMR, TDH, and prisons), hospitals and clinics run by public universities; specialty services (HIV/AIDS), Federally Qualified Health Centers (FQHCs), rural health clinics, free clinics, private physicians, and local health departments. Together these entities provide roughly $4.3 billion in uncompensated health care annually. While this figure also captures bad debt amounts, it is a good indication of the extent to which these other resources are contributing to indigent care in Texas. Their funding comes from a variety of sources. For private hospitals, revenue comes primarily from payers—out-of-pocket payers, insurance companies, DSH, and Medicare, and Medicaid. The state facilities are funded through these same means but also through state general revenue funds. Special facilities and community and rural health centers/clinics are largely funded through federal money (Title V, Title X, Ryan White, block grants) along with the state matching dollars. Local health departments rely on federal, state, and local funding sources for their programs. Free clinics on the other hand rely on fundraising and volunteers, while private physician's contributions to the indigent are from their own earnings.[24]

Texas counties and these other health care sources together spend at least $5 billion annually on safety-net healthcare.[25] The question remains: are we maximizing the use of these healthcare dollars? Another important question, given that the number of uninsured is growing, the cost of health care is rising, Texas is in a budget crisis, and local entities have finite resources (counties are limited in the amount of tax they can collect) is: should counties be responsible for indigent health care in the first place?

Funding a Health Coverage Expansion

The most fiscally savvy way for Texas to finance improvements and expansions to their current healthcare system is by drawing more federal funds into the state. Drawing down such federal matching funds returns money Texans spend on federal income tax to Texas. However, without the state's initial infusion of dollars, no expansion or improvement option to take advantage of federal dollars is available. Determining how to come up with the state portion of a match is quite a challenge for state funding experts. The first part of this section will describe the importance of accessing available federal dollars for expansion purposes as well as possible costs of a waiver. The remainder of the section will describe the current constrained financial landscape of the state.

Funding an Expansion with Federal Dollars

Many states have increased health care coverage for additional groups of children, but most have failed to significantly impact the number of uninsured adults. The cost of caring for uninsured individuals is much greater than the cost of preventative and maintenance care, as uninsured individuals tend to receive less preventive medical care and to rely more on emergency department care than their insured counterparts. This strains state and local public resources, such as public hospitals and clinics that provide care to the uninsured.[26] One of the primary recommendations by the National Governors Association for states attempting to shore up their safety-net programs that provide health care to indigents is to "take full advantage of federal grant programs and matching funds available to states and communities."[27]

The best alternative for counties and the state to get the most for each healthcare dollar spent is through a federal matching program. A number of options exist for expanding healthcare coverage to the uninsured by accessing federal funds, through Medicaid and SCHIP waivers for example. Such options enable the state to expand coverage to a number of groups including: pregnant women, parents, and adults without dependents below a given income. By expanding Medicaid and SCHIP coverage, states are building on existing, proven programs with "public accountability and a defined basic benefit."[28] Short of a straight-out general revenue-funded coverage expansion, which some states have done, most states will rely on available federal dollars to help extend coverage to those not currently eligible for coverage. With such expansions, states can take advantage of a federal match, allowing them to pay only about one-half to one-third of the cost of expanding coverage to families. In doing this, the state effectively exports a significant amount of the cost of expanding health care coverage.

States have several key options available for expanding Medicaid coverage. The first of these is an expansion through Section 1931 of the Social Security Act (SSA), which was made possible as part of the Welfare Reform Act of 1996. Section 1931 allows the expansion of Medicaid coverage to the optional population of low-income parents. Texas currently covers low-income parents up to 24 percent of the FPL. Coverage for these individuals can be achieved through a state plan amendment to increase income and resource disregards as allowed through Section 1931.States may also expand to additional populations through 1115 waivers, which authorize research, pilot, or demonstration projects to test new, innovative, or more efficient methods for achieving program goals. Many states utilize 1115 waivers to expand services to optional populations such as parents or non-disabled, childless adults. As a contingency of the waiver, budget neutrality must be maintained, thus an extensive expansion with this population can be difficult.

However, budget neutrality *can* be achieved by using a *hypothetical* Section 1931 expansion coupled with a Health Insurance Flexibility and Accountability (HIFA) Section 1115 waiver. HIFA is the Bush Administration's new approach to Section 1115 research and demonstration waivers for the Medicaid and SCHIP programs. HIFA waivers are intended to reduce the number of uninsured by allowing states to cover additional low-income populations with savings from a limited benefit package to optional and expansion populations, or by increasing cost sharing to these groups. HIFA waivers must result in an increase in the number of individuals at or below 200 percent, and state-wideness and budget neutrality must be maintained.A hypothetical section 1931 expansion uses the Section 1931 optional population expansion possibility as part of the budget neutrality equation, as a benchmark. Texas can apply for a HIFA to provide a reduced set of benefits, with or without cost sharing, to parents of children on, or eligible for, MCD/CHIP. By spending less for this population than would otherwise be spent under a real Section 1931, the state achieves cost-savings in the eyes of the federal government and can then use that savings to expand coverage to childless adults, also with a reduced set of benefits and cost sharing. For Texas to expand at all to this 1931 population would be contingent on it being allowed as a HIFA. This option varies in the number of individuals that can be covered and the cost of the expansion depending on funding.[29] Table 9.2 outlines estimated costs of the various coverage and cost sharing levels.

Table 9.2
Estimated Cost of a HIFA Waiver

FPL of Parents/ FPL of Childless Adults: Cost-sharing Imposed	Percent of Benefits Package in relation to Mandated TANF Adult	Per Member per Month Premium	Amount of State Revenue Needed over Five Years	Amount of State Revenue Needed for the Next Biennium	Number of Uninsured Texans Covered
100/50: 0%	54.05%	$136.75	$958,482,000	$360,197,000	290,419
150/50: 0%	65.87%	$166.64	$1,572,433,000	$590,920,000	390,966
200/50: 0%	71.90%	$181.90	$2,084,811,000	$783,472,000	474,879
200/100: 0%	60.83%	$153.89	$2,084,811,000	$783,472,000	561,325
100/50: 2%	54.05%	$136.75	$643,756,000	$241,924,000	195,058
150/50: 2%	65.87%	$166.64	$1,056,112,000	$369,887,000	262,589
200/50: 2%	71.90%	$181.90	$1,400,246,000	$526,212,000	318,948
200/100: 2%	60.83%	$153.89	$1,400,246,000	$526,212,000	377,010
100/50: 5%	54.05%	$136.75	$243,197,000	$91,393,000	73,688
150/50: 5%	65.87%	$166.64	$398,976,000	$149,935,000	99,200
200/50: 5%	71.90%	$181.90	$528,982,000	$198,792,000	120,492
200/100: 5%	60.83%	$153.89	$528,982,000	$198,792,000	142,426

Source: Leah Kegler, "Utilizing Federal Waiver Flexibility: Expanding Through Section 1931" (Professional Report, Lyndon B Johnson School of Public Affairs, The University at Texas at Austin, 2002), pp. 19-58.

While these cost figures are estimates, they do provide some idea of the amount of money the state will need to generate to implement this type of expansion program. The first column in the table explains what populations according to FPL the waiver expands to and the amount of cost sharing involved. The second column explains what percentages of benefits these individuals will receive in comparison to the current mandated Medicaid package. A variety of coverage options are available to the state depending on the amount of funding available.

Limited Funds for Health Care Expansion

One of the ongoing issues that Texas faces, in its efforts to decrease the number of uninsured, is ongoing budgetary constraints. Not only is Texas limited in the way it raises money through taxes, but also it is currently confronted with potentially very large budget problems both in this biennium and the next.

Possible Shortfalls for the 2002-2003 Budget

While the Comptroller has certified the 2002-2003 budget,[30] it does appear that Medicaid could have difficulty staying within appropriated funds. Interestingly, while caseloads and premium costs are expected to rise,[31] general revenue appropriations are projected to decrease slightly from 2002 to 2003.[32] The decrease may be due in part to an error in the 2002-2003 FMAP projections during the appropriations process, which estimated the rate higher than it will actually be.[33] The federal match rate is now expected to decrease in 2002-2003, lowering the total amount allocated for Medicaid and worsening HHSC's chances of getting by on appropriated funds.[34]

A primary concern with Medicaid in 2002-2003 is the implementation of cost containment strategies and the consolidation of the agencies that oversee Medicaid operations. HHSC has been mandated to implement cost containment measures to stay within the appropriated amount of funds for the 2002-03 biennium. A large piece of the cost containment efforts involving the migration of the Medicaid Health Care Financing operations at TDH to HHSC was included in the vetoed piece of legislation, Senate Bill 1156. Governor Perry ordered the transition to take place without the legislation and the move is nearing completion. Other cost containment pieces of SB 1156 are less certain; although Rider 30 in the General Appropriations Bill did reduce the amount appropriated to Medicaid by $205 million in general revenue. This will reduce the federal funds for Medicaid by an estimated $274.9 million unless additional state matching funds are found.[35]

2004-2005 Potential Budget Problems

Several bills from the 77th Legislature (see Table 9.3) will give rise to a reduction in available general revenue of about $58.6 million for the 2004-2005 biennium. Many of these bills were written so that they would have no effect on the current budget, but they will impact future budgets. Some of these bills would have to be renewed by the 2003 Legislature before they would affect 2004-2005 revenue, but others will affect future revenue even after their expiration date.[36]

Table 9.3
Bills from 77th Texas Legislature

Bill	Description	2002-2005 Cost
SB 248	Property tax exemption for leased cars	$37.4 million
SB 601	Insurance premium tax credits for certain investments	$10.4 million
HB 2686	Increase tax credits for enterprise zone investments	$6.4 million
SB 63	Franchise tax credit for hiring certain individuals with disabilities	$2.4 million
SB 1096	Incentive to bring Breeders' Cup horse race to Texas	$2.0 million

Adapted from: Center for Public Policy Priorities, *Where Will the Money Go?: A Revenue Preview* (May 9, 2001). Online. Available: www.cppp.org/products/policypages/111-130/111-130html/PP129.html. Accessed: September 12, 2001.

Current statutory provisions could also cause a reduction of cash surplus that would be available to fund the 2004-2005 budget. For example, the Education Code Sec. 42.2522 directs that any money appropriated to the Foundation School Program in 2003-2004, but not needed to fund school-finance formulas, be used to benefit certain school districts that offer the optional percentage homestead exemption. This one obscure provision could reduce General Revenue available for appropriation in 2004-2005 by more than $300 million.[37]

Medicaid funding could also have specific problems. If enrollment estimates are accurate for the Medicaid Simplification Bill impact, Medicaid costs will increase by at least $350 million in general revenue over current appropriations.[38] The federal match rate is also expected to decrease in 2002-2003 and may continue to decrease for 2004-2005.[39] The federal matching rate is adjusted annually according to the state's average income per person compared to the average per capita in the U.S. The more the average income in Texas rises relative to average nationwide income, the more revenue Texas has to appropriate to receive the same amount of federal funds.

Texas is facing a potential $5 billion dollar shortfall for the next biennium, as pointed out by Comptroller Carole Rylander in June 2001.[40] The fiscal concerns are driven by the fact that there are a number of issues that will cause the 2004-2005 budget to increase beyond $61.7 billion. These issues include the following: 1) the Teacher's Health Insurance Plan, enacted in the 77th Legislative Session, was only funded for one year in the 2000-2001 session and will need to be funded for two years in the next—a projected cost of at least $1.4 billion more than what was allocated in the current budget;[41] 2) the movement of the last month of Medicaid payments--$161 million—from the 2002-2003 biennium to the 2004-2005 budget;[42] 3) the 2002-2003 budgets are relying on a projected $2.9 billion surplus from the previous biennium; and 4) the 2002-2003 budget had an additional $800 million funded by one-time measures that cannot be repeated during the next session.[43] Texas has many commitments that will be impacted by these financial constraints.

Tax System in Texas

Expanding healthcare coverage to currently uninsured individuals will be difficult under these financial circumstances. The current tax system in Texas inhibits the states ability to generate sufficient funds for existing obligations, making it difficult to consider funds for the expansion of health coverage to uninsured individuals. More than 75 percent of Texas' state and local tax load is due to only two taxes, the property tax and the sales tax. The local property tax is the largest tax paid by most Texans, accounting for more than 40 percent of total state and local tax burden. State and local sales taxes account for one-third of taxes paid by Texans.

Approximately half of all taxes in Texas go to the state government. The other half goes to local governments, primarily to school districts. Three-fourths of state taxes go to pay for public and higher education and health and human services. Local taxes go to support public education and to fund city, county, and special district services.

The total tax load for Texans is light compared to other states, although the property tax burden is heavier than the average state. Property and sales tax rates are among the highest in the country, since most state government revenue comes from these two taxes alone. Unlike other states who avoid high property and sales taxes by distributing the tax burden onto a third major tax, Texas does not have a personal income tax with which to do so. According to Dick Lavine of the Center for Public Policy Priorities, "the current Texas state and local tax system fails to provide a stable source of adequate revenue from a balance of sources."[44]

The purpose of the state and local tax system is to provide an adequate revenue stream. In other words, taxes should provide enough to cover spending needs. One measure of the adequacy of a tax system is its ability to keep up with the growth of total personal income in a state. Personal income growth reflects both inflation and population changes, and roughly parallels the increase in the cost of providing the same level of services year after year. Personal income also reflects the ability of a state's residents to pay taxes.

Since 1994, Texas' state and local tax revenue has fallen steadily as a percentage of personal income. If tax revenue had kept up with the growth of personal income since 1994, an additional $9.8 billion would have been available to appropriate for the 2002-2003 budget. In the early 1990s, state and local tax revenues as a percent of personal income was fairly constant at 9.6 percent, but began to fall in 1994. By 2003, state and local taxes are projected to equal only 8.35 percent of personal income.[45]

Funding Options Available

While these state and county funding issues are a reality, so is the growing number of uninsured individuals in the state. With the consideration of fiscal constraints in the state of Texas, it is important to look to other methods to finance the current system and a possible expansion. There are a number of methods of financing that would not only help the state to use its funds more efficiently, but would also generate new funds. The next few sections will provide a description of these methods and their potential to raise funds for the state. The next section will describe the use of current county and hospital district indigent health care funds to bring federal matching dollars into the state to insure additional individuals. Where existing indigent health care funds fall short, new revenue sources may be needed. New revenue options are described in later sections.

Expanding Coverage through Existing Funds

This section will explore options for and implications of the use of existing safety-net expenditures to fund a health coverage expansion. In funding an expansion using existing safety-net expenditures, there are several ways to go about it: 1) utilizing current expenditures by local entities on individuals below 21 percent of the FPL, 2) using large hospital district funding only, and/or 3) relying primarily on large urban hospital district unmatched funding in addition to county and other hospital district funds. Currently most county and hospital district programs only cover individuals at or below 21 percent of the FPL. By utilizing the current expenditures on this population to draw down federal matching funds, the state could extend the level of coverage to a higher FPL, possibly covering individuals up to 50 percent of the FPL. Local entities are an obvious place to look for funds because many public hospital and CIHCP administrators recognize that current expenditures are not being used as efficiently as they could. They also recognize that by serving individuals below 21 percent of the FPL only a fraction of individuals needing care are being served. Furthermore, although some concerns were raised, much interest was generated at the county and hospital district level in 1995 with Senate Bill 10. This section will include a presentation of results from a survey of Texas CIHCP managers, county judges, and hospital district administrators, from stakeholder interviews, and from a review of related documents, reports, and legislation.

Safety Net Shortcomings

An ideal safety-net system at the county level would ensure that all counties have adequate funds to provide basic health care services to their indigent population. In the current system, the failure by one county to fund an adequate level of care can lead to a "spillover effect." A county rationing indigent health care by under funding the program may force indigent individuals to go to other counties. To ensure an adequate level of care for all eligible individuals, the burden of funding needs to be spread fairly among the counties.

Estimates of the uninsured in Texas demonstrate the enormity of the burden the current system places on counties. In 2000 about 4.5 million Texans did not have health insurance. Sixty percent of these individuals are located in the counties served by hospital districts, and over 1.5 million are located in the 138 counties served by CIHCPs or CIHCP hybrids. Though the uninsured are dispersed around the state, the financing mechanisms that fund the bulk of the care are relatively concentrated. The hospital districts raised over $1 billion in SFY 2000. The 138 counties that operate CIHCP spent $67 million in SFY 2001, with the top three counties representing 20 percent of the expenditures.[46]

This difference between the hospital district funds and CIHCP funds is a reflection, in part, of the financing mechanisms. CIHCP funds come from the general revenue of the county. This forces local officials to balance the need for indigent health care with all of the other county responsibilities faced by the counties. Because hospital districts are special revenue districts created solely to pay for hospital operations, a dedicated revenue stream better protects the funding for indigent care from competition with other local priorities. However, this does not mean that hospital districts necessarily have adequate funds for indigent care. Hospital district taxes are used to fund the broad range of a hospital's operating costs.

The numbers in Table 9.4 suggest that current programs are serving only a small fraction of the uninsured population. The majority of the uninsured population is above the eligibility levels required by the indigent care act. Though an exact figure is difficult to compute because eligibility levels vary across the state, over 90 percent of uninsured individuals have incomes over 50 percent of the FPL leaving them ineligible for many of the local assistance programs in Texas.

Table 9.4
Uninsured in Texas by Level of Income, 2000

Income as a percent of Federal Poverty Level	Number Without Health Insurance	Percent without health insurance	Percent of income group without coverage
Under 50%	466,670	10%	39%
51-99%	744,113	17%	40%
100-149%	787,617	18%	37%
150-199%	647,229	14%	30%
200-249%	551,401	12%	26%
Above 250%	1,289,019	29%	11%

Adapted from: U.S. Department of Labor. *2001 March Current Population Survey*. Online. Available: http://www.bls.census.gov/cps/cpsmain.htm. Accessed: April 8, 2002.

The strains of the current system are evident in the difficulties experienced by counties in funding their programs. The 138 counties with CIHCPs illustrate the diversity of circumstances present in the state. In SFY 2001, 29 counties qualified for state matching funds, 75 counties reported spending amounts below the spending threshold, and 6 reported no spending at all. However, qualifying for state funds did not guarantee that a county received them. The high number of counties that qualified overwhelmed the state-appropriated matching funds. In a move to ration the limited available funds, the state stopped payments to seven high-spending counties. The end of matching payments forced Atascosa, Callahan, Johnson Cameron, Medina, Tom Green, and Hidalgo counties to close or curtail their programs.[47]

Since the matching funds were created, only 30 percent of the 138 counties with CIHCPs have qualified for state funds.[48] The state has disbursed $48 million since 1989, about 40 percent of which went to Hidalgo County. The top three recipient counties, Kleberg, Johnson, and Hidalgo, have received 60 percent of the total funds disbursed. Focusing these funds has significantly helped these high spending counties, but it reduces the number of counties that can receive state assistance.

The limited state assistance funds and the subsequent curtailment of services demonstrate the dire funding situation that many counties find themselves in. For counties with large indigent populations who can access state assistance and thus spread the cost, an adequate level of care can be better ensured. When a county does not have access to needed funds, it may stop providing care altogether and pass the costs on to other programs. Strengthening the county safety net requires a more stable source of matching funds.

Legislative Groundwork

Senate Bill 10

Senate Bill 10 (SB 10) was passed by the 74th Texas Legislature in 1995 to establish a new framework for Medicaid financing and service delivery in Texas.[49] It was passed in part as a reaction to concerns regarding the potential instability of DSH funds and the general level of federal funding in future years. SB 10 in essence laid the groundwork for a local entity contribution system, as it was intended to provide for the development of a statewide Medicaid managed care system funded with local entity (funding entity) dollars and the federal demonstration waiver match money. The funds used by the funding entities were to come from resources and funds already being spent on indigent care; and were to provide the state match for the federal demonstration dollars. In turn, the funding entity would receive back at least as much as it contributed. With SB 10, counties operating CIHCPs were not required to make resources available for matching, but were encouraged to do so. The state planned to rely most heavily on money available from hospital districts in large urban areas, medical schools, and state-owned teaching hospitals.[50]

The legislation sought to make possible a Medicaid expansion to include children, and initially parents, through cost-savings arrived at as a result of statewide managed care. SB 10 included in it an option for local entities to operate the health care delivery system within their areas, with a focus on Primary Care Case Management (PCCM), and partially or fully capitated systems, and it attempted to recognize the unique situations for differing medical populations as well as differing geographic areas. Specifically it built in a stipulation regarding special payments to rural hospitals, who were the sole providers in a community and/or who served a large population of Medicaid and charitable care individuals, as well as special payments to DSH hospitals. SB 10 also intended for the system to build in cost sharing as well as an option for Medicaid buy-in for individuals within higher FPLs.[51]

There has been much deliberation since the initial passing of SB 10 and the subsequent waiver attempts regarding the intended "intergovernmental initiatives," or IGIs, and regarding the legality of a "transfer" of funds by local entities. IGIs were the mechanism in SB 10 in place to allow counties to network with large urban hospital districts for the provision of services and management of Medicaid dollars, and some would argue that they are less controversial today. Through these deliberations however many have come to understand how a more purposefully-designed local funding structure might possibly benefit all parties involved. The need for local entities to maximize their existing expenditures on safety net care is as important today as it ever has been. The design of a system that "to the extent that it is cost-effective to the state and local governments, maximize(s) the financing of the state Medicaid program by obtaining federal matching funds for all resources and other funds available for matching and expand(s) Medicaid eligibility to include persons who were eligible to receive indigent health care services through the use of those resources or other funds available for matching before expansion of eligibility" [52] is indeed *imperative* for today's health care and economic landscape.

SB 10 differed in a number of ways from current waiver considerations; however, there are considerable lessons to be learned from it. New waiver considerations also examine the practicality of using existing local dollars to fund a state match to draw down federal funds, and thus maximize the potential of local expenditures. As with SB 10, a new waiver model could rely predominantly on hospital districts (in addition to medical schools and teaching hospitals) as major funders, especially those in large urban areas with higher percentages of uninsured, and other entities (CIHCPs) could be allowed to participate if desired. For counties/hospital districts that do contribute, they could have the option to manage the newly generated Medicaid dollars. For those not contributing, while they would reap the benefit of additional covered individuals in their county, the state would mange the Medicaid dollars, either through managed care or through traditional Medicaid operations.

A difference between SB 10 and a new waiver attempt is that any new waiver would not need to rely on DSH funds to accomplish budget neutrality. A new waiver could rely on cost-savings established through a hypothetical Section 1931 expansion and a HIFA Section 1115 Waiver, which allows states to expand Medicaid coverage with a reduced benefit package and with cost-sharing.

Due to the veto by Governor Perry of Senate Bill 1156 of the 77th Legislature, which would have recodified SB 10, SB 10 sunsetted on September 1, 2001. As a result, important statutory authority that may have facilitated a local contribution funded waiver was lost. A thorough review of SB 10 and existing legislation will be required as part of a new waiver development process to determine if corollary legislation is necessary in the development of a new waiver.

SB 1156 – HIV/AIDS Waiver

Senate Bill 1156 (SB 1156) of the 77th Texas Legislature also included in it provisions for several waiver demonstration projects utilizing local contribution funding to draw down federal dollars. These projects included demonstration waivers to address HIV/AIDS, mental health, women's health, and expanded coverage for low-income adults, and would have sought to maximize current unmatched, over-tapped spending for these populations.[53] Despite the veto of SB 1156, most of these projects are still in varying stages of development. One of the most advanced of these projects is the HIV/AIDS Section 1115 waiver.

In an interview, King Hillier, Director of Legislative Relations for Harris County, explained that the HIV/AIDS waiver is important because it is a local-entity-initiated waiver to be funded solely through local match money. The involved participants to date include the following: Harris County Hospital District, Dallas County Hospital District, Parkland Public Hospital, John Peter Smith Hospital (Tarrant County), R.E. Thompson Hospital (El Paso), Bexar County Hospital, and UTMB Galveston. These entities have worked in conjunction with the State Medicaid Officer at HHSC and the Governor's Office on this project. The waiver addresses individuals with HIV/AIDS primarily in urban areas, as 75-80 percent of the HIV/AIDS population in Texas resides in urban areas, but would permit other counties to participate. This waiver, unlike the waiver proposed in SB 1156, hopes, in addition to expanding Medicaid prescription services to the HIV/AIDS population, to offer medical services as well to adults (ages 18-64) up to 200 percent of the FPL.[54]

The financing details of the HIV/AIDS waiver are still being conceived and discussed. The group will be working with an actuary to guide this process. Local contributions will likely be made based on costs incurred at each institution. Once the contribution is known, each entity's match can be determined. When the total dollar amount is known, the actuary can determine what services can be covered, and whether or not enrollment will need to be capped.

The funding structure for the waiver match is potentially a very instructive component of the project. The funding contributions, per Mr. Hillier, will be provided through a "funding certification process"—based on proof of level of expenditures for the population—and will not involve a literal transfer of funds. Such a *certification* process will require that the participants establish Exclusive Provider Organizations (EPOs), to manage the Medicaid dollars, in effect utilizing the county/district dollars first, and then the federal dollars. Mr. Hillier stressed that the previous SB 10 waiver attempt did not have a well-established EPO structure in place. Because an actual transfer of funds to the state was required under SB 10, the concern for participants (counties/hospitals) became how do we make sure the entity gets its money back, which also became a constitutional tax issue raised by commissioner's courts. At the time, the Health Care Financing Administration (HCFA), now the Center for Medicare and Medicaid Services (CMS), was emphasizing "freedom of choice," but has since become more supportive of the use of EPOs. Furthermore, in Texas, the use of EPOs for the rural areas has been addressed, according to Mr. Hillier, through the Rural Community Health System (described below), supporting rural counties/hospitals in their efforts to organize to form EPOs.[55]

According to Mr. Hillier, CMS has not to date approved a waiver allowing such a certification process. However, there are examples of such a process in the education funding system. He explained that the School Health and Related Services (SHARS) funds that schools receive for school health efforts are matched in this manner. The State Medicaid Director for Texas has indicated to the HIV waiver developers that such certification is allowable (by CMS). The HIV waiver certification process would not necessarily mimic the SHARS process, but would likely be some newly created process unique to the hospital districts' needs.[56] In this respect, the HIV/AIDS Waiver could serve a very useful role, functioning in essence as a pilot project for similar, even statewide, projects funded locally through a certification process. As of early May 2002, the HIV/AIDS waiver concept paper has been submitted to CMS.

SB 1246

Senate Bill 1246 was passed in 1997 by the 75th Legislature,[57] revised in 1999 by the 76th Legislature and, again, in 2001 by the 77th Legislature. It was originally intended to help rural counties prepare for the inevitable growth of health maintenance organizations (HMOs) by allowing the creation of a statewide rural HMO. The legislation developed through an alliance of various stakeholders: Texas Medical Association (TMA), Texas Organization of Rural and Community Hospitals (TORCH), Texas Academy of Family Physicians, Texas Hospital Association (THA), and others. With the goal of responding to "unique problems" faced by rural communities (non-urbanized counties or counties with fewer than 50,000 inhabitants), this law was developed "as an alternative to the urban-based Medicaid HMOs that overlap into rural Texas."[58] Rural physicians, hospitals, and communities are allowed under legislation to form a private, non-profit rural health care system to be governed and managed by themselves, and thus, "preserve access to local services, clinical autonomy, and health care dollars within rural communities."[59]

The encroachment of urban HMOs was causing significant concern to rural communities and providers due to the threat to the "long-term viability of rural health care delivery systems because of insufficient reimbursement, network exclusion and loss of patients and health care dollars from rural markets to urban centers."[60] The Rural Community Health System (RCHS) was developed as a result of this legislation to allow risk to be born and shared by "a single state-wide entity that will support local community health networks which will retain administrative function over and responsibility for quality and utilization within their local communities."[61] RCHS has evolved somewhat from the intent of the original legislation. Rather than serving as a statewide HMO itself, through the direction of subsequent legislation, RCHS has focused on being more of an umbrella supportive and regulatory entity, facilitating the networking required for local entities, individually or together, to develop their own networks in support of an EPO insurance model. The RCHS is to be granted at least "one of any state contract awarded to provide health care services to beneficiaries of a governmental health program so long as it satisfies contractual and licensure requirements imposed by the state on such arrangements."[62] Additionally, the RCHS can spread risk further by contracting with other private and public insurance programs.[63]

The RCHS Board is made up of eighteen members: rural hospital directors, rural physicians, and rural leaders. Although the RCHS was not funded by the Legislature, they are currently working on pursuing a pilot project "for a rural managed care EPO model as an alternative to the state mandated rural PCCM."[64] Despite the lack of funding, according to a Texas HHSC report, "the RCHS Board, supported by rural health advocacy groups, is continuing to meet and discuss grant funding, collaboration with existing rural health networks, and participation in the CHIP program. The board members recognize the value and the need for a statewide entity to coordinate rural health network efforts, regardless of the status of Medicaid managed care."[65]

Local Entity Perspectives

Survey Results

On November 16, 2001, and again on December 17, 2001, surveys were disseminated by mail to county judges and program/hospital administrators in all 254 Texas counties. The second survey was modified only slightly from the first and was sent in an effort to increase the response rate (see Appendix J for a copy of the surveys). A total of 108 surveys were returned, representing 95 unduplicated counties. The survey was conducted in an effort to gain insight from local officials and program administrators regarding the existing safety-net health care system.

Of the 53 respondents answering the survey question regarding their description of the ideal indigent care system for counties, over half answered that the system should be one in which the state has a larger role, i.e., is ultimately responsible for the safety-net system. Most responders pointed to the fact that the state has vaster resources, especially than many rural, economically challenged counties. One responder made the following comment expressing the difficulty of meeting the state mandate: "this is a real hardship on counties that are rural, lower economic status counties yet are in a corridor where they catch a lot of indigent health patients."

The majority of respondents suggested that the system should be one that builds on the existing Texas Medicaid structure. Many also suggested that the system should expand coverage to a higher FPL. Specifically, one responder offered the following:

> The Medicaid program could be expanded to cover indigents. Potentially, the monies now spent by counties and hospital districts on indigent care could be used to provide the extra match monies the state will need to draw down the additional match federal Medicaid funds that will be needed to cover these additional enrollees.

Several respondents supported the idea that the federal government should play a bigger role in the provision of indigent care at the local/state level. For instance, one respondent stated that "every county should have a primary health clinic available...It should provide services on a sliding fee scale for gap patients (over Medicaid and IHC guidelines) but unable to provide for medical care (and) should be funded by federal and state funds."

Few respondents expressed that they feel the current county system is adequate to meet the needs of their county. Other suggestions by counties included: making the system uniform and statewide, decreasing gaps in service, placing health department or primary health clinics in each county, and one responder suggested the use of sales tax instead of property tax to fund the system.

When asked whether or not counties should be responsible for providing indigent health care (IHC), the strongest response was that they should not. Out of 75 respondents answering this question, 47 answered that counties/hospital districts should not be solely responsible for providing IHC. Among these respondents, about one-fifth of them suggested that it should be a joint responsibility. One responder suggested that the program be provided for "in conjunction with state and federal (funds), but ... counties should control and audit the funds." The biggest concern expressed by respondents regarding the IHC mandate was cost. As one responder put it, "counties have no funds plus tax rates are going up." Some responders expressed frustration regarding the fact that the state mandated the service provision but did not provide any funding to counties. Several responders pointed out that meeting the mandate is especially difficult for counties that are "rural (and) have little funds." Other responders stressed that there is significant lack of consistency by having IHC at the county level—"each county has a different program with different rules, no uniformity...the base to get revenue from also varies too much from each location."

One county commissioner was moved to write the following in a letter accompanying the questionnaire:

> I retired from the private practice of medicine after my own surgery eleven years ago. Admittedly, I still carry the personal bias that private practice imposed on me. I work to see that indigent patients get the best possible care. It's tough. Money gets in the way here at the courthouse more than it ever did in my office. I can no longer treat people for free simply because the patient needs it that way. I have to deny care to deserving people because of the monetary restraints. I believe we have a decent system in [our] County that puts caring back in the mix of indigent patient care. Still, we remain a system that is only a safety net for the poorest of the poor. Contrast what we are able to do in this mid-sized county with what is—or is not—available in the poorer, less populated counties, and you see one of the basic problems with the Texas system. Care is uneven or lacking in our smallest counties, and the approach in others may be one of saving money rather than saving patients. We need to institute equality of access and administration of care for all our indigent patients. The bottom line, after all, is good and decent patient care for all our people, not local control or maintaining political power. The only answer I see to make our care even throughout our population is for the state to take it over. This would necessitate a revision of the state constitution, but that can be done.

In contrast, a few respondents expressed a belief that localities are actually better positioned to determine indigent needs within local area. And, they feel that without the county level service "many would go without necessary medical treatment."

<u>Local Control</u>

In an interview, Sue Glover, a Legislative Analyst with the Texas Association of Counties, stated that to maximize county involvement in a local contribution-funded waiver, "local control" over program decisions as well as the flow of dollars would need to be factored in. Increased local control would help to minimize uncertainty regarding county contribution requirements and would allow for a guarantee of a return on the dollar invested. In the previous 1995 SB 10 waiver attempt, there was much ambiguity/uncertainty regarding how counties could be assured that funds would be returned to their communities and about how the county contribution would occur. Ms. Glover explained that this contributed significantly to the counties ultimately not being "bought-in" to the waiver concept. A new waiver, in her opinion, might need to consider safeguards against this source of county angst.[66]

Related to the uncertainty and concerns on the part of the counties seems to be the lack of information dissemination and explanation provided to counties throughout the waiver development process. Ms. Glover explained that counties were not really brought into the loop, into the discussions until after the bill passed. Getting the county stakeholders around the table, educating them, and gathering their input along the way is a key part of a new waiver development process.[67]

Funding Logistics

In helping to fund the state match for a Medicaid expansion, a key question counties will have, according to Ms. Glover, is "What are the logistics involved in counties putting up match money?" Ms. Glover stated that a local contribution structure based on a "certification" of current expenditure level, versus an actual transfer of funds, like the structure planned by the HIV/AIDS waiver, would likely be most attractive for counties. In such a structure, the county demonstrates, through expenditure receipts, that it has spent "x" amount of money providing health care services to individuals in their county who fall below a given FPL. A funding system that requires a literal transfer of funds becomes more complicated and thus less attractive to counties.[68] This is also true for the hospital districts, although it does not appear to be a "deal breaker." In a transfer of funds situation, counties/districts are faced with the concern that they may not receive back the level of funds that they contributed. This issue also concerns many county commissioners/attorneys

Flexibility

Flexibility with regard to whether or not a county participates in the funding is another important consideration. Because of the diversity of counties and county interests, a new waiver design might consider providing an option for counties regarding participation, as was the case in SB 10, Ms. Glover pointed out. Counties with CIHCPs for instance may choose not to contribute funds toward the expansion. While the county would benefit from the Medicaid expansion by having more insured residents, they would have no control over utilization. In this case, services could be provided as they currently are for Medicaid recipients in non-managed care areas, or the state could choose to operate services through a managed care entity in that area. A county that does choose to participate in the funding effort could be given the option to operate an EPO. Flexibility achieves two basic goals: 1) for the counties who have developed a health care product that they wish to continue, it allows them to manage and deliver services, and 2) for counties/hospital districts concerned about contributed dollars returning to them, it provides this assurance. In developing their own provider networks, or EPOs, counties/hospital districts could choose to either ally with an urban/public hospital center that develops its own EPO system, or they could organize independently or by region (with other counties). Counties in rural areas might be more interested in such an alliance by region, through RCHS for instance.[69]

This issue of flexibility along with the issue of local control will be central to discussions regarding a local-contribution-funded expansion waiver, especially for the rural counties.

Hospital Districts

In the local-contribution funding option, which relies heavily on hospital district funds, especially those of large urban hospital districts, there are several important considerations. It is first important to understand the current role of DSH dollars, with regard to these entities, and their potential role in a Medicaid expansion.

The state match for federal DSH funding comes largely from hospital district tax dollars, specifically, nine large urban hospital districts. The state uses these funds, along with state hospital funds, to draw down the available federal DSH dollars. Because there is a federal cap on the total disproportionate share dollars that can be brought into the state (since the Balanced Budget Act 1997), there is a significant amount of local tax money that is not currently being "matched." These unmatched hospital district tax dollars are used for many healthcare-related purposes within a district, a significant portion of which is uncompensated health care. The cost of uncompensated care is indeed a heavy burden for these hospitals due to the especially high numbers of uninsured in large urban areas.

While it appears that these large urban hospitals may be interested in a matching scenario, there are important implications to be considered regarding the reallocation of these funds. Of primary importance to these entities, like with counties, is how and when their funds will be returned to them and what will be the return on their investment. The greatest benefit to these entities will be the increased number of Medicaid-covered individuals, individuals who are currently costing them large sums of money in uncompensated, costly emergency room and hospital care. Although these hospitals have significant unmatched tax dollars, these funds are likely "spoken for" and thus any contribution on their part would require them to leverage these funds in some manner. Such leverage would likely require some form of guarantee that the contributed funds would be returned within a reasonable timeframe. The funding return can be ensured in part by the design of EPOs in which the entity controls service utilization of covered individuals. The other potential assurance could be an increase in the entity's DSH allotment. Most of the urban hospital districts are relatively below their DSH cap, and could thus receive an enhanced DSH payment in return for a hefty upfront match contribution.

However, a DSH increase for these big urban hospitals could mean a reduction in the DSH funds available to other hospitals. This reduction might be justified if it results in a larger pool of insured individuals. Additionally, as the result of a Medicaid expansion, the number of uninsured would decrease, and this decrease could lower the federally-imposed caps to hospitals that can receive DSH payments. In other words, a decrease in the number of uninsured individuals for a hospital could affect that hospital's overall DSH allotment, but this would be the case only if that hospital was at its DSH cap. Because the DSH allotments may soon change (from 0.5 percent for Medicaid and low-income inpatient days to 0.75 percent for uninsured and 0.25 for Medicaid) with regard to the weight given for low-income inpatient numbers versus Medicaid inpatient numbers, a hospital that now has fewer uninsured and more Medicaid recipients could potentially lose DSH dollars. Most hospital district hospitals are not near their DSH cap however and thus have sufficient numbers of uninsured to preclude a significant change in their DSH allotment (other than what will take place without the expansion). Such a decrease would not affect all hospitals the same. The few hospitals that are currently at their DSH cap would have a decrease in their DSH dollars, but they are still gaining dollars through an expanded Medicaid program. To the extent that capped DSH hospitals would lose DSH money, DSH funds could be freed up to make the enhanced payments to the big urban hospital districts making the initial intergovernmental transfers without having to reduce the DSH allotments to other hospitals.[70] Table 9.5 demonstrates where the large urban hospitals are with respect to their cap.

It is important to note that while the threat to the federal DSH funds has been ongoing for some time, it is no less real today. There is something to be said for the benefit gained by all involved in having a more stable source of federal dollars flowing into these entities, via insured individuals. While a Medicaid expansion may mean that a few hospitals receive no net benefit in funds, the possibility remains that DSH funds could be gone tomorrow and to the extent that these entities have "weaned" themselves from DSH and become more reliant on alternative, more stable sources of funds, the better off they will be in the long run.

Table 9.5
Federal DSH Caps on Urban Hospital Districts

Hospitals and Hospital Districts	Estimated 2002 DSH dollars	SFY 2002 Adjusted DSH Limit	At Cap Test 0 = Cap	% Cap Amount
Bexar Co. H.D.	$74,074,581	$132,144,969	-$58,070,388	56.06%
Dallas Co. H.D.	$150,924,447	$232,380,649	-$81,456,202	64.95%
Med. Ctr. H.D.	$15,072,669	$23,682,730	-$8,610,061	63.64%
El Paso H.D.	$39,386,851	$54,101,901	-$14,715,050	72.80%
Harris Co. H.D.	$141,400,505	$256,767,177	-$115,366,672	55.07%
Lubbock Co. H.D.	$22,808,910	$34,427,798	-$11,618,888	66.25%
Christus Mem. CC	$43,276,063	$43,276,063	$0	100.00%
Tarrant Co. H.D.	$46,391,507	$168,901,657	-$122,510,150	27.47%
Brackenridge Hosp.	$41,439,691	$41,442,067	-$2,376	99.99%

Adapted from: Email from Henry Welles, Program Specialist, Texas Department of Health, "RE: Data you Requested," to Sara Stout, February 25, 2002.

In an interview, Steve Scarborough of Health Data Partners confirmed that in essence there are a fair amount of hospital tax dollars that are indeed "unmatched," and are a potential source for a match. The amount is most likely somewhere between $300 and $600 million. Mr. Scarborough added that just because the money may be there on paper does not necessarily make it easily accessible by these entities and does not mean that the decision-making authorities for these entities would be willing to do so. He also reiterated that these entities would have to be assured that the money would be returned in a reasonable amount of time. Mr. Scarborough did point out that there is a Hospital Payment Advisory Committee (Technical Advisory Committee) through HHSC made of representatives from the hospital industry, including the large urban hospital districts, and that they had discussed the possibility of putting up $48.5 million dollars for federal match to help the state meet the Medicaid shortfall. This arrangement has since been submitted as a proposal to HHSC and is being discussed and refined at this time by both industry and state officials. In this case, as would be the case in a local-contribution

Medicaid expansion waiver, these entities will be getting their money back in the form of an increased DSH payment. As was the case described above, these enhanced payments will be in the context of overall DSH allocations, and thus would result in reduced payments to other hospitals.[71]

John Umphress of the Texas Association of Public and Nonprofit Hospitals (TANPH) responded similarly, in an interview, regarding potential match contributions by big urban hospitals. Mr. Umphress stated that while these hospitals would likely be willing to contribute their unmatched money, he believed that they are constrained constitutionally from sending it out of the county without a guarantee of it coming back. He also believed that their willingness would likely depend on the rate of return. Mr. Umphress stressed that these hospitals would be looking to participate out of necessity, not desire, as it is "bad policy" for the counties because funding such safety-net care should be a *state* function.[72]

Rural Entities

When considering a statewide waiver it is important to consider that there are 254 different counties in Texas. Six counties have populations of 500,000 residents or more, and they account for more than 40 percent of the state's population. Conversely, 95counties have populations of less than 10,000 residents and account for only 3 percent of the state's population.

Complicating the design of a new waiver is the complexity of the community landscape in Texas. What works for large, densely populated urban communities may not work for sparsely populated, rural communities. Consider the following facts provided by an HHSC Report:

- Of Texas' 196 rural counties, 62 have no hospital, 106 have one hospital, 23 have two hospitals, and five have three hospitals;
- Texas led the nation in hospital closures in the late 1980s and has seen several closures of rural hospitals in the last few years: one in 1997, two in 1998, three in 1999, and one by mid-year 2000;
- Three of Texas' 196 rural counties had *no* primary care physician as of January 2000, and an additional 19 counties had only *one* healthcare practitioner;
- 172 (88 percent) of rural Texas counties are designated as medically underserved areas (MUAs); and
- 203 counties in Texas are outside of managed care, 23 of them urban; 86 hospital districts are in counties outside of Medicaid managed care; while these counties are required to provide indigent care, they also are the main provider of care to the Medicare and Medicaid patients.[73]

Such economic challenges led Texas Organization of Rural and Community Hospital (TORCH) leaders, in an interview, to indicate that the potential economic development resulting from increased Medicaid-insured individuals would be a positive selling point for their constituent group. In their view, rural and community hospitals would likely be quite interested in a Medicaid expansion, especially if it did not *require* a contribution on their part. Rural and community hospitals operate "hand-to-mouth" they explained, and thus contributing upfront money is difficult for small hospitals. If they had to pay, they would likely need some *assurance* that the money would be returned to them. They stated that if a provider-controlled mechanism was in place, it would likely help with this issue. They agreed that this could be accomplished potentially through the work of the RCHS. TORCH leaders did not believe that a potential loss of DSH dollars, associated with an expansion, would matter much to rural and community hospitals, as they receive nominal amounts of DSH funds.[74]

Sue Glover with TAC also stressed the importance of economic development possibilities for counties as a selling point, especially with rural communities that have seen the disappearance of healthcare providers. She believed that the influx of increased Medicaid/SCHIP dollars into these communities would definitely help to revitalize local health care providers and thus local economies.[75]

Considerations

Designers of a local contribution waiver will have the task of considering the concerns of all of the above stakeholder groups. One possible incentive for counties, specifically counties with CIHCPs, is that in the case of an expansion that extends Medicaid coverage up to 50 percent of the FPL, counties would benefit from the 21 to 50 percent that they did not have to fund. Additionally, it has been suggested that rescinding the state mandate would likely have positive effects on the interest of counties in participating. Counties with CIHCPs that provide coverage above 21 percent of the FPL would likely need to be allowed to contribute at the 21 percent expenditure level, and also allowed to continue generating local revenue to provide services up to the desired FPL. They would also need to retain adequate funds to cover other non-waiver targeted populations, such as undocumented residents. Again, allowing funding contribution by counties with CIHCP to be optional, as was the case with SB 10, will positively affect the projects appeal. Additionally, the new waiver proposal should strive to avoid rural versus urban battles on any related issues.

As described in an interview by Caton Fenz, Legislative Director for State Representative Garnet Coleman, for hospital districts and counties to be willing to come to the table regarding a new waiver there are two key ingredients: 1) the state must show counties a financial benefit or cost-neutrality; and 2) the contributing hospitals must know how DSH will be affected—what the ramifications would be for Medicaid revenue and DSH loss versus maintaining existing levels of DSH. Historically, county-state relations are somewhat strained and thus counties are somewhat leery of being required to do something on behalf of the state. A waiver development process needs to be respectful of that distrust he suggested.[76]

Mr. Fenz added that while rural counties are not likely the "lynchpin" in planning/ funding, they must be onboard politically with the plan, as rural interests often dominate the legislature. He reiterated that stressing the economic development importance of such an expansion could strengthen this effort. Mr. Fenz did believe that any contention on the part of rural counties/hospitals would have less to do with getting additional individuals on Medicaid than it will about increasing reimbursement rates (a big issue for rural counties). In the total financial picture of a statewide 1115 waiver, only a small amount of funding could come from the rural counties. In other words, their financial contribution is not crucial to the deal. However, the benefit of increased inflow of dollars could help them economically.[77]

It is apparent that any funding scenario that relies heavily on the big hitters, i.e., hospital districts, medical schools, and teaching hospitals, will need to include an enhanced payment system for those contributing entities, most likely through DSH. The biggest implication regarding the willingness of large urban hospitals to participate, according to TAPNH staff, is what are the potential Upper Payment Limit (UPL) effects, as against the Medicaid shift relative to DSH. The UPL is essentially the amount that Medicaid pays an entity versus what reasonably would have been paid at the Medicare level. It is important to note accordingly that hospitals do still have room within the UPL to come up—to receive an enhanced rate—even given the new federal UPL requirement.

A final implication, expressed by a TAPNH member with regard to large urban hospitals, is that costs are increasing for hospitals due to inappropriate ER utilization and trauma care for the uninsured. Public hospitals are at risk of closing as a result, so the need to intervene is an economic development issue. Essentially, a symptom of the current situation, i.e., a result of the status quo, is a collapse of the ER systems, and thus he believes large urban hospital districts are ready to come to the table.[78]

In general, the new waiver could build on three essential incentives for county participation: 1) counties spend money on health coverage more efficiently by expanding the covered population to plus or minus 50 percent of the FPL without increasing current outlays; 2) the headache regarding administration of the current program is alleviated if desired; and 3) counties have the opportunity to maintain some control if desired. For hospitals, the benefit is simply in the expanded pool of insured versus uninsured individuals served.

The following are possible waiver components for consideration during design:

- Counties contribute money based on current level of expenditures for population at or below 21 percent of the FPL (versus a set percentage of GRTL);
- Waiver extends Medicaid-covered population to plus or minus 50 percent (whatever the current expenditure plus the match allows for) for childless adults, in addition to low-income parents;
- Contribution requirement is met through "certification" of existing expenditures process; otherwise, counties transfer funds to the state on an annual, quarterly, or monthly;

- Counties can continue to levy taxes to provide services at a level above what is to be covered by the waiver and to cover population (i.e., ineligible immigrants) that are eligible economically but who Medicaid cannot cover;
- Hospital districts and interested counties can, individually or together, form "exclusive provider organizations" to manage the Medicaid dollars for their district/county; and
- The state funds currently used to provide relief to counties with CIHCPs exceeding 8 percent of their GRTL in approved expenditures is added into the overall state match.

Planners would also need to decide whether or not the state could/should rescind the 21 percent mandate in order to garner county support. Additionally, planners may want to consider whether or not a "phased-in" structure would be beneficial, with large urban hospital districts coming on board first, possibly as a pilot, then counties, then others.

Hospital districts have indicated their interest in beginning discussions about a local-contribution funded Medicaid expansion. Simultaneously, efforts are underway by Representative Coleman and Senator Lindsay to explore these possibilities. Furthermore, Sue Glover with the Texas Association of Counties believes that such an expansion is a "do-able" project from the county perspective. With these stakeholders willing to come to the table and with the RCHS making considerable headway, it does appear that there is real potential for developing a local-contribution funded Medicaid waiver that, while not without some compromise by each party, provides a benefit to all parties involved, most especially indigent residents of Texas.

Waiver Implications for Local Entities

The primary challenge for waiver developers is designing a waiver that protects the fiscal interests of the hospital districts and counties and still meets the requirements for the Medicaid program. Counties and hospital districts will want to ensure that their funds are used to provide care locally, and not used to subsidize care in other counties. The requirements of the Medicaid program can make this difficult to guarantee, but a waiver to expand Medicaid in Texas is likely to be difficult without county cooperation.

Because some counties have large indigent health care programs and others provide only minimal services, how a waiver would affect counties varies. Counties will have to consider whether the costs of participation are within their budgets and whether or not the fiscal burden is fair. A critical point for counties is in understanding how the population currently served by county programs can be shifted into the Medicaid program.

Different laws govern the state indigent care program and the federal Medicaid program with regard to eligibility. Chapter 61 of the Texas State Code defines who is eligible for medical assistance under the indigent health program, while Title 19 of the United States Code governs the parameters for basic eligibility for Medicaid. In Texas, the eligible indigent population includes any resident of a county who is not insured, not eligible for public assistance, and who has an income below the threshold set by that county. In practice this means the counties cover very low-income adults who are not eligible for Medicare or Medicaid and low-income children not eligible for Medicaid (primarily believed to be non-citizen children of undocumented workers). Eligibility is not contingent on whether an adult is also a parent. Medicaid by contrast has more complex eligibility rules.[79]

Medicaid law splits the population into three categories: mandatory, optional, and expansion populations. Under Medicaid law the uninsured adults served by county programs would be both optional and expansion population. This is because under Medicaid law adults are split into two different population categories. Parents are an optional population and childless adults are classified as an expansion population. Additionally, some populations served by county programs would be difficult to add to a waiver and likely would remain in county programs. Documented residents who have been in the country for less than five years, undocumented adults, and undocumented children cannot be covered under Medicaid. These populations could not be included in a waiver, and under current law counties would still have to provide care to this population.

How much would a waiver cost?

Using the "hypothetical" Section 1931 and HIFA Section 1115 waiver model discussed briefly in the second section (and described in detail in Kegler, 2002), the state could expand coverage to both low-income parents and childless adults. Based on this model, an expansion in Texas could cost between $91.3 million and $783 million in state general revenue during the first biennium of a five-year phase in of different options. In the first, less expensive option example, the waiver would just cover parents up to 100 percent of the FPL and childless adults up to 50 percent of the FPL, with a cost-sharing of 5 percent of annual income and a benefit package costing 54 percent of the mandated TANF Medicaid package. In a second option the waiver could cover up to 200 percent of the FPL for parents and 100 percent of the FPL for childless adults, with no cost sharing and a benefit package equal to 60 percent of the TANF benefit package. These estimates depend on a number of assumptions but they do provide ballpark estimates. These options suggest that the state would have to come up with an annual amount of extra GR of $45-392 million to fund this initiative; but greater sums than this are currently being spent by hospital districts and counties, and could be used more efficiently as a match if the right approach could be worked out. If these options were initiated they would draw down an additional $136 to $1,175 million in federal funds in the first biennium. Subsequent years would require additional funds as the five-year phase in took place, and for that additional funds would have to be found.

How would counties participate in a waiver?

The current structure of the indigent health care system suggests that counties should help fund any expansion that includes the population they serve. Counties would need to weigh how much they are currently spending and who they are currently able to serve with the conditions of a waiver. The lower the cost of county participation, and the larger the population included in the waiver, the better the value to the county.

The cost of a waiver that expands coverage to parents *and* to childless adults could require funds far beyond the current level of fiscal effort by counties. Areas that operate CIHCPs are only required to cover individuals up to 21 percent of the FPL. Other revenue options would likely be needed to reduce the fiscal load on counties with more modest means, i.e., larger contributions from large urban hospital districts, the state indigent health care matching funds, or new revenues.

Policymakers at the state and local level have developed an array of programs and funding mechanisms to deliver care to the low-income uninsured. However, the cost of indigent care is a burden that does not have to be born solely by local taxpayers. Medicaid funds offer the potential for more stability and greater health care spending in Texas counties. Reconciling the divergent interests of the counties would be the greatest challenge. Given the intricacies of the current system of funding, the conditions of any waiver will have to represent good politics as well as good policy.

New Revenue Options

Given the state's current fiscal stress and the amount of funds required, it is evident that the reallocation of existing funds may not be sufficient to cover the costs of an expansion. Other sources of revenue may be required. One obvious method of generating additional funds is through new taxes and fees. To justify new taxes, the report focuses on taxes within the healthcare arena, on providers that would benefit from a health coverage expansion, and taxable items that have a connection to increased costs in health care.

Health Care-Related Taxes

A provider tax is one way to generate revenue to help fund an expansion or to increase reimbursement to providers. This method of revenue generation allows providers who stand to benefit from an expanded pool of insured individuals, and who are currently paying in other less efficient ways for uninsured care, to help fund expanded coverage. With the high levels of uninsured individuals in the state, there is a high cost for the uncompensated care that hospitals and physicians are currently facing as well. In 1998, Texas spent approximately $2 billion on charity health care.[80] A large portion of these dollars can be attributed to the high number of uninsured individuals in the state. By investing a portion of this money up front through a tax or fee, the funds can then be used to expand existing health coverage programs. This investment will bring federal dollars into the system through the Federal Matching Assistance Program (FMAP), thus allowing the funds to stretch further and decrease the number of uninsured in Texas. Without coverage, individuals are often times forced to receive care in its most expensive form. This reallocation of funds could possibly decrease the often-avoidable costs associated with uncompensated care. The expansion of healthcare coverage programs would allow these individuals to receive needed care at an earlier, less costly time or even preclude this need through preventative care.

While states have used provider tax funds to reduce state general fund contributions to Medicaid and to fund non-Medicaid expenditures,[81] the use of such funds to expand Medicaid services to uninsured individuals and to increase reimbursement rates is the most fiscally sensible use for Texas. If the funds generated by the tax were simply substituted for current state general revenue, no additional federal dollar funds would be generated, and thus no benefit from decreased uncompensated care costs would be realized.

Tax Burden

There are many policy implications that must be addressed in the effort to generate money for the state through a provider tax. One concern with a health care related tax is the incidence of the tax burden. While these taxes can be a good investment through the addition of federal dollars that can be brought to a state, it is very difficult to assess whether the tax is not hurting the individuals in need of care. Many times these taxes are characterized as "sick taxes" because of the perception that the tax will fall only on individuals who are ill. While this tax can be seen as regressive, the perception of how burden will fall is not as clear. Verdier asserts that the ultimate burden of these taxes will be distributed in some way among healthcare providers, insurance companies, employers, workers, and healthcare recipients depending on the characteristics of the specific markets and market power.[82] While the majority of the burden appears to fall on the healthcare providers, it is possible that the funds will be replaced by the decrease in cost of uncompensated care. It is also possible for the tax's burden to be shared by the hospital or physician, the third-party payer, or the individual seeking health care. One of the original and continuing arguments for the Minnesota provider tax was that it was not intended to be absorbed by providers but rather to be collected by them and passed through to health plans of all types.[83] The 1992 legislation for the Minnesota provider tax allowed providers to pass the tax through to all third-party payers, which were then required by law to reimburse the money to hospitals and doctors.[84] Another way to decrease the burden is to distribute the tax among the different health care classes. Shifting cost along all health care consumers will also decrease the burden. The more classes that are added to the group, the smaller the assessment is on each class and the perception of equity between classes are apparent. Another consideration in this policy decision is the taxes that health care providers are already burdened with. If the providers are exempt from most taxes within the state, the burden of the implementation of a tax will not be as great.

Creating a New Tax

Another aspect of a provider tax that would affect the state of Texas is the fact that it would be the creation of a new tax. This is a very important factor in a state that has been hesitant to raise taxes or create any new taxes in the past. However, a provider tax is not always seen as an ordinary tax because of its ability to be returned as payment to the providers who paid the tax through patient services. In 1991, Illinois imposed a provider tax on hospitals, nursing homes, and centers for the mentally ill and the developmentally disabled. The system was developed as a way to attract more federal dollars to pay Illinois hospitals and nursing homes. The tax passed the Illinois House and Senate easily and was signed by the Governor Jim Edgar. The Edgar administration insisted that the tax did not break the "no new taxes pledge for four years" because it was not an ordinary tax. Those who paid the tax would soon get it back.[85] It is important to remember that provider taxes can serve an important purpose because of their ability to help states fund existing health coverage programs that provide health coverage to uninsured individuals.

Implementation of a Provider Tax

A provider tax also has a substantial ability to generate money for health care. Beginning in 1993, Minnesota implemented a provider tax that applied to all hospitals and surgical centers that provide inpatient and outpatient services in the state. In 1994, the state included physician services and sales on wholesale drug distributors. Many states focused on cigarette taxes at that time for health care reform because of the public acceptance of a relationship between smoking and health outcomes. Minnesota, however, was able to tap a somewhat larger base in the provider tax.[86] Another attribute to any tax, including a provider tax, is the ability to keep the administrative cost low. In Minnesota, the Department of Revenue reported the provider tax to be one of the easiest and most efficient to administer, costing about 80 cents for every 100 dollars collected.[87]

With health-related taxes, there is the choice of how to structure the tax and to choose what class of health care provider to tax. If the tax is developed with a fixed revenue goal in mind, it is possible to find a way to distribute the burden and administer the tax so no one health care provider or consumer is hurt by the tax. There are also distribution methods that may help the tax to be more politically viable. One is to apply it to classes that serve a high proportion of Medicaid businesses. They would increase incentive because of their interest to keep the program adequately funded and the possibility of incentives like an increase in total reimbursement. The other side is by applying the assessment to a provider class with a smaller portion of Medicaid patients. They have the fortune of not having to worry about cost sharing and the burden will not be as great. By distributing it to both of these types of classes it would lower the overall burden. Some options to consider when deciding on how to administer the tax are whether or not to apply the tax as a percentage of gross revenue, as a flat fee per day, or as a one-time fee per heath care service. All three have the potential to generate new funds for the state. To the extent possible a tax, to avoid controversy, should not overburden the sickest individuals. A fee or tax that is not based on the length of time an individual is in the hospital or the amount of cost an individual incurs would help to avoid this situation.

Provider Tax Provisions

Through the last two decades a number of provisions have been made that apply to provider taxes being able to bring down these federal dollars. In 1985, the Health Care Financing Administration (HCFA) issued a rule allowing states to receive donations from private medical care providers to draw down federal matching funds. During this time, states began using provider taxes or donation programs to bring down matching dollars. Provider taxes and donation programs proved to be financially advantages to states because it allows states to draw down federal money without the use of general revenue funds.[88] Many states took advantage of these funds. Some of these states were even seen as abusing finances to capture federal dollars.[89] In 1991, the Medicaid Voluntary Contribution and Provider-Specific Tax Amendments of 1991(P.L. 101-234) was passed to restrict the use of provider-based taxes as a means of generating federal matching funds. It also banned the use of provider donations for these funds. [90]

- Under the 1991 legislation, federal dollars would not be available for "health care related taxes" if the taxes were not broad based and if they contained a "hold harmless provision."[91]
- It is considered a health care related tax if 85 percent of the burden falls on healthcare providers. Even if the tax is not related to health care items or services, it is a health care related tax if it provides for different treatment for individuals or entities that are providing, or paying for healthcare items or services.[92]
- The tax is considered broad-based if it meets two criteria. First, the tax must apply to all items or services within the same class or providers. Second, it must apply uniformly. It is considered uniform if it is imposed on the providers within a class consistently. If is based on a licensing fee, the amount imposed must be the same for every provider in that class. If is imposed on the number of beds, the amount must be the same for each bed within the class of providers. If the tax is based on revenues, it must be imposed at the same rate on all gross revenue, or net operating costs within a class.[93] The tax may exclude revenues from Medicare and Medicaid and still meet the uniformity test.[94]
- The amendments also established that the tax could not be combined with any measures that could hold providers harmless for the tax they paid. It does not however prevent the use of the tax to reimburse health care providers. The provision does not prevent states from relying on the reimbursement to justify or explain the tax in the legislative process.[95]
- A state may submit an application for a waiver for the broad-based requirement. Waivers may include the exemptions of the tax to rural or sole community hospitals.[96] The waiver is subject for approval if the state can prove that the tax is "generally redistributive in nature."[97]

Provider Classes

There are eight main provider classes that were developed as a result of the Medicaid Voluntary Contribution and Provider-Specific Tax Amendments of 1991. These classes could be taxed at the state's discretion in accordance with the provider tax provisions. The provider classes included inpatient and outpatient hospital services, nursing homes, intermediate care facilities for the mentally retarded, physician services, home health services, outpatient prescription drugs, health maintenance organizations, and any other classification of health care items or services that may be established by regulations.[98] The National Governors' Association negotiated a number of other provider classes that could be taxed under the new legislation. These classes included dentistry, podiatry, chiropractic, optometry, psychological, therapeutic, nursing, laboratory, and radiology services. The amount of the provider tax could be different for different classes, but they were required to be uniform within each class and cover every provider in the class.[99]

Hospital Tax

Hospital taxes are one possible way to apply the tax to inpatient and outpatient services. This revenue can then be used to bring down federal matching funds. There are a number of ways that hospitals can be taxed. One way is to base the tax on gross revenue, while another is to place the fees or taxes on occupied beds only. Another way to apply the tax is through an admit fee. The provision of a provider tax on a hospital will have positive impacts on expansion. Hospitals typically deal with the high costs of uncompensated care: many times this is due to the number of uninsured individuals that are forced to use the emergency room as their primary source care. Hospitals are usually prepared not to receive a certain amount of payment due to uncompensated care every year. In theory, the implementation of a provider tax would reallocate a portion of the funds that hospitals use for uncompensated care for expansion. In return the hospitals would see a decrease in the number of uninsured that need care and a decrease in the cost of uncompensated care. It is also possible to use a portion of the funds to increase reimbursement levels. This would off set the cost-sharing burden the hospital must face due to an increase in the number of patients who would now be covered by Medicaid or SCHIP.

Currently in the state of Texas, hospitals are not heavily burdened with taxes. In theory, hospitals that are lightly burdened from other taxes would not be as burdened from the implementation of a provider tax. These hospitals would also see the return of the funds paid out for the tax though payment received for patient care.

This tax could be implemented on general revenues through various rates. The rates that were found in other state hospital taxes typically ranged from 1 to 2 percent on general revenues. Minnesota has a tax on hospitals for revenue purposes of the Minnesota Care Tax. These taxes are based on gross revenue for patient services that are provided by the hospital.[100] The tax was part of the Health Care Access Fund (HCAF), which financed MinnesotaCare. The tax has ranged from 2.0 percent,[101] to the most recent 1.5 percent,[102] accounted for the majority of HCAF revenues.[103] There is also a Hospital Surcharge, a Tax of 1.56 percent, is placed on the net patient revenues of each Minnesota hospital, and then collected for the general fund.[104] This application of the tax in Minnesota has proven to be an effective way to raise money for health care coverage.[105]

Another state that has also participated in a similar tax is Utah. In the early 1990s, Utah hospitals pursued an improvement in Medicaid match rate by voluntarily participating in a taxing arrangement. After donations were prohibited by the federal government, Utah hospitals continued the collection of the tax under a mandated statement. Starting in 1998, the hospital tax was extended to help pay for the states match for the State Children's Health Insurance Program. The assessment, which is based on patient revenues, had been scheduled to expire, but the Utah Association of Health Care Providers, an association made up of various healthcare providers including hospitals, agreed to continue the tax to ensure a stable and reliable source for the state match.[106] Once the tobacco settlement allocation became available, Utah hospitals believed these new funds should be used in replacement of the hospital tax.[107] While these taxes were eliminated, they did work to expand coverage and increase reimbursement.[108]

A tax that is attached to the amount of cost that is incurred or to the number of days is many times characterized as sick tax; a fee or tax that is not based on the time length a person is in the hospital or the amount of cost an individual incurs would help to avoid this situation. It would be a flat fee that would be placed on certain health services. The fee would be an admit fee for inpatient, outpatient (including physician office visits), and emergency room services. An admit fee would have to include provisions for prevention of duplicated fees (for individuals seen in the emergency room and admitted during the same visit). When compared to a tax rate it would not cause the majority of burden to be shifted those who are sick and must stay in hospitals for extended periods of time. The tax could also be applied to the admission process.

Table 9.6
Funds Generated from Hospital Taxes

General Revenue Hospital Tax	1999 General Revenue	0.5% Tax	1% Tax	1.5% Tax	2% Tax
Hospital inpatient	$30,606,354,227	$153,031,771	$306,063,542	$459,095,313	$612,127,085
Hospital outpatient	$14,423,194,125	$72,115,971	$144,231,941	$216,347,912	$288,463,883
Inpatient and outpatient	$45,029,548,352	$225,147,742	$450,295,484	$675,443,225	$900,590,967
Bed tax/fee	Patient Days	$ 1 bed fee	$3 bed fee	$5 bed fee	
Inpatient	10,945,507	$10,945,507.00	$32,836,521.00	$54,727,535.00	
Admit tax/fee	Admission #	$1 admit fee	$3 admit fee	$5 admit fee	
Outpatient admits	26,957,113	$26,957,113	$80,871,339	$134,785,565	
Inpatient admits	2,206,887	$2,206,887	$6,620,661	$11,034,435	
Total admits	29,164,000	$29,164,000	$87,492,000	$145,820,000	

Adapted from: Texas Department of Health, *Hospital Survey Data on Diskette* (Austin, Tex.: Office Of Health Information and Analysis, 1999) (Database on disk).

Physician Tax

The same types of taxes can be applied to physician services. These taxes can be placed on gross general revenue. It can be imposed as a fee per physician visit. Many of the same arguments for the implementation of the provider tax also apply to taxing physician services. Physicians are not burdened by many state taxes including a franchise tax or a state income tax. These health care providers would receive the benefits that the tax would create though the decrease in the number of uninsured and a possible increase in reimbursement. It is true in theory, that there is not as much uncompensated care in physician office services compared to the cost of uncompensated care in hospitals. Uninsured individuals are usually forced to use free clinics or the emergency room for care, rather than physician offices. Another possible benefit for physicians is the increase in patients who can services. Physicians who see a disproportionate number of Medicaid patients or who provide care in underserved areas could benefit from these new consumers along with an increase in what the state can provide in reimbursement.

Table 9.7
Funds Available from Physician Tax

	Total Office Visits	$ 1 visit fee	$3 visit fee	$4 visit fee
Physician Visit Fee	121,842,054.40	$121,842,054.40	$365,526,163.20	$609,210,272.00

Calculated from American Medical Association, *Physician Socioeconomic Statistics* (Chicago, IL, Center for Health Policy Research, 2000-2002), p. 49 ; Texas State Board of Medical Examiners, *Physicians In and Out of State* (January 2002). Online. Available: http://www.tsbme.state.tx.us/demo/docs/d2002/0102/inout.htm. Accessed: February 22,2002.

A state that has effectively implemented a provider tax on physician services is Minnesota.[109] The physician tax was created to fund MinnesotaCare, a subsidized health care coverage program that was passed in 1992.[110] The initial tax setup was similar to the hospital tax and was part of the Health Care Access Fund (HCAF), which financed MinnesotaCare. The 2 percent tax on gross revenues, physicians, and other healthcare providers[111] was decreased to 1.5 percent in 1998, due to a surplus and was scheduled to return to 2 percent in 2002.[112] While Minnesota has shown a percentage tax on physician services to be a beneficial way to raise health care funds,[113] it is possible to implement the tax as a small fee that is the same for every health care consumer. This could be implemented similar to the admit fee for hospital services. It would then be rendered for each patient bill for physician services. The fee would be nominal when compared to the medical bill, and could be a small as a few cents and could remain as small at a few dollars.

While it is possible to keep the burden of a tax on physician services small, it is usually very controversial to implement a tax on physicians. In West Virginia, the provider tax was first enacted in 1993 to be used for federally matched funds in the Medicaid program.[114] Medical doctors paid 2 percent of their gross earnings in taxes while dentists, podiatrists, chiropractors, and the other practitioners paid 1.75 percent.[115] The 2001 legislature in West Virginia repealed the provider tax. The tax is now being phased out over the next ten years.[116] The provider tax in West Virginia was a controversial issue that was opposed by many healthcare providers. There were approximately 31,000 individual health care practitioners including doctors, nurses, optometrists, podiatrists, chiropractors, physical therapists, psychologists, and massage therapists who pay quarterly to support the state's Medicaid program. While these providers did not want to hurt the state Medicaid program, they voiced concern that the tax has been a burden on the community, making it difficult to recruit health care professionals into the state, thus causing a healthcare access crisis.[117] While they voiced this concern they were never able to show that it was causing problems with keeping providers in the state.

Pharmaceutical Tax

It is also possible to implement a tax at the pharmaceutical level. This tax encompasses many of the same implications as the other healthcare related taxes. The main concern is the effect it will have on the individuals purchasing these medications. It can easily be seen as a regressive tax. However is the tax remains small, the burden will remain small for the individuals purchasing the pharmaceuticals. The state of Alabama had very little opposition when it initiated a pharmacy tax in the early 1990s. It kept their tax small at 10 cents per filled prescription. With the initiation of the tax it also increased the dispensing fee to pharmacies to keep them happy with the plan.[118] It is also possible to offset the cost to the consumer by requiring third-party payers to also share in the burden. A pharmaceutical tax has the potential to increase the funds available for healthcare and could ease the fiscal stress the state has with medication reimbursement.

Table 9.8
Funds Available though a Pharmaceutical Tax/Fee

Retail Pharmaceuticals	Total Retail Rx	$.50 Tax	$1.00 Tax
Pharmaceutical Fee/Tax	189,540,397	$94,770,198.50	$189,540,397.00
Retail Pharmaceuticals Dollars	Total Retail Rx Dollars	0.5% Tax	1% Tax
Pharmaceutical Revenue Tax	$9,033,409,467	$45,167,047.34	$90,334,094.67

Calculated from: Novartis, *Texas Summary2000.* Online. Available: http://www.novartisvin.com/content/ Statefacts/state_result.asp?State=TX&date=2000. Accessed: February 22,2002.

Nursing Home Bed Tax

Another type of provider tax is the application of a tax on nursing facilities, either though a bed tax or a revenue tax. The nursing home bed tax would not be as beneficial of a tool for expansion within that service type because of the lack of need for expansion. However, if utilized, it is one way to increase reimbursement payments to nursing facilities without using additional state general revenue dollars. With the additional increases in spending of state Medicaid dollars, Texas would also be able to bring down additional federal Medicaid dollars to help ease the fiscal tension of the state to make Medicaid payments. There was a previous attempt to implement this tax during the 77th Texas Legislature. The nursing home bed tax or quality assurance fee was presented as a way to increase funding to nursing homes. Early versions of Senate Bill 1839 (SB1839) contained the fee. The bed tax, also known as the Quality Assurance Fee, had a $5.25 per day tax levy.[119] These funds would then be used to bring down additional Medicaid dollars to increase reimbursement to nursing homes. The fee would be revised by the HHSC in six months to determine if the amount was cost feasible. The bill establishes the quality assurance fund as a fund outside the state treasury held by the Texas Treasury Safekeeping Trust Company. The bill specified that subject to legislative appropriation and these provisions, fees combined with federal matching funds would support or maintain an increase in Medicaid reimbursement for institutions.[120] HHSC or DHS would have been required to devise the formula by which amounts received will increase the reimbursement rates. HHSC would have been required to ensure that the formula provides incentives for nursing homes to increase direct care staffing and direct care wages and benefits.[121] Opposition to the fee now dubbed as the "sick tax" grew. The final versions of the bill did not include the fee for nursing facilities but did keep the fee for ICF/MRs.[122]

This shows that the implementation of a tax that has any perception of burdening the sick will have difficult passage. This is an easy characterization to develop with the passage of a healthcare related tax. It is important to see the implications that can occur without the tax. In Texas, 80 percent of the nursing home population receives Medicaid services; these individuals would not feel the burden of this tax.[123] The 20 percent of the population that would have felt the burden of the additional $5.25 a day would possibly have to see these types of increases in cost anyway. This cost increase would be due to the nursing home industry's need to implement cost sharing as a result of the disproportionate number of Medicaid patients. With this possibility in mind, it would be more reasonable to pay the $5.25 fee a day to the state so it can matched by federal dollars to offset the cost of the nursing home industry and increase reimbursement payments.

Arkansas is one of the many states that have passed a nursing home bed tax recently to help increase reimbursement to the nursing home industry; this tax was passed in March 2001. At that time 15 other states had a similar bed tax. The state passed the tax to help fund the growing number of nursing home residents who were primarily Medicaid patients. The bed tax allows the state to bring down additional federal funds through the Federal Medicaid Assistance Program. The bed tax has adopted the name of the quality assurance fee, and levies a tax of $5.25 per day on occupied beds. The rate of the fee can be adjusted in the future according to the needs of the nursing homes. The Arkansas governor favored the tax because it would help the financial problems the state faces with nursing homes and the fact that it was self-imposed by the industry.[124] Supporters of the bill believed it was necessary to provide nursing homes with money to hire additional staff that is more qualified. Opponents to the bill state that the fee penalizes nursing home residents who pay their own costs and do not receive Medicaid benefits.[125]

Medical Services Sales Tax

A source of new funding for health care coverage in Texas could come from establishing a sales tax for medical services. Currently medical services are exempt from sales tax in Texas. One estimate of the possible revenue generated by creating a sales tax for medical services puts the figure at $583.8 million for physician's services, $187.8 million for dental services, and $312.8 million for other health care services.[126] This would generate revenue totaling over $1 billion, all with a strong tie to health care. The drawback of this type of tax is that it is a tax on sick people. People utilizing more medical services will pay more tax, and unfortunately they are not always able to afford that increase. In addition, a tax of this type, like all sales taxes, is regressive in that the less an individual makes, the higher percentage of his/her income goes to pay sales tax. Advocates are quick to point out that the "sick tax" is their least favorite of funding options.[127]

The Franchise Tax

Altering or replacing Texas' franchise tax could increase revenues collected by the state and provide a source of funding for increasing health care coverage. The franchise tax serves as Texas' primary business tax. Considered a privilege tax, corporations pay the tax in exchange for certain advantages granted by the State of Texas. These privileges include access to the state's legal system, the right to accumulate property separate from any individual's property, and a limitation of personal financial liability for officers of the corporation.[128]

The tax is imposed on corporations that are chartered in Texas or have a certificate of authority to do business in the state. In addition, non-Texas corporations doing business in the state without a certificate of authority are also liable. The term "corporation" includes limited liability companies, S corporations, banks, state limited banking associations, savings and loan associations, and professional corporations.

The tax is calculated by computing a corporation's "net worth" (taxable capital) tax base and "earned surplus" tax base. The corporation pays a tax on the higher of the two tax bases. " Net worth" is defined as the firm's total assets minus debts. It is equal to a corporation's stated capital (capital stock) plus surplus, where stated capital is the par value of the firm's outstanding shares of stock, and surplus is the remainder of the firm's net worth. The total net worth tax base is apportioned according to the share of the firm's total business done in the state and is measured in terms of their gross receipts. The tax on net worth is levied at $2.50 per $1,000 of taxable capital. "Earned surplus" includes federal net taxable income plus compensation paid to officers and directors of a corporation. The earned surplus tax base is also apportioned according to the share of the firm's total business done in the state and is measured in terms of their gross receipts. The tax rate for earned surplus is 4.5 percent of the apportioned tax base.[129] A tax deduction can be granted to a firm, allowing it a subtraction from its tax base or its apportionment computation. Because the deduction is applied before the application of the tax rate, the reduction in tax liability is usually less than the deduction amount.[130]

Inequities

Criteria that are recognized as standards for evaluating taxation systems include equitable distribution of the tax burden, economically efficient taxes, and stable revenue sources.[131]

The franchise tax has been criticized for being inequitable, as it favors some business sectors at the expense of others. Because it is disproportional, it has also been criticized for being economically inefficient. Additionally, the franchise tax has been criticized for being an unstable revenue source, as it is largely based on income.[132] The burden of the franchise tax is unequally distributed and a variety of exemptions allow certain entities to not pay franchise taxes. "The burden of the franchise tax liability among the sectors of the Texas economy does not correspond to the contribution each makes to the gross state product."[133] The service sector accounts for a greater percentage of gross state product than the manufacturing sector, but pays a smaller percentage of the tax.[134] Exemptions to the franchise tax exist under both federal and state regulations. Statutory exemptions grant full waivers from all franchise tax liability and reporting to certain types of firms. Insurance companies, for example, are granted full waivers because they must pay separate taxes on their gross premiums.[135] Overall, non-corporate business entities are exempt from the franchise tax. These entities include limited partnerships, partnerships, sole proprietorships, and professional associations.

Value of Exemptions

The comptroller estimates that the value of franchise tax exemptions to profit-making and non-profit corporations in fiscal year 2002 will be $662.2 million. By fiscal year 2006, that estimated value increases to $792.3 million (see Table 9.9).[136]

Table 9.9
Cost of Franchise Tax Exemptions Fiscal Year 2002 to 2006
(in millions of dollars)

	2002	2003	2004	2005	2006
Exemptions: For-Profit Corps	361.1	380.7	403.0	427.6	454.1
Exemptions: Non-Profit Corps	301.1	309.4	318.7	328.4	338.2
Total Exemptions	**662.2**	**690.1**	**721.7**	**756.0**	**792.3**

Adapted from: Texas Comptroller of Public Accounts, *Tax Exemptions and Tax Incidence Report.* (January 2001). Online. Available: http://www.window.state.tx.us/taxinfo/incidence/table19.html. Accessed: November 20, 2001.

Repealing Franchise Tax Exemptions

There are currently 1,050 health-related businesses exempt from the franchise tax.[137] In addition, 12,375 health-related businesses are currently paying a total of $36,023,868 in franchise tax.[138] Health-related is defined as the following categories of the 1987 Standard Industrial Classification Manual published by the federal Office of Management and Budget: accident and health insurance, hospitals and medical service plans, pension, health and welfare funds, insurance agents, brokers, and services, offices and clinics of doctors and medicine, offices and clinics of dentists, offices and clinics of doctors of osteopathy, offices and clinics of chiropractors, offices and clinics of optometrists, offices and clinics of podiatrists, offices and clinics of health practitioners, skilled nursing care facilities, intermediate care facilities, nursing and personal care facilities, general medical and surgical hospitals, psychiatric hospitals, specialty hospitals, medical laboratories, dental laboratories, home health care services, kidney dialysis centers, specialty outpatient facilities, health and allied services, residential care, and administration of public health programs. The amount of franchise taxes currently paid by health-related businesses combined with the amount generated from repealing exemptions in health-related businesses could be used for health coverage expansion purposes. The revenue generated from repealing exemptions to non-health-related businesses would go into general revenue.

Replacing the Franchise Tax

Another possibility for increasing state tax collections is to replace the current state franchise tax with a new business tax. One example of a previous proposal is the Business Activity Tax (BAT). Former Texas Governor George W. Bush proposed this replacement tax, modeled after Michigan's Value Added Tax, in 1997. If the BAT was again proposed and implemented, it would apply to all forms of business, including corporations, limited liability companies, limited partnerships, partnerships, trusts, estates, and sole proprietorships. It would be levied at 1.25 percent of sales in Texas and would cover only business activity, not investment activity. It would include federal taxable income, plus wages and other compensations, such as depreciation and costs for retirement and health insurance programs. In order to adjust the tax base for each business, the cost of new capital investments and a standard deduction of $500,000 would be subtracted. The Texas Governor's Office estimated that the BAT would have raised approximately $1 billion more than the franchise tax in fiscal years 1998 and 1999.[139]

Proponents of the BAT say it would grow with increased business activity, be economically efficient because of the low rate levied on a broad base, and be equitably applied to all business. They also say it would be a stable source of revenue compared to taxes based on income, be relatively simple to calculate and administer, and be essentially a consumption tax that could be passed on to customers. Opponents of the BAT say it would be a hardship on companies in bad business years because, unlike a tax based on profits or income, it would be levied regardless of ability to pay. Additionally, they say it would unfairly shift the tax burden to companies with high labor costs and potentially inhibit employment, salary, or benefit increases. Some observers have argued that the BAT could be viewed as an income tax since it would impose a tax on sole proprietors, as well as individual partners in a partnership, and could thus be challenged in the courts. Others, however, say that the BAT could not be considered an income tax because the basis on which the taxes are calculated are very different. Depreciation that is allowed under an income tax would not be allowed under BAT. Additionally, the BAT would include compensation and employee benefits and would deduct the costs of new capital investments.[140]

Application and Benefits

A tax on health-related businesses, applied either through repealing exemptions to the current franchise tax or through a replacement business tax, would essentially be a provider tax. Service-oriented industries, such as these health related businesses, have historically supported the franchise tax and thus may initially be opposed to any changes to its current form. However, the benefits these businesses would receive in return are greater than their original loss through taxes. The money generated through a provider tax would be used for a federal Medicaid match.

Excise Taxes

Implementing new excise taxes would provide new revenue that could either go into the general fund or be earmarked for specific health insurance expansion purposes.

Nutritional Factors and Obesity

One category of excise taxes that have been implemented in a number of states are small taxes on food with low nutritional value, such as soft drinks and snack foods. These taxes are based on the knowledge that dietary factors contribute significantly to number of preventable illnesses and premature deaths in the U.S.[141] An estimated 61 percent of adults in the U.S. are overweight or obese, based on body mass index (BMI). BMI is calculated by dividing an individual's weight in kilograms by height in meters squared (a BMI between 25.0 and 29.0 is considered overweight, and a BMI above 30 is considered obese). The prevalence of obesity has nearly doubled is the past two decades. Approximately 13 percent of children are seriously overweight, a prevalence which has nearly tripled in the past two decades.[142, 143]

Nutritional factors are associated with four of the ten leading causes of death: coronary heart disease, certain types of cancer, stroke, and type 2 diabetes.[144] According to the Surgeon General, 300,000 deaths a year in the U.S. are associated with obesity.[145] Spending on hospital and outpatient care is 36 percent higher and medication costs are 77 percent higher for individuals who are obese than for individuals in a normal weight range.[146] Of the total cost of health care in the U.S., approximately 8.9 percent is spent on conditions related to obesity.[147, 148] Assuming Texas' health care expenditures on obesity-related conditions are of similar proportion, the states' direct cost of obesity is approximately $6.1 billion a year.[149] A recent study shows that health care costs linked to obesity and obesity-related conditions are larger than costs associated with smoking and problem drinking.[150] Texas currently addresses the problems of smoking and drinking by taxing tobacco products and alcohol, but does not address the more significant problem of obesity. Obesity-related conditions and costs could be addressed by implementing a tax on soft drinks.

Consumption of food with low nutritional value is largely connected to the problems of obesity, and thus the cost of health care. Soft drinks, in particular, can be linked to these problems and costs. Soft drinks are the leading source of added sugar in one's diet and Americans are consuming twice as much soda as they did 25 years ago.[151, 152] According to researchers at the Harvard School of Public Health, each can or glass of soft drink consumed by a child increase his/her risk of obesity by 1.6 times.[153] Additionally, children who drink soda tend to take in more calories than those who do not.[154] For these reasons, it can thus be argued that the revenue from a soda tax should be earmarked for health purposes, such as expanding health care coverage. This would help to decrease the direct health care costs associated with obesity.

Soda Tax: Current Examples

Excise taxes on soft drinks and snack food can be levied at the wholesale or retail level, and can be levied as a fixed tax per volume of product or as a percentage of sales price. Small excise taxes on widely consumed foods can raise significant revenues. Arkansas' tax on soft drinks generates approximately $40,435,799 a year in revenues. These revenues are dedicated to the state's Medicaid Program Trust Fund.[155] The tax is paid by every distributor, manufacturer, or wholesale dealer on the first sale in the state and is levied on soft drinks as well as syrups and powder bases used to manufacture soft drinks.[156] The rates of the tax in Arkansas are as follows:

- On soft drink syrup or simple syrup: $2.00 per gallon;
- On canned or bottled soft drinks: 21 cents per gallon; and
- On powders or other base products: 21 cents per gallon.[157]

These taxes translate into a 2 percent tax per 12 ounces of soda.

In West Virginia, revenues from its soft drink tax, which total approximately $12,539,000 annually, are used to support medical, dental, and nursing schools.[158] The tax is levied on the sale, use, handling, or distribution of bottled soft drinks, syrups, and powder bases. The tax is paid through the purchase of tax stamps or tax crowns by wholesale or retail dealers, manufacturers, distributors, or any other person who is the original consignee of soft drinks, syrups, or powders. Tax crowns are symbols that are permanently applied by manufacturers to bottle caps, can lids, cartons, or labels. The tax is collected only once on any bottled soft drink or soft drink product sold, distributed, or manufactured by the state. The rates of the tax in West Virginia are as follows:

- On bottled soft drinks: 1 cent on each 16.9 fluid ounces or any fraction of that amount, or 1 cent on each half-liter or any fraction of that amount.
- On soft drinks syrup: 80 cents on each gallon and, on each fractional part of a gallon, the same fractional part of that part of 80 cants, or 84 cents on each 4 liters and, on any fractional part of 4 liters, the same fractional part of 84 cents.
- On dry mixture used for making soft drinks: 1 cent on each ounce or any fraction of that amount, or 1 cent on each 28.35 grams or any fraction of that amount.[159]

Soda Tax: Potential and Feasibility in Texas

The annual per capita consumption of 12-ounce soft drinks in the U.S. is 566.[160] Therefore, for Texas' populations of approximately 20.85 million, the annual supply is approximately 11.8 billion 12-ounce soft drinks.[161] A one-cent tax on each 12 ounces of soda, levied either at the wholesale or retail level, could therefore generate approximately $118 million a year. This tax could also be applied as 2 percent per every 12 ounces of soda.

According to a report in the American Journal of Public Health, small taxes are unlikely to have a substantial impact on the price or consumption of food, and are thus unlikely to be strongly opposed by consumers. A nationally representative opinion poll revealed that taxes of one cent per pound of soft drinks, chips, and butter that produced revenues dedicated to health education programs were supported by approximately 45 percent of adults surveyed. "This appears to be remarkably great support for a tax that would affect most adults and that has not been discussed in the media."[162] A soda tax in Texas could generate substantial revenues for health coverage expansion at very little cost to consumers.

Cigarette Tax

A source for additional revenue for the State of Texas lies in increasing the state cigarette tax. Currently the state imposes a $0.41 tax on each pack of cigarettes purchased in the state. Texas ranks 23rd in the nation on the amount it charges in cigarette tax, and is above the national average of $0.34.[163] It is estimated that Texas will bring in almost $474 million from the cigarette tax in 2003.[164] Just a $0.04 increase in the tax per pack would generate an additional $46,225,951 to the state general revenue and represent less than a 10 percent increase in the tax and less than an 2 percent increase in the cost of a pack of cigarettes.

Several other states already link money generated by the cigarette tax to health care. This in many ways seems a natural link to raise money for health care by taxing a product that is detrimental to health. Arkansas and Florida use a portion of their cigarette tax to fund their state's portion of the Medicaid match. Connecticut is considering raising their cigarette tax by $0.61 (it is currently $0.50)[165] in order to deter smoking and help offset health care costs.[166]

Advocates for smokers say the tax is discriminatory, and puts too harsh of a penalty on smokers.[167] Advocates for the tax say that the tax has an added benefit of deterring young people from starting the addicting habit.[168] The American Medical Association has recently advocated that states should raise cigarette taxes to deter smoking and cure budget shortfalls.[169] One problem with the tax is that in increasing the price per pack of cigarettes, some individuals will give up cigarettes, which may be good for their personal health, but this effect aggregated would mean a decrease in overall cigarette sales, and possibly a reduction in the amount of tax collected. It should be noted that a reduction in the purchase of cigarettes could lead to a more than commensurate decrease in health care cost associated with smoking, and offset the decrease revenue. Several states have raised the cigarette tax without experiencing any decrease in revenue. In 1999, California increased its cigarette tax by 50 cents, which resulted in a 90 percent increase in new revenue at the same time decreasing cigarette consumption by almost 19 percent.[170] States like Washington and New York have a tax of over $0.80 per pack,[171] but still bring in money from the tax and have just recently voted to raise the cigarette tax to more than $1.40 per pack.[172] Others against the tax say that the tax is regressive, in that like any sales tax, poorer individuals pay a larger portion of their income on the tax. One could argue that if individuals find it an undue burden to pay an increase in cigarette tax, they should not be purchasing a luxury item such as cigarettes in the first place. However, cigarettes are addictive and the fact remains that some people will spend more than they reasonably can afford to purchase them, rather than give them up.

If an increase in the cigarette tax is instituted, the state of Texas will need determine how much of a tax increase would correspond to an increase in general revenue, factoring in the possible drop in sales resulting from the tax. The increase in revenue could be designated to health care spending, in some ways pacifying the smoking advocates that may feel the tax unfair. By linking the tax to health care spending, it is taxing people more likely to need health care.

Income Tax

One untapped source of funding in the state would be implementation of a state income tax. Texas remains one of one a handful of states in the nation that does not currently have an income tax. Even traditionally no-tax states like Tennessee and New Hampshire have recently instituted an unearned income tax to obtain more general revenue for the state.[173] Historically, implementing an income tax in Texas has been difficult to say the least. Texas is currently collecting the majority of its general revenue dollars from property and sales taxes. There are concerns that the state's tax system has not kept pace with the economy and it's growth.[174] Some believe that the growing pressure from opponents of Texas's "Robin Hood" school funding mechanism will bring the issue of Texas's tax structure to the forefront of the 2003 legislative session.[175]

Looking at a redesign of the tax system in Texas is not new. Recent attempts include plans from Bill Hobby, Bob Bullock, and George W. Bush.[176] Despite several attempts to reform the tax system in Texas, only small changes have been implemented. The atmosphere in Texas has never been one to obtain broad-based support for a state income tax. After a tough legislative session in 2000-2001, some legislators are proposing income tax legislation.[177] Most support for tax restructuring is fueled by the need to change educational funding. Forty-six percent of education cost is funded through property taxes. Many school districts in Texas have reached the upper limit of $1.50 per $100 valuation that is set by state law for maintenance and operations of schools. In addition, some wealthier school districts have filled lawsuits challenging the way in which educational tax dollars have been distributed.[178] Legislators are looking for ways to restructure the tax system.

Implementation

There has been little support from the general public for tax restructuring. A 1997 poll indicated that only 5 percent of Texans polled would support an income tax. Twenty-three percent of people polled in Texas would support a new sales tax.[179] This is interesting to note, especially because income taxes are considered to be "fairer" or more progressive taxes. The comptroller's office reports that the poorest families in Texas pay 10.7 percent of their income on sales tax while the richest Texans spend only 1.6 percent.[180] Currently sales taxes make up 55.3 percent of the state's revenue. Texas also has one of the lowest tax burdens in the nation, ranking 48th for amount of tax collected per capita in 1999. Not surprisingly, Texas is also has high rates of child poverty, high rates of uninsured, and poor teacher health benefits.[181]

In 1993, Texas passed a constitutional amendment, making it impossible to implement a state income tax without a majority popular vote. This alone may be the biggest impediment to Texas implementing a state income tax. Another problem arises when considering using the revenue from the state income tax for health care coverage for Texans. As it stands right now, the Texas constitution mandates that if an income tax is implemented, one-third of the tax must be used for education, and the remaining two thirds of the tax be used to reduce property taxes.[182] This would mean that first Texans would have to approve an income tax, and then vote to change the Constitution allowing the revenue from the tax to be used for human services. Another possibility would be to vote to modify the Texas Constitution, allowing the legislature to approve an income tax and giving the legislature the ability to designate how it can be spent.

Since the Texas Legislature does not even have the right to give itself a raise without a majority popular vote, there is little hope for giving the legislature such discretion in distributing income tax revenue. It is more likely, as with the state lottery in Texas, that once more funds are available for education through an income tax, general revenue dollars from the state's sales tax would be available for other uses such as health care coverage.[183] Estimates put the revenue generated by a state income tax (a simple tax such as one currently implemented in Kansas) at $17 billion dollars, which would mean a net increase of just under $6 billion dollars for state revenue.[184]

Other Potential Sources of Revenue

Several other state-controlled areas are worth mentioning as potential sources of additional revenue generation, either as a match, or simply as savings. These areas include: state-owned teaching hospitals and medical schools, unclaimed lottery funds, and SCHIP cost sharing.

State-Owned Teaching Hospitals and Medical Schools

In an effort by the state to maximize its own dollars spent on health care for the indigent, the state might examine how it is currently allocating its own resources within state institutions, specifically state-owned teaching hospitals and medical schools. The state dollars that are currently transferred to these entities are fairly substantial in amount and are unmatched. It would benefit these entities to have both an expanded pool of health care covered individuals that it serves and possibly an enhanced reimbursement rate. By virtue of reducing the number of uninsured for whom care would be provided, the institutions' fiscal health would be improved. Texas' teaching hospitals and medical schools currently receive federal and state funding to assist in the provision of health care services through resident clinics. Funds are transferred to these entities to help pay for supervising physicians of the residents and to encourage their continued participation. This money does not appear to have any stipulations attached to it, and in theory, the state funds could be used to draw down matching funds to assist in coverage of additional Texans.

Texas operates four state-owned teaching hospitals: The University of Texas Medical Branch at Galveston (UTMB-Galveston), the University of Texas M.D. Anderson Cancer

Center, the University of Texas Health Science Center at Tyler (UTHSC-Tyler), and the Harris County Psychiatric Center. These hospitals provide both inpatient and outpatient care, and in 1998, $561 million of that care was unreimbursed. Texas also has eight medical schools, seven public and one private institution: Southwestern, Baylor, UTMB, Texas Tech Health Science Center, UTHSC-San Antonio, University of North Texas, Texas A&M Health Science Center, M.D. Anderson, UT-Tyler, and the Texas A&M University College of Dentistry. All eight operate a University Physician Practice Plan (UPPP) and all provide health care services to patients in a variety of settings, both inpatient and outpatient, providing hands-on training for students and residents. In 1997, these medical schools provided $284 million in unreimbursed care (amounts for Baylor College of Medicine and the Texas A&M College of Dentistry are not included).[185]

Any potential match of these state funds would be best served by the cooperation of all involved entities. The Health Science Centers would not likely wish to give up any portion of their current state funding without some guarantee that the money would be coming back to them. Because they are state entities, a guarantee could be worked through legislation and budget execution authority. Medicaid patients have the freedom of choice to see any doctor that accepts Medicaid reimbursement as a form of payment. HSC would only be able to re-coup their portion of funding used for a Medicaid match if they: 1) were guaranteed a set population of Medicaid patients to treat and/or 2) received a higher reimbursement rate in the form of an add-on payment for the Medicaid patients they do treat. The first of these guarantees could be addressed in a waiver, limiting the freedom of choice of Medicaid patients in the areas surrounding the HSC through an EPO arrangement. The second guarantee would require the state to make a special provision for higher reimbursement rates for HSC doctors. The state should also consider an examination of the tobacco endowments for these entities as a source of potential match.

Teaching hospitals and medical schools appear to have themselves recognized the need for expansion. As evidenced by the Academics for Access to Health Care initiative, spearheaded by the Association of Academic Health centers (with nine Texas members), which simply put endorses health coverage for all Americans, specifically through an expansion of Medicaid to include parents of children covered by Medicaid/SCHIP programs or to low-income adults without children.[186]

The state might also discover substantial amounts of unmatched money within all state agencies, currently being expended on potential expansion populations. It would be worthwhile to determine whether or not this money could be made available for a match. For instance, how many individuals are currently receiving services provided by TDMHMR who would be eligible for Medicaid coverage under an expansion. How might general revenue dollars currently unmatched and spent on these individuals for care be better spent? In FY 1998, TDMHMR spent $1.9 billion in non-Medicaid funds, $1.2 billion in Medicaid dollars (another $72 .4 million was spent by local MHMR Authorities).[187] HHSC has been instructed by the 77th Legislature to conduct just such an examination of current expenditures to determine whether or not federal dollars are being maximized.

Unclaimed Lottery Dollars

Another source of funds that the legislature has set up for use in healthcare services for indigent individuals is the statewide program for unclaimed lottery prizes. Currently these dollars are allocated to teaching hospitals that serve the needy and provide high-level trauma services, pediatric surgery and cancer treatment. This program was set up by the 76th Legislature. It accumulated $57.2 million dollars in the first 24 months. This year is the first year the program has paid out.[188]

According to the Texas statutes no more than $40 million in prize money each biennium will be appropriated to the TDH state-owned multi-categorical teaching hospital account. Any prize money in excess of the $40 million is deposited in the tertiary care facility account.[189] This year, the first $40 million went to the University of Texas Medical Branch at Galveston; 90 percent of the remaining funds went to trauma centers and hospitals providing specialized care, 5 percent went to emergency rooms that had been in extreme circumstances, and the last 5 percent went to the state's County Indigent Health Care Program.[190]

Unclaimed lottery funds are an example of a source of funds that has been set aside to help counties and hospitals with their indigent-care burden. The accumulation of these funds does help the hospitals that receive them, and the application of these funds to indigent care costs is crucial. However, if the funds were invested in a Medicaid expansion program, these state dollars could ensure that each dollar spent was being used more efficiently.

Cost Sharing/SCHIP

The cost-sharing option of revenue generation is at once provocative and sensitive. The practice of cost sharing is surrounded with contentious issues, and yet it seems to be growing in popularity as a cost-containment tool by states with shrinking resources and growing budgets. In the context of the State Children's Health Insurance Program or Medicaid, cost sharing is defined as the mechanisms, such as annual enrollment fees, monthly premiums and co-payments, by which states require beneficiaries to share in the cost of the provision of health care. States generally use family caps that define the maximum cost sharing required by families and sliding scales that are based on family size and income. Cost-sharing mechanisms are used to reduce the total health spending by the state and the federal government.[191] This reduction occurs through increased revenue generation from premiums, which go directly to the state, and through cost-savings achieved by using co-payments to deter overuse of more costly services (emergency) in exchange for preventive and maintenance services. There are a number of federal requirements that guide states use of cost sharing for cost savings. These requirements have to do with the total amount of co-payments and the types of cost sharing that can be used at various federal poverty levels. One of the most important stipulations for consideration here is that states are prohibited from using cost-sharing collections as *matching* money.[192]

Important Considerations

There are a number of issues that must be kept in mind when considering an increase to cost-sharing amounts. Of utmost importance is that states must carefully set co-payments at levels that do not deter utilization of appropriate services. Cost-sharing requirements, which *can* often deter families from enrolling and utilizing services, may conflict with a program's overarching objective to provide services to low-income individuals, and therefore must be carefully designed. States must pay especially close attention to setting co-payments at levels that do not deter utilization of preventive services, but *would* assist in controlling the improper use of other services such as emergency room utilization. This "price sensitive" cost-sharing with moderately priced cost-sharing mechanisms can serve to instill a sense of responsibility in participants, and help to deter the welfare stigma that is often associated with public programs. Some states have learned that participants attached a welfare stigma to a free program, and thus cost-sharing can instill a sense of responsibility in participants without creating a barrier to enrollment, by allowing parents to feel that they are paying for their children's health care through a monthly premium.

"Price sensitivity" also refers to levels of premiums and co-payments that families perceive to be affordable. It is important to note that price sensitive requirements may not be what families can afford, but rather what they are willing to pay for health care services. Related to issues of price sensitivity is the decision of whether to implement a flat fee premium for all participants or one that is based on a sliding scale. While a flat-fee may be administratively appealing because it is simpler to administer, designing premiums on an income-based sliding scale may encourage greater participation. Some states found that cost-sharing amounts that are too high did result in decreased enrollment. State program representatives felt that premiums at a lower level (between $5-10) were a viable means of evoking a sense of responsibility in participants by making public insurance comparable to employer-sponsored coverage.

The use of cost sharing to raise revenues through premiums and help offset costs, and the use of co-payments to affect utilization of services, have proved effective. Higher co-payments for emergency room services, which are generally viewed as costly and often inappropriately utilized, to encourage families to seek preventive and primary care services can deter utilization.

In addition to countering welfare stigma, cost-sharing mechanisms are seen as a way of helping acclimate participants to the requirements of employer-sponsored insurance, thus building a bridge between conditions of uninsurance and private insurance. Several states have identified the affordability of employer-sponsored insurance as an important consideration in the implementation of mechanisms to limit crowd out. As research has suggested that substitution is most commonly seen in higher income ranges, substitution of state-funded programs for private insurance coverage has become a substantial concern. Families are making difficult decisions which may directly impact individually based substitution. While families may opt to substitute a separate state program for private insurance or for Medicaid, it is important to understand that family decisions are based upon affordability of plans, comparability of the benefit packages, and health status of children.

State and national research has not produced conclusive evidence that employers are dropping coverage, at least not yet, although there is evidence that employer-based coverage is declining. Several states have suggested that the coverage issue, in most cases, is not employers dropping coverage, but rather individuals are choosing to opt out of private insurance coverage for state subsidized programs. The extent to which states deliberately institute mechanisms limiting substitution varies by program and state.

State mechanisms to limit individual-based substitution primarily target those dynamics that prompt family decisions to opt out of private coverage, such as the cost comparisons of co-payments and premiums, the affordability of private coverage, and the comprehensiveness of benefits. The primary mechanisms utilized by states include the following: 1) evaluating affordability of private coverage; 2) requiring periods of uninsurance; 3) providing subsidies; and 4) limiting the scope of benefit packages. These mechanisms are effective ways to curb substitution by making state-sponsored health insurance comparable to employer-sponsored coverage.[193]

Administrative burdens on the program or its providers to collect premiums or co-payments cannot be overlooked. Many programs have shifted the burden of collecting co-payments to providers in order to reduce the administrative costs to the program. However, it has been suggested by some states that, in many cases, providers have either been unable or unwilling to collect co-payments from beneficiaries who were incapable or unwilling to pay for services rendered. This becomes a concern for providers who collect co-payments from patients as a portion of their reimbursement under the program. For these providers, the inability to collect co-payments may result in an overall decrease in their total reimbursement by the program. This could ultimately affect their willingness to participate in the program.[194] CMS guidance has suggested that it is easier to track a family's cumulative cost-sharing maximum if the cost sharing is simply done through premiums and enrollment fees. This mechanism alleviates the administrative burden for providers and for the family attempting to keep track of the amount.

Allowed amounts

In general, states are prevented from implementing annual cost sharing in excess of 2.5 percent of a family's annual income (in the year under consideration) for families at or below 150 percent of the FPL, and 5 percent for families above 150 percent of the FPL. This maximum amount is referred to as the cumulative cost-sharing maximum.

The state recently submitted an amended state Children's Health Insurance Program State Plan to the Center for Medicare and Medicaid Services (CMS) seeking approval of its cost-sharing increases. The changes were to go into effect March 1, 2002. Although Texas is increasing some cost-sharing amounts, with a focus on altering utilization, a gap still remains between what is currently being received in the form of cost-sharing and what is federally allowable. The table in Appendix K demonstrates Texas' previous cost-sharing amounts and the recently implemented changes, as well as the federal allowables and differences among the amounts. The cost-sharing slack remaining, following the changes, would likely only minimally provide for additional cost-savings. Texas appears to have increased cost sharing in areas where the state hopes to deter utilization (emergency rooms and brand name drugs) and has lowered cost sharing or left it the same in other areas. Texas however did not alter any of the premium or enrollment amounts.

Using current SCHIP enrollment numbers, broken down by FPL, as well as various potential cost-sharing increases, revenue gains could be projected for additional cost-savings. Because only the premiums and enrollment fees are paid to the state, not co-payments, etc., this is the only amount that could be projected. However, the use of co-payment amounts to deter more acute forms of service in favor of lesser costing forms of care can ultimately provide for cost-savings as well, albeit less concretely. While cost-sharing revenue cannot itself be used as a match, it is possible that premium-generated revenue and cost-savings from avoidance of costly service utilization could free up money from other budget areas to be used as a match. Whether or not it is used as a means for drawing down federal money, it may be useful to continue to examine this option for cost-saving possibilities. However, in doing so, it is important to be mindful of any potential drop in the participation rate as a concurrent event. Continued work in this area will need to focus on determining actual numbers (revenue), determining the viability of using cost-sharing for decreasing overall program expenditures in Texas, examining possibilities for decreasing administrative burdens associated with cost-sharing, particularly for providers, and in particular, giving consideration to more reliance on premiums and enrollment fees versus co-payments.

Conclusion

> *To develop and prosper, community members must have access to basic health services and must believe these will be sustained in the foreseeable future.*[195]

In a waiver development process clear goals are vital to determine, as a state, why expansion is necessary. Expansion is important for Texas for a number of reasons. First,local entity resources are stretched thin. The cost of caring for uninsured individuals is much greater than the cost of preventative and maintenance care—uninsured individuals tend to receive less preventive medical care and to rely more on emergency department care than their insured counterparts. The uninsured are also more likely to be hospitalized for avoidable conditions. Thus, this reliance on last-minute care can severely strain state and local public resources, and limits the effectiveness of each local tax dollar spent.

Expansion is also important because the primary stewards of our emergency and trauma care services, hospital districts and public hospitals, are facing the very real fear of closure as the result of overwhelmed systems. These entities have come to recognize the wisdom in pooling various local resources to expand health care coverage. Such a cooperative exercise is commonly viewed as a necessity to preserve the existing emergency and trauma systems.

Additionally, a health care expansion in Texas has significant potential impact on economic development. This impact takes two important forms: 1) an insured work force is a healthier, more productive work force, and 2) creating a larger federal Medicaid draw down can bring millions, possibly billions, more dollars into the state, serving to help stabilize provider systems, and in some cases, whole communities.

Finally, expansion is important because the incentive to do something more efficient is at hand. Our survey of county programs and hospital districts reveal that increases in the numbers of uninsured individuals and health care costs are causing local entities to focus their attention on ways to maximize their current expenditures. Counties recognize their fiscal limitations to meeting the indigent care needs of their residents single-handedly. Many local entities are interested in an indigent health care system that builds upon the existing Medicaid structure. Some, in fact, have begun to express an interest in a county-match arrangement. Thus, local entities are beginning to understand that they could spend more efficiently by having a larger number of individuals with coverage, utilizing more appropriate services.

Once the state has recognized the need for expansion, it must address funding. States that have had success decreasing their number of uninsured have done so primarily by expanding Medicaid/SCHIP eligibility to additional populations, usually parents within a range of FPLs. Options to fund an expansion can be found by maximizing state leveraging of existing available federal dollars and by building on the state's existing public health care system. Texas could first utilize current expenditures on safety-net care by local entities, state-owned teaching hospitals, and medical schools, and then could focus on preventative and maintenance care, versus emergency care services, for the newly insured. Where existing dollars fall short, Texas could generate additional revenue from providers that stand to benefit from an expanded pool of insured patients, e.g., doctors, hospitals, and nursing homes. The state could revisit the viability of a provider tax, taking care to spread the burden equitably among providers who stand to benefit from an expansion, as well as among providers, insurance companies, and individuals. The franchise tax loophole, which is receiving much attention currently by state officials, could also be repealed. Additional new funds could be generated through taxes on potentially-health-damaging products such as sodas and cigarettes. In all cases, revenue generated could be earmarked for expansion purposes.

In planning an expansion that utilizes local entity funding, there are important considerations to be addressed in the funding design. For instance, local entity differences, in the areas of geography, taxing ability, mandate, number of uninsured, and percentage of population below a given federal poverty level could all be built into the structure to the extent possible. The degree of local control allowable would also need to be considered. In other words, can a local entity choose not to contribute, especially a county with a CIHCP, and do counties have the option to develop a locally controlled provider organization. Another very important design consideration is whether or not a local entity can simply certify a given level of expenditure versus actually transferring funds to the state. Consideration might also be given to whether or not there is any benefit to a phased-in funding system, beginning with large urban hospital districts, for example, and then counties and others.

Texas is not new to the area of local contribution arrangements. Texas, to some extent, has actually laid some of the legislative groundwork for a local entity contribution structure. Senate Bill 10, for instance, mandated the development of a federal expansion waiver utilizing funding primarily from hospital districts, medical schools and teaching hospitals, but also from counties with indigent health care programs if they chose to participate. Senate Bill 1156 of the 77th Legislature contained several demonstration waivers that were to be designed using local funding. Additionally, SB 1246, which created the RCHS, provided a mechanism for local entities to network together and design a provider-controlled organization.

While SB 10 has been sunsetted, and SB 1156 was vetoed, they have lasting impacts. These pieces of legislation served to provoke much discussion and much interest in local contribution efforts to pull federal dollars into the state. This interest is shared both by state officials and many local entities. As a result, a number of smaller local contribution efforts have continued to be discussed and developed, such as the HIV/AIDS waiver. Such local efforts can potentially serve to instruct planners regarding the implementation of a locally-funded contribution system. This is especially true with the "certification of funds" finance method that the HIV/AIDS waiver could pilot.

The next step for Texas is dialogue, the facilitation of a discussion with all of the pieces of the funding and expansion puzzle on the table at one time and with all interested parties present. This discussion to the extent possible should strive to involve all stakeholders and take into account issues unique to each, in order to facilitate buy-in of all entities. While state and local funding constraints are a stark reality, so is the growing number of uninsured individuals in the state. It is indeed because localities and the state are facing budget shortfalls that the state needs to consider other potential funding sources to finance a health coverage expansion in Texas.

Notes

[1] Caton Fenz, *Providing Health Care to the Uninsured in Texas: A Guide for County Officials* (Boston, MA: The Access Project, August 9, 2000), p. 3.

[2] U.S. Department of Labor, *2001 March Current Population Survey*. Online. Available: http://www.bls.census.gov/cps/cpsmain.htm. Accessed: April 8, 2002.

[3] Ibid.

[4] Ibid.

[5] Texas Comptroller of Public Accounts, *Texas Health Care Spending* (Austin, TX, March 2001). Online. Available: http://www.window.state.tx.us/specialrpt/hcs/pg33.html. Accessed: November 15, 2001.

[6] Caton Fenz, *Providing Health Care to the Uninsured in Texas: A Guide for County Officials* (Boston, MA: The Access Project, August 9, 2000), pp. 3-8.

[7] Ibid.

[8] Caton Fenz, *Providing Health Care to the Uninsured in Texas: A Guide for County Officials*, pp. 12-31.

[9] Texas Department of Health, Indigent Health Care Division, *Summary, Indigent Health Care Program, August 2000* (Austin, Tex., October 3, 2000), p. 1.

[10] Texas Comptroller of Public Accounts, "Hospital District Taxes for State Fiscal Year 2000" (Austin, Tex., 2002) (Excel file).

[11] Caton Fenz, *Providing Health Care to the Uninsured in Texas: A Guide for County Officials*, pp. 12-31.

[12] Ibid.

[13] Ibid.

[14] Telephone interview by Evan Christman with Rose Marie Linan, Team Leader, Indigent Health Care Division, Texas Department of Health, Austin, Texas, September 19, 2001.

[15] Caton Fenz, *Providing Health Care to the Uninsured in Texas: A Guide for County Officials*, pp. 12-31.

[16] Ibid.

[17] Ibid.

[18] Ibid.

[19] Texas Department of Health, Office of Policy and Planning, *Agreement Regarding the Disposition of Tobacco Settlement Proceeds* (June 8, 1999). Online. Available: http://www.tdh.state.tx.us/dpa/tobsett.htm. Accessed: January 31, 2002.

[20] Ibid.

[21] Texas Association of Counties, "Tobacco Reimbursement Funds will be Distributed Later this Month," *TACNews*, vol. 9, no. 54 (April 6, 2001). Online: Available: http://www.county.org/resources/TACnews/news04061.html. Accessed: January 31, 2002.

[22] Ibid.

[23] Charlotte Huff and Kelly Melhart, "Tobacco Fund Loss Troubles Hospitals," *Fort Worth Star Telegram* (February 21, 2002). Online. Available: http://www.dfw.com/mld/startelegram. Accessed: February 30,2002.

[24] Caton Fenz, *Providing Health Care to the Uninsured in Texas: A Guide for County Officials*, pp. 22-31.

[25] Ibid.

[26] National Governor's Association. *Health Insurance Coverage and Financing.* Online. Available: http://www.nga.org/center/topics/1,1188,D_355,00.html. Accessed: November 15, 2001.

[27] Ibid.

[28] Families USA, *Five Good Reasons for States to Expand Coverage* (April 2000). Online. Available: http://www.familiesusa.org/index6.htm. Accessed: April 15, 2001.

[29] Leah Kegler, "Utilizing Federal Waiver Flexibility: Expanding Through Section 1931" (Professional Report, Lyndon B Johnson School of Public Affairs, The University at Texas at Austin, 2002), pp. 19-48.

[30] Texas Comptroller of Public Accounts, *Comptroller Rylander Certifies Budget; Warns of Potential $5 Billion Shortfall Next Session* (June 6, 2001). Online. Available: http://www.window.state.tx.us/news/1060bud.html. Accessed: October 2, 2001.

[31] Texas Legislative Budget Board, *Text of Conference Committee Report, Senate Bill. 1* (May 23, 2001). Online. Available: http://www.lbb.state.tx.us/Publish_AppBills_LBEs.htm. Accessed: October 4, 2001.

[32] Ibid.

[33] Texas Legislative Budget Board, *Summary of Conference Committee Report on Senate Bill 1* (May 23, 2001). Online. Available: http://www.lbb.state.tx.us/Publish_AppBills_LBEs.htm. Accessed: September 18, 2001.

[34] Texas Legislative Budget Board, *SP 43 Enrolled Version Fiscal Note,* 77th Regular session (May 22, 2001). Online. Available: http://www.capitol.state.tx/tlo/77rfiscal/SB00043.htm. Accessed: September 30, 2001.

[35] Texas Senate Bill 1, 77th Legislature, regular session (2001).

[36] Center for Public Policy Priorities, *Where Will the Money Go?: A Revenue Preview* (May 9, 2001). Online. Available: www.cppp.org/products/policypages/111-130/111-130html/PP129.html. Accessed: September 12, 2001.

[37] Ibid.

[38] Texas Legislative Budget Board, *77th Regular session SP 43 Enrolled Version Fiscal Note,* (May 22, 2001). Online. Available: http://www.capitol.state.tx/tlo/77rfiscal/SB00043.htm. Accessed: September 30, 2001.

[39] Ibid.

[40] Texas Comptroller of Public Accounts, *Comptroller Rylander Certifies Budget; Warns of Potential $5 Billion Shortfall Next Session* (Online).

[41] Ibid.

[42] Texas Senate Bill 1, 77th Legislature, regular session (2001).

[43] Texas Comptroller of Public Accounts, *Comptroller Rylander Certifies Budget; Warns of Potential $5 Billion Shortfall Next Session* (Online).

[44] Center for Public Policy Priorities, *Texas Taxes* (April 1999). Online. Available: http://internationalbudget.org/cdrom/papers/tax/TexasTaxes.htm. Accessed: September 12, 2001

[45] Center for Public Policy Priorities, *Why Isn't There Enough Money?* (March 14, 2001). Online. Available: http://www.cppp.org/products/policypages/111-130/111-130html/PP117.html. Accessed: September 12, 2001

[46] Texas Department of Health, Indigent Health Care Division, *Summary, Indigent Health Care Program, August 2000* (October 3, 2000), p. 1.

[47] Telephone interview by Evan Christman with Rose Marie Linan, Team Leader, Indigent Health Care Division, Texas Department of Health, Austin, Texas, April 19, 2001.

[48] Texas Department of Health, *Summary of Indigent Healthcare Program Matching Grants*, Online. Available: http:/www.tdh.state.tx.us/hcf/ihcp. Accessed October 15, 2001.

[49] Texas Senate Bill 10, 74th Legislature, regular session (1995). Online. Available: http://tlo2.tlc.state.tx.us/ cgi-bin/tlo/textframe.cmd?LEG=74&SESS=R&CHAMBER=S&BILLTYPE=B&BILLSUFFIX=00010 &VERSION=5&TYPE=B. Accessed: April 15, 2002.

[50] Ibid.

[51] Texas Health and Human Services Commission, *1995 Texas Medicaid Legislation*, 74th Texas Legislature, regular session (March 25, 1999). Online. Available: http://www.hhsc.state.tx.us/medicaid/ med_info/medleg_74.html. Accessed: April 15, 2002.

[52] Texas Senate Bill 10, 74th Texas Legislature, regular session (1995). Online. Available: http://tlo2.tlc.state.tx.us/cgi-bin/tlo/textframe.cmd?LEG=74&SESS=R&CHAMBER=S&BILLTYPE= B&BILLSUFFIX=00010&VERSION=5&TYPE=B. Accessed: April 15, 2002.

[53] Texas Senate Bill 1156, 77th Texas Legislature, regular session (2001). Online. Available: http://tlo2.tlc.state.tx.us/cgi-bin/tlo/textframe.cmd?LEG=77&SESS=R&CHAMBER=S&BILLTYPE= B&BILLSUFFIX=01156&VERSION=5&TYPE=B. Accessed: April 15, 2002.

[54] Telephone interview by Kristie Kimbell with King Hillier, Director, Legislative Relations, Harris County, Houston, Texas, February 4, 2002.

[55] Ibid.

[56] Ibid.

[57] Texas Senate Bill 1246, 75th Texas Legislature, regular session (1997). Online. Available: http://tlo2.tlc.state.tx.us/cgi-bin/tlo/textframe.cmd?LEG=75&SESS=R&CHAMBER=S&BILLTYPE =B&BILLSUFFIX=01246&VERSION=5&TYPE=B. Accessed: April 15, 2002.

[58] State Bar of Texas Health Law Section, *Medicaid Legislation, Rural Community Health Systems* (SB 1246, Summer 1997). Online. Available: http://www.texhealthlaw.org/Public/archive/s7medicaid.pdf. Accessed: April 15, 2002.

[59] Texas Medical Association, *Status Report: Rural Community Health Systems*. Online. Available: http://www.texmed.org/pmt/pay/rhh/ruralleg.asp. Accessed: April 15, 2002.

[60] State Bar of Texas Health Law Section, *Medicaid Legislation, Rural Community Health Systems* (SB 1246, 1997). Online. Available: http://www.texhealthlaw.org/Public/archive/s7medicaid.pdf. Accessed: April 15, 2002.

[61] Ibid.

[62] Ibid.

[63] Ibid.

[64] Texas Organization of Rural and Community Hospitals, *TORCHNet: Frontline.* Online. Available: http://www.torchnet.org/fl11-08.html. Accessed: April 15, 2002.

[65] Texas Health and Human Services Commission, *Medicaid Managed CareReport, Chapter13 – Medicaid Managed Care in Rural Areas.* Online. Available: http://www.hhsc.state.tx.us/medicaid/mmc_htm/c13_rural_managed_care.htm. Accessed: April 15, 2002.

[66] Interview by Jamie Dudensing and Kristie Kimbell with Sue Glover, Legislative Analyst, Texas Association of Counties, Austin, Texas, February 1, 2002.

[67] Ibid.

[68] Ibid.

[69] Ibid.

[70] Interview by Jamie Dudensing, Kristie Kimbell, and Dr. David Warner with John Umphress, Executive Director, Texas Association of Public and Nonprofit Hospitals; King Hillier, Director, Legislative Relations, Harris County; and Rick Peters, Steve Scarborough, and Steve Svadlenak, Partners, Health Data Partners, L.L.P., Austin, Texas, February 6, 2002.

[71] Interviewed by Jamie Dudensing and Kristie Kimbell with Steve Scarborough, Partner, Health Data Partners, L.L.P., Austin, Texas, February 28, 2002.

[72] Interviewed by Jamie Dudensing and Kristie Kimbell with John Umphress, Executive Director, Texas Association of Public and Nonprofit Hospitals, Austin, Texas, February 28, 2002.

[73]Texas Health and Human Services Commission, *Medicaid Managed CareReport, Chapter13—Medicaid Managed Care in Rural Areas.* Online. Available: http://www.hhsc.state.tx.us/medicaid/mmc_htm/c13_rural_managed_care.htm. Accessed: April 15, 2002.

[74] Interview by Jamie Dudensing, Kristie Kimbell, and Dr. David Warner, with John Boff, President/CEO, Texas Organization of Rural and Community Hospitals and Kevin Reed, Legal Counsel, Texas Organization of Rural and Community Hospitals, Austin, Texas, February 20, 2002.

[75] Interview by Jamie Dudensing and Kristie Kimbell with Sue Glover, Legislative Analyst, Texas Association of Counties, Austin, Texas, February 1, 2002.

[76] Telephone interview by Kenneth Apfel, Jamie Dudensing, Kristie Kimbell, Laura Koenig, and Dr. David Warner with Caton Fenz, Legislative Director, Texas State Representative Garnet Coleman, Austin, Texas, February 4, 2002.

[77] Ibid.

[78] Interview by Jamie Dudensing, Kristie Kimbell, and Dr. David Warner with staffers and one member, Texas Association of Public and Nonprofit Hospitals, Austin, Texas, February 6, 2002.

[79] Jennifer M. Ryan, "Health Insurance Family Style: Public Approaches to Reaching the Uninsured." *Issue Brief No. 767* (Washington, D.C.: National Health Policy Forum, September 24, 2001), p. 7; Center for Medicare and Medicaid Services, *Medicaid Eligibility*. Online. Available: http://hcfa.hhs.gov/medicaid/meligib.htm. Accessed: September 5, 2001; and John Holahan, "Restructuring Medicaid Financing: Implications of the NGA Proposal" (Washington, D.C.: The Henry J. Kaiser Family Foundation, 2001), p. 3.

[80] Carole Keeton Rylander, *Texas Health Care Spending* (Austin, Tex.: Texas Comptroller of Public Accounts, March 2001), p. 7.

[81] James M Verdier, "State Provider Assessments to Fund Medicaid," *National Tax Journal,* vol. 46, no. 3 (1993), pp. 377-383. Online. Available: http://www.ntj/tax.org. Accessed: January 8, 2002.

[82] Ibid.

[83] Jan Malcolm, "The Minnesotacare provider tax debate," *The Medical Journal of Allina,* vol. 6, no..3 (1997), pp. 1-5. Online. Available: http:// www.allina.com/Allina_Journal/Summer1997/malcolm.html. Accessed: November 20, 2001.

[84] Citizens' Council on Health Care, *Distribution, Utilization and Impact of the Minnesota Provider Tax*, (January2000). Online. Available: http:// www.cchconline.org/publication/providertaxsumm.php3, Accessed: November 20, 2001.

[85] Anthony Man, "State's Medicaid funding, or fingers in the dike," *Illinois Issues,* vol, XVII, no. 6 (August/September 1991). Online. Available: http://www.lib.niu.edu/ipo/ii910833.html. Accessed: February 1, 2001.

[86] Eric Cook and Michael Vlaisavljevich, "Implications of Health Reform for State and Local Fiscal Policy," *National Tax Journal*, vol. 47, no. 3 (1994), pp. 639-654. Online. Available: http://www.ntj/tax.org. Accessed: January 30, 2002.

[87] Citizens' Council on Health Care, *Distribution, Utilization and Impact of the Minnesota Provider Tax*, (January 2000). Online. Available: http:// www.cchconline.org/publication/providertaxsumm.php3. Accessed: November 20,2001.

[88] Teresa Coughlin and David Liska, *The Medicaid Disproportionate Share Hospital Payment Program: Background and Issues* (Washington, D.C.: The Urban Institute, October 1997), pp. 1-10. Online. Available: http://newfederalism.urban.org/html/anf14/html#tab1. Accessed: November 20, 2001.

[89] Karen Matherlee, *Issue Brief: the Federal-State Medicaid Match: An Ongoing Tug-of War over Practice and Policy* (Washington, D.C.: National Health Policy Forum, George Washington University, December 2001), pp. 1-10. Online. Available: http://www.nhpf.org/pdfs/8-760+(web).pdf. Accessed: November 20, 2001.

[90] Coughlin and Liska, *The Medicaid Disproportionate Share Hospital Payment Program: Background and Issues*, pp. 1-10..

[91] Social Security Act, ch.19, sec 1903(w)(3)(A).

[92] Social Security Act, ch.19, sec 1903 (w)(3)(A).

[93] Social Security Act, ch.19, sec 1903 (w)(3)(C)(i).

[94] Social Security Act, ch.19, sec 1903 (w)(3)(D)(ii).

[95] Social Security Act, ch.19, sec 1903 (w)(4).

[96] Social Security Act, ch.19, sec 1903 (w)(3)(E)(i).

[97] Social Security Act, ch.19, sec 1903 (w)(3)(E)(ii).

[98] Social Security Act, ch.19, sec 1903 (w)(7)(A)

[99] James M Verdier, "State Provider Assessments to Fund Medicaid," *p*p. 377-383.

[100] Minnesota Department of Revenue, *Minnesota Revenue Notice Number 00-07,MinnestoaCare Tax-Hospital Gross Revenues*. Online. Available: http://www.taxes.state.mn.us/rnotices/00_07.html. Accessed: November 20, 2001

[101] Jan Malcolm, "The Minnesotacare provider tax debate," *The Medical Journal of Allina,* vol. 6, no.3 (1997), pp. 1-5. Online. Available: http:// www.allina.com/Allina_Journal/Summer1997/malcolm.html. Accessed: November 20, 2001.

[102] Minnesota Department of Revenue, *Reforming the tax system: Health Care Tax Reform Team*. Online. Available: http://www.taxes.state.mn.us/reform/stdygr/healarch.html. Accessed: January 30, 2002.

[103] Jan Malcolm, "The Minnesotacare provider tax debate," pp. 1-5.

[104] Minnesota Department of Revenue, *Reforming the tax system: Health Care Tax Reform Team* (Online).

[105] Eric Cook and Michael Vlaisavljevich, "Implications of Health reform for state and local fiscal policy," pp. 639-654.

[106] Bureau of National Affairs, "Utah: Legislature Approves Bill to Provide Matching Funds for Children's Health," *State News,* vol. 6, no. 10 (Washington, D.C.: Health Care Policy Report, March 9, 1998). Online. Available: http://pubs.bna.com/ip/BNA/HCP.NSF/a21f0cc38764582574300db37c/2156d566eb172c11853565bf00785edf?OpenDocument. Accessed: November 11, 2001.

[107] Email from Bruce Murray, Executive Vice President, UHA Hospitals and Health Systems Association, "Utah Medicaid Tax," to Jamie Dudensing, November 26, 2001.

[108] Email from Roy Dunn, Utah Department of Health, "Using Tax Revenues for Medicaid," to Jamie Dudensing, January 24, 2002.

[109] Minnesota Statutes 2001, *Table of Chapters, Table of contents for Chapter 295.* Online. Available: www.revisor.leg.state.mn.us/stats/295/52.html. Accessed: November 23, 2001

[110] Jan Malcolm, "The Minnesotacare provider tax debate," pp. 1-5.

[111] Ibid.

[112] Citizens' Council on Health Care, Distribution, *Utilization and Impact of the Minnesota Provider Tax* (January 2000). Online. Available: http:// www.cchconline.org/publication/providertaxsumm.php3. Accessed: November 20,2001.

[113] Eric Cook and Michael Vlaisavljevich, "Implications of Health reform for state and local fiscal policy," pp. 639-654.

[114] Bureau of National Affairs, "West Virginia, Legislature passes Tobacco Tax Measure Bill to Eliminate Health Care Provider Tax," *State News,* vol. 9 (Washington D.C.: Health Care Policy Report, April 23, 2001). Online. Available: http://pubs.bna.com/ip/BNA.NSF/a21f6df0cc387645256743006db37c/0e9098e8031a8852563400833386?opendocument. Accessed: November 11, 2001.

[115] Ibid.

[116] Ibid.

[117] T. Michael Murdock, Huntingtonnews.net, *Provider Coalition Formed to Phase Out Healthcare Services Tax.* (January 10, 2001). Online. Available: http://www.huntingtonnews.net/state/Provider Coalition1.html. Accessed: November 23,2001.

[118] Email from Terry Bryant, Alabama Medicaid Director, Alabama Medicaid Agency, "Re: Healthcare Finance Questions," to Kristi Kimble, February 12, 2002.

[119] Texas Office of House Bill Analysis, *SB 1839 Bill Analysis,*77th Texas Legislature, Regular Session (Austin, Tex., May 16, 2001). Online. Available: http://tlo2.tlc.state.tx.us/cgi-bin/tlo/textframe.cmd?LEG=77&SESS=R&CHAMBER=S&BILLTYPE=B&BILLSUFFIX=01839&VERSION=3&TYPE=A. Accessed: November 4, 2001.

[120] Ibid.

[121] Texas Office of House Bill Analysis, *SB 1839 Bill Analysis* (Online).

[122] Texas House of Representatives, House Research Organization, *SB 1839* (May 22,2001), pp. 1-16. Online. Available: http://www.capitol.state.tx.us/hrofr/frame2.htm. Accessed: November 4, 2001.

[123] Ibid.

[124] Arkansas Department of Human Services, *Nursing Home Rate Study* (July 2001). Online. Available: http://www.medicaid.state.ar.us/arkansasmedicaid/nhstudy.overvw.htm. Accessed: November 20, 2001.

[125] Bureau of National Affairs, "Arkansas: House Passes Bill to Levy 'Bed Tax" On Nursing Homes to Raise Medicaid Funds," *State News,* vol. 9, no. 6 (Washington, D.C.: Health Care Policy Report, February 12, 2001). Online. Available: http://pubs.bna.com/ip/BNA/HCP.NSF/a21f6d0cc387645256743006db37c/d1976c858f09ce1a852569ee0079cfda?OpenDocument. Accessed: November 7, 2001.

[126] Telephone interview by Laura Koenig with Dick Lavine, Senior Fiscal Analyst, Center for Public Policy Priorities, Austin, Texas, January 29, 2002.

[127] Ibid.

[128] Texas Comptroller of Public Accounts, *Franchise Tax.* Online. Available: http://www.window.state.tx.us/taxinfo/frantax.html. Accessed: November 14, 2001.

[129] Ibid.

[130] Ibid.

[131] Japonica Partners, *Free Cash Flow: A Better Value Indicator?* Online. Available: http://www.japonica.com/network/freecashflow.html. Accessed: January 31, 2002.

[132] House Research Organization, *The Tax System and Public School Financing in Texas* (March 24, 1997). Online. Available: http://www.capitol.state.tx.us/hrofr/focus/taxes.pdf. Accessed: November 10, 2001.

[133] Ibid.

[134] Ibid.

[135] Texas Comptroller of Public Accounts, *Franchise Tax.* Online. Available: http://www.window.state.tx.us/taxinfo/frantax.html. Accessed: November 14, 2001.

[136] Texas Comptroller of Public Accounts, *Tax Exemptions & Tax Incidence Report* (January 2001). Online. Available: http://www.window.state.tx.us/taxinfo/incidence/table19.html. Accessed: November 20, 2001.

[137] Email from Teresa Comer, Texas Comptroller's Office, "Re: Texas Franchise Tax", to Kate Brodsky, February 15, 2002.

[138] Email from Teresa Comer, Texas Comptroller's Office, "Re: Texas Franchise Tax", to Kate Brodsky, February 14, 2002.

[139] House Research Organization, *The Tax System and Public School Financing in Texas* (March 24, 1997). Online. Available: http://www.capitol.state.tx.us/hrofr/focus/taxes.pdf. Accessed: November 10, 2001.

[140] Ibid.

[141] Food and Drug Administration, National Institute of Health, *Healthy People 2010: Nutrition and Overweight,* vol. II (November 2000). Online. Available: http://www.health.gov/healthypeople/Document/HTML/Volume2/19Nutrition.htm#_Toc490383116. Accessed: January 31, 2002.

[142] National Center for Chronic Disease Control and Prevention and Health Promotion, *Obesity and Overweight: A Public Health Epidemic* (September 12, 2001). Online. Available: http://www.cdc.gov/nccdphp/dnpa/obesity/epidemic.htm. Accessed: January 31, 2002.

[143] Office of the Surgeon General, *Overweight and Obesity: At A Glance.* Online. Available: http://www.surgeongeneral.gov/topics/obesity/calltoaction/fact_glance.htm. Accessed: January 31, 2001.

[144] Food and Drug Administration, National Institute of Health, *Healthy People 2010: Nutrition and Overweight,* Vol. II (Online).

[145] Office of the Surgeon General, *Overweight and Obesity: At A Glance* (Online).

[146] Rhonda Rundle, "Obesity Tops Smoking for Medical Costs," *The Wall Street Journal* (March 12, 2002), p. B7.

[147] Texas Comptroller of Public Accounts, *Texas Health Care Spending* (March 2001). Online. Available: http://www.window.state.tx.us/specialrpt/hcs/intro.html. Accessed: February 1, 2002.

[148] American Obesity Association, *Report on AOA Cost Study* (1999). Online. Available: http://www.obesity.org/cost_report.htm. Accessed: January 31, 2002.

[149] Texas Comptroller of Public Accounts, *Texas Health Care Spending* (March 2001). Online. Available: http://www.window.state.tx.us/specialrpt/hcs/intro.html. Accessed: February 1, 2002.

[150] Rhonda Rundle, "Obesity Tops Smoking for Medical Costs," p. B7.

[151] David S. Ludwig, Karen E. Peterson, and Steven L. Gortmaker, "Relation between Consumption of Sugar-Sweetened Drinks and Childhood Obesity: A Prospective, Observational Analysis," *The Lancet*, vol. 357, no. 9255 (February 17, 2001), pp. 505-508. Online. Available: http://www.thelancet.com/search/search.isa. Accessed: January 31, 2002.

[152] Center for Science in the Public Interest, "Soft Drinks Undermining Americans' Health," October 21, 1998 (press release). Online. Available: http://www.cspinet.org/new/soda_10_21_98.htm. Accessed: November 20, 2001.

[153] Ludwig, Peterson, and Gortmaker, "Relation between Consumption of Sugar-Sweetened Drinks and Childhood Obesity: A Prospective, Observational Analysis," pp. 505-508.

[154] Marion Nestle, *Soft Drink "Pouring Rights": Marketing Empty Calories* (Department of Nutrition and Food Studies, New York University, 2000). Online. Available: http://www.asu.edu/educ/epsl/Archives/CERU%20Archives/cace-00-03/cace-00-03.htm. Accessed: January 31, 2002.

[155] Michael F. Jacobson and Kelly D. Brownell, "Small Taxes on Soft Drinks and Snack Foods to Promote Health," *American Journal of Public Health*, vol. 90, no. 6 (June 2000), pp. 854-857.

[156] Arkansas Department of Finance and Administration, *Miscellaneous Tax Section.* Online. Available: http://www.state.ar.us/dfa/taxes/misc_tax/index.html. Accessed: November 19, 2001.

[157] State of Arkansas, *Soft Drink Tax.* Online. Available: http://arkleg.state.ar.us/data/TAXBOOK/TAXES/SOFTDR~1.htm. Accessed: November 19, 2001.

[158] Michael F. Jacobson and Kelly D. Brownell, "Small Taxes on Soft Drinks and Snack Foods to Promote Health," pp. 854-857.

[159] State of West Virginia, *Excise Taxes.* Online. Available: http://www.state.wv.us/taxrev/97taxlaws/9761_excise.pdf. Accessed: November 19, 2001.

[160] Marion Nestle, *Soft Drink "Pouring Rights": Marketing Empty Calories* (Online).

[161] U.S. Bureau of the Census, *U.S. Bureau of the Census, Texas Metropolitan Statistical Area Population Estimates: 1900 to 2000.* Online. Available: http://www.cpa.tx.us/ecodata/popdata/msa1. Accessed: January 31, 2002.

[162] Michael F. Jacobson and Kelly D. Brownell, "Small Taxes on Soft Drinks and Snack Foods to Promote Health," *American Journal of Public Health*, vol. 90, no. 6 (June 2000), pp. 854-857.

[163] Federation of Tax Administrators, *State Excise Tax Rates On Cigarettes.* Online. Available: http://www.taxadmin.org/fta/rate/cigarett.html. Accessed: January 23, 2002.

[164] Texas Comptroller of Public Accounts, *2002-2003 Biannual Revenue Estimate.* Online. Available: http://www.window.state.tx.us/taxbud/bre0203/tablea3.html. Accessed: February 1, 2002.

[165] Federation of Tax Administrators, *State Excise Tax Rates On Cigarettes* (Online).

[166] Connecticut's Attorney Generals Office, *Attorney General's Statement Regarding Increasing Cigarette Tax by $.61* (January 24, 2002). Online. Available: http://www.cslib.org/attygenl/mainlinks/tabindex4.htm. Accessed: February 1, 2002.

[167] The Independent Institute, *Book Summary Taxing Choice: The Predatory Politics of Fiscal Discrimination.* Online. Available: http://www.independent.org/tii/content/briefs/BriefTaxingChoice.html. Accessed: January 29,2002.

[168] Campaign for Tobacco-Free Kids, *Higher Cigarette Taxes Reduce Smoking Save Lives Save Money.* Online. Available: http://tobaccofreekids.org/reports/prices. Accessed: January 29, 2002.

[169] American Medical Association, *News Releases and Statements: January 28, 2002—States Look to Cigarette Taxes to Reduce Smoking, Help Cure Ailing Budgets.* Online. Available: http://www.ama-assn.org/ama/pub/article/3880-5846.html. Accessed: March 2, 2002.

[170] Ibid.

[171] Federation of Tax Administrators, *State Excise Tax Rates On Cigarettes* (Online).

[172] American Medical Association, *News Releases and Statements: January 28, 2002—States Look to Cigarette Taxes to Reduce Smoking, Help Cure Ailing Budgets* (Online).

[173] State of New Hampshire Department of Revenue Administration, *NH State Tax Forms—2002.* Online. Available: http://webster.state.nh.us/revenue/forms/index.htm. Accessed: December 16, 2001.

[174] Dave McNeely, "Income tax on verge of Texas Horizon," *Abilene Reporter News (*April 15, 2001). Online. Available: http://www.reporternews.com/2001/opinion/tax0415.html. Accessed: November 18, 2001.

[175] Ibid.

[176] Ibid.

[177] Lisa Falkenberg, "Lawmakers: Prosperity of state depends on overhauling tax structure," *Abilene Reporter News* (April 9, 2001). Online. Available: http://www.reporternews.com/2001/texas/tax0409.html. Accessed: November 20, 2001.

[178] Ken Ellsworth, "State income tax resurfaces," *Abilene Reporter New (*May 8, 2001). Online. Available: http://www.texnews.com/1998/2001/local/tax0508.html. Accessed: November 21, 2001.

[179] Ibid.

[180] Lisa Falkenberg, "Lawmakers: Prosperity of state depends on overhauling tax structure" (Online).

[181] Ibid.

[182] The Texas Legislature Online, *The Texas Constitution, Article 8-Taxation and Revenue, Section 24 - Personal Income Tax; Dedication of Proceeds.* Online. Available: http://www.capitol.state.tx.us/txconst/sections/cn000800-002400.html. Accessed: November 16, 2001.

[183] Telephone interview by Laura Koenig with Dick Lavine, Senior Fiscal Analyst, Center for Public Policy Priorities, Austin, Texas, January 29, 2002.

[184] Ibid.

[185] Texas Comptroller of Public Accounts, *Texas Health Care Spending* (March 2001). Online. Available: http://www.window.state.tx.us/specialrpt/hcs/pg33.html. Accessed: November 15, 2001.

[186] Association of Academic Health Centers, *Academics for Access to Health Care Initiative.* Online. Available: http://www.ahcnet.org/pdf/aahci.pdf. Accessed: April 10, 2002.

[187] Texas Comptroller of Public Accounts, *Texas Health Care Spending* (Online).

[188] Leigh Hopper, "Lottery Winners' loss is poor patients' gain: Area Hospitals get $46 Million in Unclaimed Funds," *Houston Chronicle* (April 5, 2002). Online. Available: http:www.chron.com/cs/CDA/prinstory.hts/topstory2/1343438. Accessed: April 5, 2002.

[189] Texas Government Code Annotated, ch. 466, sec. 466.408.

[190] Leigh Hopper, "Lottery Winners' loss is poor patients' gain: Area Hospitals get $46 Million in Unclaimed Funds" (Online).

[191] Department of Human Services, *Cost Sharing.* Online. Available: http://aspe.os.dhhs.gov/health/reports/benefits/state_approaches_to_costsharing.htm. Accessed: November 20, 2001.

[192] Texas Health and Human Services Commission, *CHIP Program Design Issues.* Online. Available:http://www.hhsc.state.tx.us/chip/cnews/PrgmDsgnIssues071801.html. Accessed: November 1, 2001.

[193] U.S. Department of Health and Human Services, *Examining Substitution: State Strategies to Limit Crowd out in the era of Children's Health Insurance* (January 10, 2001). Online. Available: http://aspe.os.dhhs.gov/health/reports/hinsubst/XSubstit.htm. Accessed: November 20, 2001.

[194] U.S. Department of Health and Human Services, *Children's Health Insurance Expansions: State Experiences in Developing Benefit Packages and Cost-Sharing Arrangements* (February 17, 1998). Online. Available: http://aspe.os.dhhs.gov/health/reports/benefits/state_approaches_to_costsharing.htm. Accessed: November 20, 2001.

[195] Management Sciences for Health, *Home Page*. Online. Available: http://www.msh.org. Accessed: February 15, 2002.

Appendix A. Expansion Using Waivers

by Laura G. Garcia

States employ a variety of options to reduce the number of uninsured residents. The options range from Section 1931 amendments to Medicaid and SCHIP programs, 1115 waivers to Medicaid and SCHIP programs and the most recent option, the HIFA waiver. This report provides a description of selected state plans and the types of options they have implemented.

The selection of the states was based on the variation of waivers that were granted and implemented and the types of expansions that were used. For example, California was selected because of the similarities to Texas in terms of population characteristics size and composition and the many approaches it has used to expand health coverage to its low-income populations. Table A.1 compares and contrasts state population characteristics.

Table A.1
A Comparison of State Demographic Profiles

States	Average percent of poverty, 1999-2000	Waivers	Percent foreign born, 2000	Personal income per capita, 1997	Percent uninsured, 1991	Percent uninsured, 2000
California	13.3	1915(b), Medicaid 1115, Medicaid 1931, Family Planning, HIFA	25.9	26,314	19.4	17.9
Minnesota	6.6	Medicaid 1115	5.4	26,243	9.3	9.0
New Jersey	7.9	SCHIP 1931, SCHIP 1115	17.8	32,356	11.0	12.5
Oregon	11.6	Medicaid 1115	8.0	23,920	14.3	13.8
Tennessee	13.3	Medicaid 1115	3.6	22,699	13.4	10.3
Texas	14.9		14.3	23,707	22.8	21.4
Wisconsin	8.9	Medicaid 1115, SCHIP 1115	4.1	24,048	8.1	7.4

Adapted from: U.S. Census Bureau, *Census 2000 Supplemental Survey.* Online. Available: http://factfinder.census.gov/home/en/c2ss.html. Accessed: April 4, 2002; Valerie Lewis, *Medicaid Waivers: California's Use of a Federal Option* (Oakland, Calif.: Medi-Cal Policy Institute, March 2000), pp. 6, 10-11; Health Care Financing Administration, *Health Insurance Flexibility and Accountability (HIFA) Initiative Fact Sheet.* Online. Available: http://www.hcfa.gov/medicaid/hifa/cafactsh.htm. Accessed: April 1, 2002; Melora Krebs-Carter and John Holahan, *State Strategies for Covering Uninsured Adults* (Washington, D.C.: The Urban Institute, 2000), p. 3; Jeanne Lambrew, *Section 1115 Waivers in Medicaid and the State Children's Health Insurance Program: An Overview* (Washington, D.C. The Kaiser Commission on Medicaid and the Uninsured, July 2001), pp. 7-8.

California

Background

California is probably the state with demographics most similar to that of Texas. Like Texas, it faces the difficult task of providing health coverage to a large immigrant and undocumented population in addition to having a small fraction of the population with employer-sponsored health insurance. One out of five nonelderly Californians lacks health insurance coverage.[1] The state relies heavily on its county indigent health centers because the counties are required to be the providers of last resort. They serve approximately 5 percent of the state's population at a cost of about $2 billion annually.[2]

California's strategy for health care for the low-income population is based on its Medi-Cal program and its support of the county based indigent health care system. Medicaid is known as Medi-Cal in California. Medi-Cal covers pregnant women and infants up to age one at incomes below 200 percent of the Federal Poverty Level (FPL) regardless of assets. California has chosen to keep documented immigrants eligible for Medi-Cal under the same rules that existed before welfare reform. About one quarter of California's Medi-Cal enrollees are non-citizen immigrants.[3]

In July of 1998, California implemented Healthy Families, the state's SCHIP program to provide health coverage to children and provide subsidies to allow families to purchase children's coverage through commercial plans.[4] The Healthy Families program covers children ages 1 through 6 in families between 133 percent and 200 percent of the FPL and children ages seven through 19 in families with incomes between 100 percent and 200 percent of the FPL.[5]

Other Publicly Funded Programs

The Access for Infants and Mothers Program (AIMS) provides subsidized health insurance for pregnant women and infants with incomes between 200 and 300 percent of the FPL. This program is funded from tobacco tax revenues and premiums from subscribers. In 1995, the average subscriber contribution for the basic service package was $630.00.[6]

Amendments and Waivers

California is administering several 1915(b) Medicaid waiver programs. One of the waivers was specifically used for its two-plan model to limit choice. The two-plan model consists of two plans: 1) a local initiative, which must contract with all hospitals and traditional providers that receive federal disproportionate share hospital funds and 2) a commercial plan. California also has a 1915(b) waiver for each of its five county-organized health systems, which represent providers, beneficiaries and local government.[7]

In addition to the 1915(b) waivers, California amended its Medicaid plan using Section 1931 in September of 1998. It allows family coverage for parents with incomes up to 107 percent of the FPL.

The State of California had a state subsidized family planning access, care and treatment program. It rolled this program into the Medi-Cal program so it could receive a Medicaid family planning waiver to cover reproductive services for medically indigent females between 100 and 200 percent of the FPL. This allowed the state to receive a federal match of 90 percent.

On April 15, 1996, Los Angeles County was granted an 1115 Medicaid waiver for the restructuring of the county's health service system. The goal of the waiver was to transform the county's large hospital based public medical care system so that it would coordinate and integrate the services of its six public hospitals and 45 health centers. It intends to rely on more primary and outpatient care. This is the only 1115 waiver that increases federal cost. This was because under the waiver Los Angeles County was allowed to receive a federal match for services provided to indigent patients that were not otherwise not eligible for Medi-Cal and it provides funding to offset reduction in disproportionate share hospital funds in recent years.[8] The waiver was to have expired on June 30, 2000, but Los Angeles County was granted an extension until June 30, 2005.[9]

California had submitted an 1115 SCHIP waiver and waited over a year for a response. During the wait, the Bush Administration U.S. Department of Health and Human Services announced the HIFA waiver and California chose to resubmit its SCHIP waiver as a HIFA waiver. California's HIFA waiver intends to expand Medi-Cal for children up to age 18 in families with incomes up to 100 percent the FPL and have the Healthy Families program cover those children with incomes between 100 and 250 percent of the FPL. Healthy Families will also expand to cover parents with incomes between 100 percent and 200 percent the FPL and parents under 100 percent the FPL that do not qualify for Medi-Cal. The HIFA waiver would expand to children first and then to parents. Parents would be required to pay co-payments for services with a yearly maximum of $250.[10] The projected implementation of the waiver is scheduled for July 1, 2002,[11] however, because of budget constraints it is unlikely that California will begin implementation as planned.

What Texas Can Learn from California

California has used a variety of options waivers and amendments to expand access to health insurance. Texas can definitely learn from California's use of the Section 1931 amendment to expand family coverage in addition to its use of the HIFA waiver. The Administration has already stated that it will no longer consider waivers targeted to special populations, a Family Planning waiver would not be an option unless it was a part of more comprehensive waiver.[12] The Center for Medicare and Medicaid Services has let it be known that county specific waivers would be considered but would have to exceptional to be granted.

Minnesota

Background

Minnesota is similar to Texas in that more than half the state's population resides in a seven county metropolitan area. As opposed to Texas, Minnesota has a substantial Medicaid program, a large subsidized state health insurance program and a high rate of coverage by employer-based health insurance. In 1992, Minnesota passed a series of legislation known as a whole as Minnesotacare. This legislation created a subsidized health insurance program known also as Minnesotacare. This subsidized health insurance program is targeted towards uninsured families with children with incomes up to 275 percent of the FPL and individuals with incomes up to 175 percent of the FPL.[13]

Waivers

Minnesota has been administering a Medicaid 1115 waiver for over 15 years. This waiver allowed a demonstration with select counties in the state to convert part of its Medicaid fee-for-service program to managed care plans. This program is known as the Prepaid Medical Assistance Program (PMAP).[14]

In 1995 Minnesota was granted another 1115 waiver and an amendment to their original waiver to expand PMAP to other counties in the state in a program know as PMAP+. PMAP+ expanded coverage to Medicaid eligible pregnant women and children up to age two with family incomes under 275 percent of the FPL. It allowed the state to receive federal matching funds for the MinnesotaCare program for children under two years old enrolled in MinnesotaCare. MinnesotaCare continued to cover uninsured families with children under 275 percent the FPL in the first phase and to extended Medicaid coverage to uninsured low-income adults without dependent children up to 175 percent of the FPL in its second phase. Some of these individuals would be required pay nominal premiums and cost sharing.

On June 13, 2001, Minnesota was granted an 1115 SCHIP waiver to enroll all parents of Medicaid and SCHIP eligible children in families with incomes between 100 and 200 percent the FPL. The state would be eligible to receive an enhanced matching rate for the parents and the parents would receive traditional Medicaid benefits and be required to pay premiums and co-payments on a sliding fee scale.[15]

What Texas Can Learn from Minnesota

Unfortunately, Texas is not eligible to apply for an 1115 SCHIP waiver and benefit from the enhanced match rate for parents. For Texas to be eligible to apply for an 1115 SCHIP waiver, it would need to change the current requirements of its SCHIP program. Texas has already begun a simplified process for Medicaid and SCHIP. However, it has not eliminated the assets test, offered 12 month continuous eligibility, simplified the renewal process or instituted presumptive eligibility for children. If Texas is able to implement at least two of those four requirements, it may become eligible to apply for an SCHIP waiver and reap the benefits of expanding to more individuals and receiving an enhanced federal match.

New Jersey

New Jersey has historically had a wide array of public programs designed to assist low-income populations. The top health priority in New Jersey is the Medicaid program. New Jersey is one of the nation's most urbanized areas and has a plentiful, well-distributed supply of doctors and hospitals.[16]

New Jersey had a major overhaul of its health care system with the Health Care Reform Act of 1992. Within this legislation, there was a subsidized insurance program for working families that became known as Health Access New Jersey. The program began in 1995 and was targeted to individuals with incomes of up to 250 percent of the federal poverty level who are not eligible for Medicare or Medicaid and have no access to health insurance through their employers. The subsidies were offered on a sliding scale based on income and the health plan selected.

New Jersey's Medicaid and SCHIP programs were housed under KidCare in 1998. KidCare was covering children in families up to 350 percent of the FPL. In July 2000, the state enacted legislation to cover uninsured parents up to 200 percent of the FPL and childless adults up to 100 percent of the FPL. Because of these expansions, KidCare became known as FamilyCare. Only state funds were used to cover childless adults between 50 and 100 percent of the FPL.[17]

The Medicaid program has mandated enrollment in fully capitated mangaged care organizations for all welfare- and poverty related beneficiaries. This mandate was done through a series of small 1915(b) waivers as opposed to one large 1115 waiver. Once the New Jersey SCHIP program was underway, Medicaid was expanded to cover children in families with incomes of up to 133 percent of the federal poverty level.

New Jersey is preserving Medicaid for legal immigrants where federal funding is available and has created a state program to encourage naturalization. The immigrant population is a significant portion of New Jersey population. The Census Bureau 2000 Supplemental Survey estimates that 17.8 percent of the state's overall population is foreign-born.[18]

Amendment and Waivers

New Jersey has applied for and received waivers and amendments to their Medicaid and SCHIP plans. In 1998, New Jersey was granted an 1115 waiver for its Medicaid program to assist in the treatment of charity care patients. Since the waiver was granted, it does not appear that there has been a move to implement the plan.

To further expand health coverage, New Jersey applied for and received a waiver and amendment to their SCHIP program in January 2001. The waiver allowed the state to receive an enhanced match for parents of Medicaid and SCHIP eligible children up to

200 percent of the FPL and for pregnant women with incomes between 185 and 200 percent of the FPL who were not insured and not covered by Medicaid. The State would receive the enhanced match for parents below 133 percent of the FPL who are eligible under Section 1931 of the Medicaid plan. Other parents up to 200 percent of the FPL who are not eligible for Medicaid would be enrolled in a state defined benefits package. In addition, families between 150 and 200 percent of the FPL would be required to share cost in the form of co-payments that would not exceed 5 percent of family income. [19] In addition, New Jersey amended its SCHIP plan through Section 1931, which allowed earning disregards from the old AFDC standard up to 133 percent of the FPL in September of 2000.

What Texas Can Learn from New Jersey

New Jersey has continued its commitment to covering families by amending their Medicaid plan to disregard income to expand coverage to more parents whose children may be already covered and to entire families. This decision to use a Section 1931 amendment allows New Jersey to expand without having to bear the burden of budget neutrality, instead it will receive a federal match for the newly covered. In addition, by receiving an SCHIP waiver, New Jersey is now reaping the benefits of expanding to more individuals and receiving an enhanced federal match.

Oregon

Background

Oregon began its campaign for universal health coverage in 1989 by enacting the Oregon Health Plan. This move towards health reform was due in part to the high cost of organ transplants, which caused them to be discontinued as a service in the Medicaid program.[20] The Oregon Health Plan (OHP) involves a series of health reforms that would affect the entire state and provide the country with a new approach to Medicaid 1115 waivers. In addition to the waiver, the OHP plan also included a high-risk pool, small business purchasing pool and various market reforms in the small employer market.[21] In the quest to achieve universal coverage, the legislation called for a creation of the Health Services Commission to rank health services according to their benefit to the entire population being served and clinical effectiveness. This Commission consisted of consumers and providers of health and social services. The Medicaid program is currently covering adults up to 100 percent of the FPL while the SCHIP program covers children in families with income up to 170 percent of the FPL.

Amendments and Waiver

Since February 1, 1994 Oregon has implemented its 1115 Medicaid waiver. This waiver expanded eligibility to individuals up to 100 percent of the FPL in addition to moving recipients into managed care plans with limited benefits. Of the approximately 745 potential services, Oregon has been able to offer 606 services. The number of services covered depends on the state budget and on the restriction of the 1115 waiver that requires budget neutrality. Overall, Oregon's Health Plan offers services more comprehensive than the mandatory services required by Medicaid.

In an attempt to further expand health coverage, Oregon anticipates requesting an amendment to its 1115 Medicaid waiver and submitting a HIFA waiver.[22] Oregon plans to restructure OHP into OHP2. This new plan would have three components, two of which relate to its current Medicaid and SCHIP programs. The first component of the plan would be OHP Plus, which would offer the current OHP benefit package to people eligible for Medicaid, people on general assistance and pregnant women and children with income up to 185 percent of the FPL. The second component of the plan would be OHP standard, which would offer a commercial package and cap enrollment. OHP standard would be available to adults not eligible for Medicaid with incomes up to 185 percent of the FPL. It would finance the expansion with unspent SCHIP, once those were depleted, it would begin using Medicaid funds.[23]

What Texas Can Learn from Oregon

Oregon has taken the Medicaid 1115 waiver to a new level of health coverage. By prioritizing services and expanding coverage to parents the state has experienced a dramatic decrease in the number of uninsured in the state. A report to the legislative assembly by the Office for Oregon Health Plan Policy and Research estimates that the percentage of uninsured adults was reduced from more than 18 percent in early 1990 to 11 percent in 1998 and the percentage of uninsured children reduced from 20 percent in early 1990 to 10 percent in 1998.

Tennessee

Background

The state of Tennessee resembles Texas in that it does not have a state income tax. This lack of additional revenue for the state may have contributed to the struggle with the cost of Medicaid services. In an effort not to increase taxes, it chose to consolidate the state and county funds it was already using towards health care so it could receive a federal match under the Medicaid program. Tennessee's reason for pursuing an 1115 Medicaid waiver was based on the state's inability to operate under a fee for service arrangement.

Waiver

The state of Tennessee began implementing expansion under a Medicaid 1115 waiver in January of 1994. The waiver for Tennessee limited the choice that Medicaid eligible individuals had when picking their providers and also capped enrollment at 1.4 million individuals. TennCare, as the Medicaid program is known, moved all Medicaid eligible beneficiaries into managed care and created near universal coverage by expanding to the uninsured and the medically uninsurable. By combining state, federal, and local funds dedicated to providing care to low-income populations and requiring cost-sharing by those individuals with incomes above the federal poverty level, Tennessee devised a means of covering over 400,000 previously uninsured individuals.[24] Tennessee was able to cover these individuals because the TennCare plan requires all beneficiaries, except those in the Medicaid eligibility group, with incomes above 100 percent of the FPL to pay a portion of the cost. This cost is in the form of premiums, deductibles, and co-payments based on income.[25]

TennCare has had to freeze enrollment to the program at least two times since its inception. In 1995, TennCare was forced to freeze enrollment to the general population at 1.3 million beneficiaries because of higher than expected enrollment and cost, however, the Medicaid eligibles and medically uninsurable were able to continue to enroll. Enrollment was once again opened in 1997 to children and dislocated workers when SCHIP funds became available. At this time, TennCare remains open to people who are Medicaid eligible or who are uninsurable as determined by an insurance company as well as children under the age of 19 whose individual family incomes are below 200 percent of the FPL.[26] The enrollment in TennCare is at dangerously high levels. State officials are expecting that by February 2002, the TennCare program will reach its cap and overspend its budget by $37.5 million by June 2002.[27] With these milestones in mind, state officials are attempting to remove ineligible members from the program.

What Texas Can Learn from Tennessee

While the consolidation of state and county funds may not be an ideal solution for the state of Texas, Tennessee's waiver indicates the kinds of aggressive strategies that the federal government was willing to support at one time. Tennessee's 1115 waiver is seen as the most aggressive use of the demonstration authority of the waiver.[28] The drawback of this type of waiver stems from the Texas' need to service a great number of immigrants who would not currently be eligible to receive services that were partly financed by the federal government.

Wisconsin

Background

The state of Wisconsin has been innovative in implementing various social policy initiatives, most recently in the area of welfare reform. Because Wisconsin has a high rate of employer sponsored health insurance, in 1995 nearly 80 percent of the state residents had employer-sponsored health insurance, health care for the low income people of the state has not been a main priority.[29] In addition, Wisconsin has the most extensive Medicaid program in the country. Its Medicaid program covers all the mandatory and optional services available in the program, indicating the state's progressive welfare policy.

BadgerCare was enacted in 1997 but was not formally begun until July of 1999. This program provides family based coverage for families above Medicaid limits and 185 percent of the FPL. Prior to the inception of BadgerCare, only children under age 6 and pregnant women under 185 percent of the FPL were covered under the Healthy Start program. Medicaid covered children between the ages of 6 and 14 up to 100 percent of the FPL and parents and older children up to the old AFDC income standard.[30] The family based approach of BadgerCare, covering both eligible children and their parents with the same services as Medicaid is based on the premise that health care is essential for working families with children and that extending health insurance to the entire family improves child enrollment, continuity of care, and the well being of the whole family.[31] Families are eligible for BadgerCare up to185 percent of the FPL and can stay enrolled in the program up to 200 percent of the FPL. In accordance with the traditional programs, children enrolled in the program are funded through SCHIP while parents are funded through Medicaid.

Other Public Health Programs

Wisconsin has a variety of services available to individuals ineligible for Medicaid and SCHIP. Immigrants that are ineligible to receive Medicaid because of their immigration status and length of time in the United States are eligible to receive services through the state funded general assistance medical program. For childless adults who have lived in the state for over 60 days, counties receive block grants to offer health care to their residents. If sufficient funds are available, the counties may be able to offer cash assistance.

Amendments and Waiver

In May of 1998, Wisconsin received approval to expand Medicaid coverage to children ages 15 through 18 in families under 100 percent of the FPL by using SCHIP funds. In a subsequent amendment and an SCHIP 1115 waiver, Wisconsin was able to expand Medicaid to parents of BadgerCare children (SCHIP) and children not eligible for Medicaid up to 185 percent. The state would receive the Medicaid match for the parents but the enhanced match for the children. In addition, the state is eligible to receive an enhanced match for both parents and children if it is cost-effective for the family to be covered under employer sponsored health insurance as defined under the SCHIP criteria.

What Texas Can Learn from Wisconsin

The relative success of the BadgerCare program can be attributed to many factors. Peggy Bartels, the administrator of the Division of Health Care Financing, Wisconsin Department of Health and Family Services, believes that the seamless integration of their SCHIP and Medicaid program has made the program more acceptable by low-income families as well as less costly to administer.[32] This seamless integration consists of a single point of entry, the same type of identification cards, access to same health maintenance organizations and same benefits packages for each member regardless of inclusion in Healthy Start, Medicaid and BadgerCare. Wisconsin covers both eligible children and their parents under the same services as Medicaid, covering the entire family improves children's enrollment and ultimately the quality of health they receive.[33]

As noted earlier, Texas is not eligible to apply for an SCHIP 1115 waiver and benefit from the enhanced match rate for parents. However, Texas can immediately begin to restructure its Medicaid and SCHIP programs to have seamless integration and a single point of entry into its public health systems. In the future Texas may become eligible to apply for an SCHIP waiver.

Conclusion

These have been approaches that states have implemented to expand access to health coverage. Their approaches can be examples that Texas can look to for guidance when it decides to expand access to health coverage. By learning from other states experiences, Texas could begin to implement changes and also adapt a combination of waiver initiatives to specifically meet its needs.

Notes

[1] Stephen Zuckerman, Teresa Coughlin, Len Nichols, David Liska, Barbara Ormond, Alicia Berkowitz, Meghan Dunleavy, Jodi Korb, and Nelda McCall, *Health Policy for Low-Income People in California* (Washington, D.C.: The Urban Institute, 1998) p. 3.

[2] Ibid.

[3] Ibid., p. 24.

[4] Department of Health Services, Projects and Initiatives, *Expansion of Healthy Families Coverage.* Online. Available: http://www.dhs.cahwnet.gov/home/projectsinitiatives/projectsinitiatives.htm. Accessed: January 23, 2002.

[5] Ibid.

[6] Zuckerman, et al., *Health Policy for Low-Income People in California,* p. 27.

[7] Valerie Lewis, *Medicaid Waivers: California's Use of a Federal Option* (Oakland, Calif.: Medi-Cal Policy Institute, March 2000), p.7.

[8] Zuckerman, et al., *Health Policy for Low-Income People in California,* p. 50.

[9] Health Care Financing Administration, *California's 1115 Medicaid Demonstration For Los Angeles County Fact Sheet.* Online. Available: http://www.hcfa.gov/medicaid/1115/lacnfact.htm. Accessed: November 29, 2001.

[10] Health Care Financing Administration, *Health Insurance Flexibility and Accountability (HIFA) Initiative Fact Sheet.* Online. Available: http://www.hcfa.gov/medicaid/hifa/cafactsh.htm. Accessed: April 1, 2002.

[11] Ibid.

[12] Jeanne Lambrew, *Section 1115 Waivers in Medicaid and the State Children's Health Insurance Program: An Overview* (Washington, D.C.: The Kaiser Commission on Medicaid and the Uninsured, July 2001), p. 10.

[13] Melora Krebs-Carter and John Holahan, *State Strategies for Covering Uninsured Adults* (Washington, D.C.: The Urban Institute, 2000), p. 18.

[14] Teresa Coughlin, Shruti Rajan, Stephen Zuckerman, and Jill A. Marsteller, *Health Policy for Low-Income People in Minnesota* (Washington, D.C.: The Urban Institute, 1997), p. 26.

[15] Health Care Financing Administration, *Minnesota Title XXI Program Fact Sheet.* Online. Available: http://www.hcfa.gov/init/chpfsmn.htm. Accessed: November 14, 2001.

[16] Randall R. Bovberg, Frank Ullman, Alison Evans, John Holahan, and Susan Flanagan, *Health Policy for Low-Income People in New Jersey* (Washington, D.C.: The Urban Institute, 1998), p. 3.

[17] Leanne DeFranxesco, Christina Folz, Madeleine Konig, and Carole Lee, *State of the States* (Washington, D.C.: State Coverage Initiatives, January 2002), p. 7. Online. Available: http://www.statecoverage.net/pdf/stateofstates2002.pdf. Accessed: January 20, 2002.

[18] U.S Census Bureau, *Quick Facts, Profile of Selected Characteristics.* Online. Available: http://factfinder.census.gov/servlet/QTTable?ds_name=ACS_C2SS_EST_G00_&geo_id=04000US34&qr_name=ACS_C2SS_EST_G00_QT02. Accessed: April 4, 2002.

[19] Health Care Financing Administration, *New Jersey Title XXI Demonstration Fact Sheet.* Online. Available: http://www.hcfa.gov/init/1115nj.htm. Accessed: November 14, 2001.

[20] Richard Conviser, The Office for Oregon Health Policy and Research, *A Brief History of the Oregon Health Plan and its Features.* Online. Available: http://www.ohppr.state.or.us/docs/pdf/histofplan.pdf. Accessed: January 21, 2002.

[21] Office for Oregon Health Plan Policy and Research, *The Oregon Health Plan and Oregon's Health Care Market, A Report to the 71st Legislative Assembly* (Salem, Ore., August 2000), p.1.

[22] Office for Oregon Health Policy, *The OHP 2 Waiver Application.* Online. Available: http://www.ohppr.state.or.us/Waiver_Application/index_waiver.htm. Accessed: February 4, 2002.

[23] Ibid.

[24] Krebs-Carter and Holahan, *State Strategies,* p. 23.

[25] Kaiser Commission on Medicaid and the Uninsured, *Daily Health Policy Report.* Online. Available: http://kaisernetwork.org/daily_reports/rep_index.cfm?DR_ID=8006. Accessed: November 13, 2001.

[26] Bureau of TennCare, *Daily Health Policy Report.* Online. Available: http://www.state.tn.us/tenncare/whatis.html. Accessed: November 9, 2001.

[27] Kaisernetwork.org, *Daily Health Policy Report.* Online. Available: http://kaisernetwork.org/daily_reports/rep_index.cfm?DR_ID=8006. Accessed: November 13, 2001.

[28] Lambrew, *Section 1115 Waivers,* p. 9.

[29] Teresa A. Coughlin, Joshua M. Wiener, Jill A. Marstellar, David G. Stevenson, and Susan Wallin, *Health Policy for Low-Income People in Wisconsin* (Washington, D.C.: The Urban Institute, 1998), p. 5.

[30] Wisconsin Council on Families and Children, *Wisconsin's BadgerCare Program.* Online. Available: http://www.wccf.org/BadgerCare.pdf. Accessed: February 3, 2002.

[31] Jeremy Albrega , *Wisconsin's BadgerCare Program Offers Innovative Approach for Family Coverage* (Washington, D.C.: Academy for Health Systems Research and Health Policy, 2001), p. 2.

[32] Ibid.

[33] DeFranxesco, Folz, Konig, and Lee, *State of the States*, p. 7.

Appendix B.
Information on Individual State Premium Assistance Programs

Premium Assistance Programs using Medicaid Funds (HIPP Programs)

The Iowa HIPP program, started in 1991, is the oldest HIPP program in the country. It enrolls about 8,500 individuals, 5,574 of which are Medicaid eligible. It is estimated to save the state nearly $3 million yearly.[1] The program is administered similar to the Texas program, but the employer is given the option of being paid directly from the HIPP program for the premium reimbursement. However, for the most part, employers choose to have the employee pay the premium and be reimbursed from the state.[2]

Wisconsin

The Wisconsin BadgerCare HIPP program did not begin enrolling families until June of 2000. Initially enrollment has been very low only around 239 individuals since the start of the program. This small enrollment is attributed to limited number of enrollees with access to employer-based coverage. Wisconsin recently lowered the employer contribution restriction from 60 percent of the cost of the plan to 40 percent of the cost of the plan. Currently, in order for a plan to be considered, employers must provide between 40 percent to 80 percent of the cost of the plan. Wisconsin uses SCHIP funds to cover eligible children whose parents have access to employer-based coverage and Medicaid funds are used to cover eligible adults.[3] Using SCHIP funds for employer-based insurance coverage will be discussed in more detail in a later section.

Premium Assistance Programs using SCHIP funds

Maryland

Overview

Maryland's SCHIP plan is a combination of Medicaid expansion and a separate SCHIP program. In November, 2000, Maryland received approval of an amendment to its SCHIP plan that established phase II of its SCHIP program. This phase expanded the program to provide coverage for uninsured children in families earning from 200-300 percent of the federal poverty level (FPL). As part of this approval, Maryland developed a premium assistance program using federal SCHIP funds.

Funding

Maryland will receive Federal SCHIP match only for the cost of the subsidy for the uninsured child.

Benefits

In order for a child to enroll in employer-sponsored health insurance, the plan must meet the standards for benchmark or benchmark-equivalent coverage. The benchmark plan is the Comprehensive Standard Health Benefits package that includes well-child care, well-baby care, and immunizations.

The cost-sharing element for the premium assistance program is the same the cost-sharing element for the public plan. Families whose incomes are 200 to 250 percent FPL are responsible for a $450 contribution per family per year. Families whose incomes are above 250 to 300 percent FPL are responsible for $562 contribution per family per year. Premium assistance beneficiaries are not responsible for any co-payments, coinsurance, or deductibles imposed by the employer plan. Providers bill the state for these fees, and providers will receive direct reimbursement for these amounts.

Crowd-Out

To avoid the possibility of crowd-out, the state will not enroll any individual who is covered or who has voluntarily refused or terminated employer-based health insurance within the preceding six months. Employers participating in the premium assistance program must pay at least 50 percent of family coverage.

Mississippi

Overview

Mississippi submitted an amendment to its state Children's Health Insurance Plan on August 4, 1998, to develop a non-Medicaid program option also known as phase II of their SCHIP program. This new plan covered uninsured children below age 19 in families with income levels between 100 to 133 percent FPL. This amendment also proposed a premium assistance program for children with access to employer-sponsored coverage. Mississippi has subsequently expanded its SCHIP eligibility to children 200 percent of the FPL.

The Mississippi premium assistance program has been put on hold indefinitely, in part because of political reasons. A premium assistance program can be administratively burdensome and expensive, and it appears that the current administration did not want to spend the money necessary to implement the program.

Funding

Mississippi would have received the enhanced federal SCHIP match for the subsidies of children enrolled in cost effective employer-sponsored health insurance plans.

Benefits

The employer-sponsored health insurance must meet benchmark coverage equivalent to the benefit package offered under the "network option" of the State and Public

Employer's Health Insurance Plan plus additional benefits such as immunizations, vision and hearing screening, and dental services. If the employer plan does not pay for immunizations, they will be available at the local health department or through the child's physician at no cost to the family.

The Mississippi plan contains a cost sharing requirements. For families at or below 150 percent of the FPL, there is no cost-sharing requirement. For families between 151 to 175 percent of the FPL, there is a co-pay of $5 per outpatient visit, $15 per emergency room visit, and an $800 out of pocket maximum. For families above 175 percent FPL, the out of pocket maximum increases to $950. Individuals enrolled in premium assistance pay these cost sharing requirements and do not have to pay co-payments, deductibles, or premiums imposed by their employer plan. Providers bill the state for these fees.

Crowd-Out

The Mississippi plan imposes a six-month period of not being insured for enrollment into the premium assistance program. In addition, employers must contribute at least 50 percent of the cost of the employer-based coverage.

Massachusetts

Overview

MassHealth aims to assist low-income employees and self-employed individuals in affording employment-based coverage. The MassHealth Family Assistance Program was originally established as part of the state SCHIP plan in 1998. The program provides premium assistance for families purchasing employer based coverage. Massachusetts was able to include families in the premium assistance program because of an earlier approved section 1115 waiver. Families at or below 200 percent of the FPL will be considered for the premium assistance program if they have access to employer sponsored coverage. As of January 2002, around 12,000 individuals have enrolled in the family assistance program and all are below 200 percent of the FPL.

Cost-Effectiveness Test

The state subtracts the amount of the employer contribution and the family contribution from the cost of the insurance plan. This contribution amount is compared with the cost effective amount—the amount that the state would have to pay to enroll only the children in the public health plan. If there is a difference, the state will provide a subsidy to the family for the cost effective amount. The family must enroll in the employer plan unless the ultimate family share exceeds 5 percent of the family's income.

Funding

Massachusetts will receive the enhanced match for the cost effective amount of families enrolled premium assistance programs.

Benefits

In the Massachusetts program there is no minimum benefit package. Any insurance package that can be sold is satisfactory. Children under 150 percent of the FPL and adults under 133 percent of the FPL receive Medicaid wrap around benefits in addition to the benefits offered under their employer plan.[4] There is a cost-sharing element to the Massachusetts premium assistance program. Families at or below 150 percent of FPL are not required to pay any part of their monthly premium, but families about 150 percent must pay a family share. This share is a flat amount based on the number of children in the family. As stated above, the entire family share cannot exceed 5 percent of income.

Crowd-Out

The employer must pay at least 50 percent of the health insurance cost. There does not appear to be a look-back period.

Virginia

Overview

The first amendment to the Virginia state plan was approved on December 22, 2000. The amendment changes the name to Family Access to Medical Insurance Security Plan (FAMIS). FAMIS covers children from birth through age 18 in families with gross incomes up to 200 percent of the FPL. This amendment also establishes a premium assistance program for children in families that meet FAMIS eligibility requirements and who have access to health insurance coverage through their parent's employer. Under the program, the state may pay the cost of family coverage including the premium of the employee if it is cost-effective (see below). Please note that this program is not mandatory for eligible populations.

Cost-Effective Test

The cost of the family coverage under the employer plan is equal to or less than Virginia's cost of providing coverage under the public program FAMIS only for the eligible low-income children.

Benefits

The benefits of the employer-sponsored coverage must be equivalent to the coverage under the FAMIS benefit package. The Department of Medical Assistance Services provides supplemental coverage if the employer plan does not provide services included in the benchmark plan.

There is a cost-sharing component for families with incomes greater than 150 percent of the Federal Poverty Level. For one child the premium is $15 per month, for two children the premium is $30 per month and for three or more children the premium is $45 per month.

Crowd-Out

The child must be uninsured for six months and the employer must contribute at least 40 percent.

Wisconsin

Overview

BadgerCare provides health insurance to families up to 185 percent of the Federal poverty level, and family members can stay on the insurance up to 200 percent. Wisconsin was able to expand coverage to the families by obtaining a section 1115 demonstration waiver that was approved in January of 2001.

Funding

All BadgerCare children are financed through state SSCHIP funds (federal match of 71 percent). Parents of BadgerCare children are usually covered under Medicaid funds with a match of 59 percent. In September of 2000, Wisconsin was approved by HCFA to use Title XXI funds to cover parents by obtaining a waiver to buy private coverage if it is cost-effective (see following explanation). The BadgerCare Premium Assistance program builds from the infrastructure already in place for the Wisconsin HIPP program. As of October 1, 2001, about 130 cases or 47 families actually qualified for the HIPP program.

Cost-Effectiveness Test

The cost-effectiveness test is the same as the test for the HIPP program. Individuals falling in the Medicaid eligible range are considered for the HIPP program if an employer sponsored plan is cost effective. It will be considered cost-effective if the cost to the state for coverage of the entire family (including employee share of premium plus wrap-around costs) is less than the cost of Medicaid HMO coverage for the family. If the family is cost-effective according to this test, then the state receives only the Medicaid federal match.

The state can receive the enhanced SCHIP match if the individual falls in the SCHIP eligibility range and the cost of covering both the children and the parents in the employer sponsored plan does not exceed the cost of covering the whole family in the BadgerCare public program. If cost-effective in this manner, the state receives the enhanced match for the entire family.

For both the SCHIP and the Medicaid premium assistance programs, the state considers administrative costs to the state in its cost-effectiveness formula.

As the BadgerCare program continues to grow, the HMOs in Wisconsin are not taking additional enrollees. The state is now paying for these individuals on a fee-for-service basis. It cost the state more money to pay fee-for-service, and it is possible that more

BadgerCare-eligible individuals will meet the cost-effectiveness test because of the additional cost for fee-for-service.

Benefits

The benefit plan of the employer must be comparable to the BadgerCare program. Benefits include the employer-sponsored plan and benefits that are not covered by the private plan but are available in the public program. These benefits are treated as wrap-around benefits and are paid for by the state.

Cost-sharing requires that families above 150 percent FPL pay a premium of no more than 3 percent of income—approximately $60 per month for a family of three at 185 percent of FPL.

Crowd-Out

Wisconsin requires the individual to be uninsured for the last six months if the employee had access to insurance with less than 80 percent employer sponsorship, and 18 months with access to employer-based coverage if the percent the employer pays greater than 80 percent. The employer must contribute between 40 and 80 percent of the cost of the plan in order for that plan to be eligible.

New Jersey

Overview

New Jersey's Section 1115 SCHIP waiver expands Medicaid coverage to parents with earned incomes up to 133 percent of FPL. The SCHIP waiver also expands coverage to parents with incomes between 134 percent and 200 percent FPL through a state-designed program and employer-sponsored insurance. Finally, the waiver expands coverage to children only in families with income ranges of 200 to 350 percent of the FPL. From September 1, 2000, until this writing, New Jersey had enrolled around 161 people into the premium assistance program, and around the same number of people are in the pipeline for premium assistance.

Cost-Effectiveness Test

For families under 200 percent of the FPL, premium assistance/employer-sponsored coverage will only be pursued if the cost to the state and family combined for the employer plan is less than it would cost the state to provide coverage for the entire family under the state-contracted plan. There is a modified cost-effectiveness test for the parents of children in the 200 to 350 percent range. The parents can be covered if the cost of covering the entire family in the employer plan is less than covering only the child in the public New Jersey plan. If it is not cost-effective to cover the adults, but it is cost-effective to cover the child, then the child can be eligible for premium assistance.

In developing the cost-effective formula, New Jersey hired the William Mercer Group, an accounting firm, to develop a computerized formula. This formula takes into account age, gender, health history, and several other factors. Once the formula is in place, the individuals determining cost-effectiveness simply plug the information into the formula.

Funding

The state obtained the enhanced match for adults between 100 to 133 percent, but if the SCHIP allotment runs out, then the state will return to the Medicaid match rate for this group. Additionally, the state obtained the enhanced match rate for the adults in the 134 to 200 percent FPL range, however, if the SCHIP allotment runs out, then New Jersey will have to fund this program with state general revenue entirely. If state money runs out, then enrollment will be capped and a waiting list established.

Benefits

Parents and children at 133 percent and below receive the same benefits as the Medicaid package. For families from 134 to 200 percent FPL, the benefits equal equivalent to the most widely sold HMO plan in the state. In the premium assistance program, for large businesses (greater than 49 employees), the employer coverage is not acceptable unless the benefit package meets or exceeds the FamilyCare Package. In smaller businesses, families will not be enrolled unless the plan is a standardized insurance plan. Wrap-around services will be provided on a fee-for-service basis only in small employers. If the employer sponsored plan is not cost-effective, but has richer benefits, the enrollee has the option of paying out-of-pocket for the difference.

For families 200 to 350 percent FPL, the adults will not receive wrap-around benefits if the modified cost-effective test is met and they receive premium assistance.

There is a cost-sharing requirement under the New Jersey plan. Families with incomes above 150 percent FPL must pay a monthly premium of $25 for the first adult and then $10 for each additional member of the family. In addition, there are also co-payments associated with the cost of the insurance. For the premium assistance program, the individual pays the cost of the co-pay stipulated in the employer plan and is then reimbursed by the state or the provider can bill the state for the difference. The state will have providers bill the state directly for preventative services co-payments.

Crowd-Out

The employer must pay 50 percent of the cost of the program and the parents and children must be uninsured and meet a six-month waiting period requirement. There are exceptions to this look-back period such as loss of job, divorce, or death of covered family member. The look-back period is also waived if the individual had previously been covered by an individual insurance plan.

Administrative Features

The New Jersey plan has several unique administrative features that allow this program to succeed. Individuals enrolled in premium assistance are reimbursed for their cost-sharing requirements and these reimbursements are processed in-house. The premium assistance program staff receives the request for reimbursement requests, and they enter the information into an online payment system. This information is sent to the treasury for the State of New Jersey. The check is then issued from the treasury. Additionally, New Jersey has started a database that keeps track of employer plan information.

Rhode Island

Overview

In February of 2001, Rhode Island created RIte Share, the employer buy-in part of their public insurance program. The government established RIte Share in response to the fiscal crisis that the state's SCHIP and Medicaid programs found themselves in after expanding the SCHIP program to adults up to 185 percent FPL. The Rhode Island Health Reform 2000 requires all individuals with access to employer-sponsored coverage to enroll in the RIte Share program.[5] Similar to other programs, the state pays the employers and providers for the cost of the employee's share of the premium and additional co-pays and expenditures for services not covered by the employer's plan.

Benefits

Rhode Island has developed broad standards for approving eligible employer health plans. Most commercial plans in Rhode Island are approved, and the benefits not covered under this plan are paid for by the state.

Cost-Effectiveness

Cost-effectiveness is assessed at the program level and based on an average family rate rather than calculated for each individual family.[6]

Notes

[1] Jennifer Sexton, *Overview of the Iowa Health Insurance Premium Payment (HIPP) Program* (Washington, D.C: Institute for Health Policy Solutions, February 2000), p. 1.

[2] Sharon Silow-Carrol, Stephanie E. Anthony, and Jack A. Meyer, *State and Local Initiatives to Enhance Health Coverage for the Working Uninsured* (New York, NY: The Commonwealth Fund, November 2000), p. 20.

[3] Ibid.

[4] Presentation by Michael Miller, Community Catalyst/ Health Care for All, at the Families USA Conference, Washington, D.C., January 17, 2002.

[5] State Coverage Initiatives, "State of the States" (Washington, D.C.: Academy for Health Care Services Research and Health Policy, 2002), p. 14.

[6] Ibid.

Appendix C. Procedures Included in Analysis of AAP Study on Medicaid FFS Rates

CPT Code	Category	Procedure
95010	Allergy/immunology	Allergen immunotherapy two or more injections
95004	Allergy/immunology	Percutaneous tests with allergenic extracts
95024	Allergy/immunology	Intracutaneous tests with allergenic extracts
95015	Allergy/immunology	Allergen immunotherapy single injection
95117	Allergy/immunology	Percutaneous tests sequential
95115	Allergy/immunology	Intracutaneous tests with biologicals
93510	Cardiology	Left heart catheterization
93501	Cardiology	Right heart catheterization
32020	Cardiology	Thorascotomy tube
92950	Cardiology	Cardio pulmonary resuscitation
93303	Cardiology	Transthoracic echocardiography
93320	Cardiology	Doppler echocardiograph
93307	Cardiology	Echocardio-graphy real time with image doc
99255	Consultations	Initial patient visit high complexity
99254	Consultations	Initial patient visit moderate complexity
99245	Consultations	Office visit high complexity
99244	Consultations	Office visit moderate complexity
99243	Consultations	Office visit low complexity
99242	Consultations	Office visit straightforward decision
36488	Critical Care	Place catheter percutaneous >2yrs
31500	Critical Care	Intubation endotracheal
36620	Critical Care	Arterial line placement
36600	Critical Care	Arterial puncture diagnostic
99291	Critical Care	Evaluation and management first hour
99292	Critical Care	Evaluation and management add'l 30 min
36489	Critical Care	Place catheter percutaneous <2yrs
99282	Emergency Care	Visit low complexity
99283	Emergency Care	Visit moderate complexity
99284	Emergency Care	Visit high complexity
12015	Emergency Care	Simple surgical repair of facial wound
10120	Emergency Care	Simple surgical removal of foreign body
62270	Emergency Care	Lumbar puncture diagnostic
36410	Emergency Care	Venipuncture >2yrs
36400	Emergency Care	Venipuncture <2yrs
92551	EPSDT-Evaluation and management	Screening test hearing evaluation
99205	EPSDT-Evaluation and management	New patient high complexity
99204	EPSDT-Evaluation and management	New patient moderate complexity
99215	EPSDT-Evaluation and management	Est. patient moderate complexity
99203	EPSDT-Evaluation and management	New patient office visit
99202	EPSDT-Evaluation and management	New patient expanded visit
99214	EPSDT-Evaluation and management	Est. patient high complexity
99213	EPSDT-Evaluation and management	Est. patient low complexity
99201	EPSDT-Evaluation and management	New patient low complexity
99212	EPSDT-Evaluation and management	Est. patient expanded visit
99211	EPSDT-Evaluation and management	Est. patient office visit
99391	EPSDT-Preventive medicine	Est. patient 18 through 39
99392	EPSDT-Preventive medicine	Est. patient 12 through 17
99393	EPSDT-Preventive medicine	Est. patient 5 through 11
99395	EPSDT-Preventive medicine	Est. patient under 1 yr
99394	EPSDT-Preventive medicine	Est. patient 1 through 4

99381	EPSDT-Preventive medicine	New patient under 1 yr
99382	EPSDT-Preventive medicine	New patient 1 through 4
99383	EPSDT-Preventive medicine	New patient 5 through 11
99384	EPSDT-Preventive medicine	New patient 12 through 17
99385	EPSDT-Preventive medicine	New patient 18 through 39
99220	Evaluation and management	Initial care low severity
99219	Evaluation and management	Initial care moderate severity
99218	Evaluation and management	Initial care high complexity
67314	Gastrointestinal	Strabismus surgery vertical
67311	Gastrointestinal	Strabismum surgery, horizontal
44389	Gastrointestinal	Colonoscopy with biopsy
43239	Gastrointestinal	Upper GI endoscopy w/biopsy
45331	Gastrointestinal	Sigmoidoscopy with biopsy
68810	Gastrointestinal	Nasolacrimal probing
99238	Hospital care	Hospital discharge under 30 min
99222	Hospital care	Initial hospitalization moderate complexity
99221	Hospital care	Initial hospitalization low complexity
99231	Hospital care	Subsequent hospitalization low complexity
99223	Hospital care	Initial hospitalization high complexity
99232	Hospital care	Subsequent hospitalization moderate complexity
99233	Hospital care	Subsequent hospitalization high complexity
99440	Newborn care	Newborn resuscitation
99431	Newborn care	Initial newborn care
99435	Newborn care	Same day admit and discharge
99433	Newborn care	Subsequent newborn care
92567	Newborn care	Tympanometry hearing evaluation
54150	Newborn care	Circumcision
42821	Otolaryngology	Tonsillectomy/adenoidectomy >12 yrs
42820	Otolaryngology	Tonsillectomy/adenoidectomy <12yrs
69436	Otolaryngology	Tympanostomy and tubes
87060	Pathology and laboratory	Throat or nose culture
87430	Pathology and laboratory	Streptococcus screen
86580	Pathology and laboratory	Tuberculosis intradermal
85095	Pathology and laboratory	Bone marrow aspiration
36510	Perinatal Pediatircs (NIC)	Umbilical vein catheterization
36660	Perinatal Pediatircs (NIC)	Umbilical artery catheterization
99297	Perinatal Pediatircs (NIC)	Subsequent NICU stable neonate
99296	Perinatal Pediatircs (NIC)	Subsequent NICU unstable neonate
99295	Perinatal Pediatircs (NIC)	Initial NICU care
42200	Plastic surgery	Cleft palate repair
40700	Plastic surgery	Cleft lip repair
90801	Psychiatry	Diagnostic exam
31622	Pulmonology	Bronchoscopy
32000	Pulmonology	Thoracentesis
71010	Radiology	Frontal chest x-ray
94010	Radiology	Spirometry including graphic record
49500	Surgery	Bilateral inguinal hernia <5yrs
28262	Surgery	Extensive clubfoot release
44950	Surgery	Appendectomy
49505	Surgery	Bilateral inguinal hernia >5yrs
50200	Urology and dialysis	Renal biopsy
90945	Urology and dialysis	Peritoneal dialysis

Adapted from: American Academy of Pediatrics, *Medicaid Reimbursement Survey, 2001: 50 States and the District of Columbia.* Online: http://www.aap.org/research/medreimPDF01/all_states.PDF. Accessed: November 13, 2001.

Appendix D. SCHIP Enrollment, Health Plans, and Rates

CSA	SCHIP Enrolled	SCHIP Eligible	Health Plans	PMPM				% Incr.
				<1	1- 5	6- 14	15-18	
CSA # 1: Panhandle Area	14,189	5,418	FirstCare Southwest Alliance	$448.37	$91.26	$59.74	$118.07	17.40
			Texas University Health Plans- Tots to Teens	$460.75	$93.86	$61.36	$121.47	23.70
CSA # 2: Dallas/ Ft. Worth Area	81,453	24,345	Amerigroup	$436.72	$88.89	$58.21	$115.81	3.00
			Cook Children's Health Plan	$529.02	$89.99	$75.21	$140.29	25.50
			Parkland Comm-unity Health Plan- KIDS*first*	$559.26	$113.83	$74.54	$148.31	31.90
CSA # 5: Austin Area	20,111	5,187	Seton Health Plan	$456.51	$92.92	$60.82	$120.21	19.00
CSA # 6: Houston/ Beaumont Area	125,609	28,106	Amerigroup	$484.57	$98.63	$64.63	$129.58	0.00
			UTMB Health Care System- Choice 1	$569.20	$115.86	$75.91	$152.21	18.00
			Texas Children's Health Plan	$627.03	$116.94	$91.87	$156.99	29.40
CSA # 7: San Antonio Area	37,901	11,940	Community First Health Plans	$445.57	$90.69	$59.34	$116.85	22.60
			Texas Universities Health Plan- Tots to Teens	$358.86	$73.41	$47.78	$94.14	0.00
CSA # 8: Corpus Christi Area	20,717	4,980	Driscoll Children's Health Plan	$181.60	$100.21	$79.14	$87.47	18.70
CSA # 10: Laredo Area	10,299	2,722	Mercy Health Plan	$425.58	$86.62	$56.68	$111.61	17.10
CSA # 11: El Paso Area	25,723	7,762	Texas Universities Health Plan- Tots to Teens	$402.26	$81.95	$53.56	$105.51	12.20
			El Paso First Health Plan	$433.94	$88.32	$57.79	$113.80	19.40
CSA # 3, 4, 9: Rural Areas	140,842	37,081	Clarendon (EPO)*	$497.11	$99.92	$63.67	$131.12	

Adapted from: Presentation by David Wilkes, SCHIP Actuary, Birch and Davis, to the SB1053/1299 Task Force, Austin, Texas, November 15, 2001.

* These rates are from 2000-2001. Clarendon no longer contracts on a full-risk basis for 2001-2002.

Appendix E. Medicaid Managed Care Rates by Service Delivery Area

				RISK GROUPS				
County and Projected Enrollment	**Average All Risk Groups**	**TANF Children**	**TANF Adults**	**Pregnant Women**	**Total Newborns**	**Expansion Children**	**Federal Mandate**	**SCHIP Phase I**
Travis SDA *598,456*	$177.97	$91.79	$194.69	$583.42	$436.67	$91.80	$60.81	$86.49
Bexar SDA 163,361	$158.04	$83.22	$203.94	$568.02	$436.33	$74.42	$55.19	$78.42
Lubbock SDA *163,361*	$159.79	$100.74	$229.53	$512.10	$432.66	$77.02	$67.84	$96.63
Tarrant SDA *760,712*	$203.91	$99.68	$228.77	$613.19	$493.31	$100.77	$68.86	$98.08
Harris SDA *1,562,797*	$207.78	$105.79	$225.28	$614.23	$634.21	$117.57	$67.51	$96.10
Dallas SDA* *885,752*	$175.51	$91.45	$220.96	$606.80	$471.65	$117.03	$57.92	$83.83
El Paso SDA* 389,019	$135.20	$97.83	$196.73	$550.28	$450.99	$86.28	$48.69	$68.99
All Areas *4,778,559*	*$184.79*	*$97.04*	*$217.21*	*$597.20*	*$520.83*	*$104.40*	*$61.91*	*$86.24*

Adapted from: Texas Department of Health, *HMO Rate Setting Methodology FY 2002* (Austin, Texas, 2001), p. 7.

* Dallas and El Paso have enhanced rates.

Note: The rates include a legislative increase of $38.53 million allocated over all geographic areas and risk groups by percentage of premium; this increase includes EPSTD Medical screen increased reimbursement from $49 to $70 per screen and $8.71 million for outpatient facility cost.

Appendix F. List of the 42 Counties in the Border Region

Atascosa County
Bandera County
Bexar County
Brewster County
Brooks County
Cameron County
Crockett County
Culberson County
Dimmit County
Duval County
Edwards County
El Paso County
Frio County
Hidalgo County
Hudspeth County
Jeff Davis County
Jim Hogg County
Kenedy County
Kerr County
Kimble County
Kinney County
Kleberg County
LaSalle County
Live Oak County
Maverick County
McMullen County
Medina County
Nueces County
Pecos County
Presidio County
Real County
Reeves County
San Patricio County
Starr County
Sutton County
Terrell County
Uvalde County
Val Verde County
Webb County
Willacy County
Zapata County
Zavala County

Adapted from: Senate Bill 1299 Workgroup, *Border Rate Workgroup on Medicaid and CHIP Final Report* (Austin, Tex., May 2000), Attachment B, p. 1.

Appendix G. Border Counties Compared to Texas as a Whole

Demographic Categories	Border Counties (43)	Entire State (254)
Population (2001)	4,289,000 (21%)	20,698,000 (100%)
Uninsured Pop under 66 yrs of age (2000)	1,178,000 (27.5%)	4,712,000 (27.8%)
Pop. in Medicaid (2001)	661,000 (15.4%)	1,847,000 (8.9%)
Pop. in SCHIP (2001)	140,000 (10%)	458,000 (7.6%)
Pop. Living in Poverty (2000)	1,065,000 (25.3%)	3,093,000 (15.2%)
Unemployment rate (2000)	124,000 (7%)	487,000 (4.2%)
Personal Income per capita (1999)	$19,790	$26,834

Adapted from: Texas Health and Human Services Commission, Advisory Committee for Senate Bill 1053 and Senate Bill 1299, *Percent of Uninsured in Adults ages 19-65 in 2000, Percent of Children Under 19 Uninsured in 2000, Population Living in Poverty in 2000, Monthly Average Rate of Unemployment* (Austin, Tex., October 26, 2001), n. p. (draft paper).

Appendix H. Health Insurance Premiums

Health Insurance Premiums	Year		
	1998	1999	2000
TOTAL Texas Health Insurance Premiums and Other Considerations for CY 1998-2000	**$17,760,010,733**	**$19,223,302,062**	**$20,620,072,071**
Short-term limited duration coverage (contracts less than 1 year)	$12,751,381	$23,203,484	$15,169,579
Accident only (including accidental death and dismemberment)	$399,179,483	$549,363,996	$430,324,250
Disability income insurance	$809,637,014	$635,505,303	$882,799,587
Dental only or vision only benefits	$532,921,713	$624,835,156	$689,635,714
Credit insurance	$194,007,966	$240,519,383	$230,619,489
Coverage for a specified disease or illness only (such as cancer-only coverage)	$184,495,577	$205,730,140	$193,505,734
Hospital indemnity or other fixed indemnity insurance	$249,891,301	$215,979,341	$187,417,306
Coverage issued as a supplement to liability insurance	$183,179	$4,733,336	$0
Insurance arising out of workers' compensation or similar law	$20,733,594	$6,154,191	$4,027,885
Automobile medical payment insurance and personal injury protection	$2,699,878	$3,324	$34,666
Insurance under which benefits are payable with or without regard to fault and which is statutorily required to be contained in any liability insurance policy or equivalent self insurance	$208,177	$218,757	$0
Medicare supplement insurance, subject to article 3.74, including medicare select	$723,067,485	$771,719,731	$838,723,702
Small employer group health insurance, subject to articles 26.01-26.76	$1,684,674,096	$1,701,516,863	$2,377,077,936
Federal employees health benefits program, 5 U.S.C. §8909	$895,581,599	$977,425,248	$1,072,912,841
Medicaid, U.S.C. Title XIX and Medicare risk, §1854(g) of the Balanced Budget Act of 1997, part c, Title XVIII, Social Security Act	$5,259,719,599	$5,696,070,498	$6,189,905,626
Civilian health and medical program of the uniformed services (CHAMPUS), 32 CFR 199	$11,682,994	$11,162,279	$9,654,862
Long term care insurance premiums (1999 was not exempted)	-	$127,368,025	$267,009,596
Total Premiums Exempt from Assessment	**$10,981,435,035**	**$11,664,141,032**	**$13,388,818,773**
Net Assessable Health Insurance Premiums Reported	**$6,778,575,698**	**$7,559,161,030**	**$7,231,253,298**

Adapted from: Steven Browning, "Health Insurance Premiums Reporting Form: Amounts Reported for Health Insurance Premiums for Texas Residents," *Board of Director and Committee Meetings—Briefing Book* (Austin, Tex.: Texas Health Insurance Risk Pool, July 2001), p. 89; Steven Browning, "Health Insurance Premiums Reporting Form: Amounts Reported for Health Insurance Premiums for Texas Residents," *Board of Director and Committee Meetings—Briefing Book*, (Austin, Tex.: Texas Health Insurance Risk Pool, June 2000), p. 68; and Steven Browning, "Health Insurance Premiums Reporting Form: Amounts Reported for Health Insurance Premiums for Texas Residents," *Board of Director and Committee Meetings—Briefing Book* (Austin, Tex.: Texas Health Insurance Risk Pool, July 1999), p. 57.

Appendix I. Online Rate Guide Website Addresses

New Jersey Individual Health Coverage Program Rates, Monthly Rates for plans A-D and HMO Plan.

- www.state.nj.us/dobi/ihcrates.htm

New Jersey 2002 Small Employer Health Benefits Premium Comparison Survey, 2000 Premium Comparisons for Plans A-E and HMO Plan, Bergen, Camden, Middlesex Counties.

- www.state.nj.us/dobi/semrates.htm

Colorado Small Employer Group Health Premium Comparison, A Survey of Costs for Colorado's Mandated Small Employer Group Health Benefit Plans for the Grand Junction and Pueblo Areas, January 2002.

- www.dora.state.co.us/insurance/pb/sg2001.pdf

Rates for Individual (Non-Group) Plans in Vermont, Managed Care and Indemnity Plans by Insurer Effective January 1, 2002.

- www.bishca.state.Vermont.us/consumpubs/hcatipsandpubs/Shop_IndivandSmallGroup/rates_individual.htm

Monthly Rates for Small Group Plans in Vermont, Indemnity, PPO, Managed Care and Common Benefit Plans by Company Effective January 1, 2002.

- www.bishca.state.Vermont.us/consumpubs/hcatipsandpubs/Shop_IndivandSmallGroup/rates_smallgroup.htm

North Dakota Department of Insurance, Small Employer Group Insurance Providers, Basic and Standard Plans by Company, Monthly Premiums as of December 1, 2000.

- www.state.nd.us/ndins/consinfo/smallins.html

North Dakota Department of Insurance, Individual Health Policy Providers, Basic and Standard Plans by Company, Monthly Premiums as of December 1, 2000.

- www.state.nd.us/ndins/consinfo/indvhealth.html

Appendix J. Surveys

Survey One

Please answer each question to the best of your ability. You may skip questions that you do not feel pertain to your position. Please attach additional sheets where needed to adequately answer the question.

Identify county: ___________________

1. Check all that apply:

Operate County Indigent Health Care Program (CIHCP) ___

Operate Public Hospital (PH) ___ Hospital District (HD) ___

2. Estimated number of uninsured in county (FY 2000)? _________________

Source:

Estimation _________ Survey data (name survey) ___________

1999 Census _________ 2000 Census ___________

Other ____

Expenditures:

3. Total amount spent by county on health care for uninsured (FY 2000)?

4. Amount of figure in question 3 not compensated by Federal or State Government?

5. How is the money spent? (types of care – physician services, home health, supplies, prescriptions, inpatient care, et cetera; provider types; amount spent on each if avail.)

6. What other sources are used by the county to fund health care (excluding public health) for uninsured individuals in your county? (grants, fund-raising, etc.)

7. Are health care expenditures (excluding public health) for uninsured by private providers recorded by the county? If so, who are the providers? How much do they spend?

8. If HD, how much of hospital tax goes for DSH match? How is the rest of the revenue spent?

Revenues:

9. What is the tax base used for funding indigent care (FY 2000)? (type and amount).

10. Identify any unmet health care needs of uninsured in the county.

11. Describe the ideal indigent care system for the county; for the state (include funding streams, program components, etc.).

12. Would the county be willing to or positioned to contribute money to increase federal matching funds for the provision of care for specific populations, i.e., pregnant women? Explain.

In addition to what it currently spends?

In place of what it currently has?

13. How many times in the last 15 years has the county had to request additional funds (tax revenue) in order to meet indigent health care demand?

14. How much tobacco money has the county received to date? How has it been/will it be used?

15. Do you think the resources in your community are adequate to fund the requirement for indigent health care in your community? Explain.

16. Should counties be responsible for providing indigent health care? Explain.

17. What is the approximate number of physicians providing indigent health care in your county?

18. Percent of FPL served. ____________________

Survey Two

Please answer each question to the best of your ability. You may skip questions that you do not feel pertain to your position. Please attach additional sheets where needed to adequately answer the question.

Identify county: ____________________

1. **Check all that apply:**

Operate County Indigent Health Care Program (CIHCP) ___

Operate Public Hospital (PH) ___ Hospital District (HD) ___

2. Estimated number of uninsured in county (FY 2000)? ________________

Source:

Estimation _________ Survey data (name survey) __________

1999 Census _________ 2000 Census __________

Other ____

3. Percent of FPL served. ____________________

4. How is indigent health care money currently spent in your county/district? (types of care – physician services, home health, supplies, prescriptions, inpatient care, et cetera; provider types; amount spent on each if available).

5. If Hospital District, how much of hospital tax goes for DSH match? How is the rest of the revenue spent?

6. Identify any unmet health care needs of uninsured in the county.

7. Describe the ideal indigent care system for the county; for the state (include funding streams, program components, etc.).

8. Do you think the resources in your community are adequate to fund the requirement for indigent health care in your community? Explain.

9. Should counties be responsible for providing indigent health care? Explain.

10. Would the county be willing to contribute existing tax funds (or a portion) cooperatively with other counties/hospital districts in order to provide matching money to draw down federal funding to expand Medicaid coverage to populations (in whole or in part) currently receiving services through counties? If the state were to absolve the county of its mandate to provide indigent heath care services, but require proportional (need-based) county contribution, would this effect the response? How?

Cover Letter

Dear Administrator,

As an Administrator of one of the State's County Indigent Health Care Programs, Hospital Districts, or Public Hospitals, you are undoubtedly aware of the dire problem in Texas of high numbers of uninsured individuals (Texas currently has the highest number of uninsured individuals per capita in the nation). We are conducting a grant-funded research project at the University of Texas – Lyndon Baines Johnson School of Public Affairs. Our mission is to evaluate funding options for decreasing the number of uninsured individuals in Texas.

Counties as a whole spend a vast amount of money on the provision of health care for the uninsured. In researching this issue in Texas, we believe that it is imperative to provide a clear understanding of the related issues facing counties, the unmet needs of counties, as well as any recommended solutions. We are therefore surveying all program administrators (County Indigent Health Care Programs, Hospital Districts, and Public Hospitals) at the county level.

We have included a survey, along with a stamped, self-addressed envelope. Your assistance in our research is crucial to our overall effort, and it is very much appreciated. We know that your time is limited and we have therefore attempted to limit the number of survey questions. Please answer the questions to the best of your knowledge. If you need additional space for your responses, please feel free to attach additional sheets of paper. If you feel that the survey would be best completed by someone else, please feel free to pass it along to that individual.

Data reported will not reflect individual responses, but may identify counties. Confidentiality and anonymity of all opinion responses will be respected. As we are working on a school calendar timeline, we would very much appreciate your response by November 20, 2001. If you have any questions regarding this survey, please feel free to contact me at any time.

Thank you in advance for your participation.

Sincerely,

David Warner
Professor
LBJ School of Public Affairs
University of Texas

Appendix K. Cost Sharing Table

Cost Sharing Type / FPL	Current Policy	Allowable Policy	Differ-ence	Comments	Amounts effective 3/1/02	Post 3/1/02 Difference
Copays, Coinsurance, Deductibles						
At or Below 100%						
Office Visit	$0	$1-3	$1-3		no change	$1-3
ER	$0	$3	$3	assumes ER cost >$50	$3	$0
Non-emergency ER	n/a	$6	$6		na	na
Generic Drug	$0	$1-3	$1-3		no change	$1-3
Brand Drug	$0	$1-3	$1-3		$3	$0
Co-pay Cap	n/a	subject to 5% cumulative cap			100	??
Coinsurance	$0	5% of payment			no change	??
Deductible, non-institutional	$0	$2 per family/month			no change	
Deductible, institutional	$0	50% of 1st day payment			no change	
101% to 150%						
Office Visit	$2					
ER	$5	$5	$3		no change	$3
Non-emergency ER	n/a	$5	$0		no change	$0
Generic Drug	$1-2 based on cost	$10	$10			Na
Brand Drug	$1-2 based on cost	$5	$3-4		0	$5
Co-pay Cap	$100	$5	$3-4		$5	$0
Coinsurance	$0	subject to 5% cumulative cap			no change	??
Deductible, non-institutional	$0	5% of payment				no change
Deductible, institutional	$0	$3 per family/month			no change	

151% to 185%						
Office Visit	$5	$10	$5	based on Health Select Plus	no change	$5
ER	$25	$50	$25	subject to cumulative 5% cap	50	$0
Non-emergency ER	n/a	?	?			
Generic Drug	$5	$5	$0		no change	$0
Brand Drug	$10	$20	$10		20	$0
Coinsurance	$0	subject to 5% cumulative cap.				
Deductible, non-institutional	$0	subject to 5% cumulative cap.			no change	
Deductible, institutional	$0	subject to 5% cumulative cap.			no change	
186% to 200%						
Office Visit	$10	$10	$0	based on HealthSelect Plus	no change	
ER	$35	$50	$15	subject to cumulative 5% cap	50	
Non-emergency ER	n/a	?	?		?	?
Generic Drug	$5	$5	$0		no change	$0
Brand Drug	$10	$20	$10		20	
Coinsurance	$0	subject to 5% cumulative cap.			no change	
Deductible, non-institutional	$50/family/ outpatient	subject to 5% cumulative cap.			0	
Deductible, institutional	$200/family /inpatient	subject to 5% cumulative cap.			0	

Adapted from: Texas Health and Human Services Commission, *Chip Cost-sharing Change Scenarios.* Online. Available: http://www.hhsc.state.tx.us/chip/cnews/prgmdsgnscen071801.htm. Accessed: April 5, 2002.; Texas Health and Human Service Commission, *Proposed CHIP Cost-sharing Changes, Request for Public Comment.* Online. Available: http://www.hhsc.state.tx.us/chip/cnews/chip_cost_sharing.html. Accessed: April 5, 2002.; and U.S. Department of Health and Human Services, "State Child Health; Revisions to the Regulations Implementing the State Children's Health Insurance Program; Final Rule." *Federal Register*, vol. 66, no. 122, June 25, 2001, pp. 33810-33824. Online. Available: http://www.hcfa.gov/init/hcfa2006.pdf. Accessed: April 5, 2002.

Notes: Preliminary analysis of allowable copays, based on nonfinal federal rules. Subject to change and federal approval. For children at or below 150%, rules only allow one type of cost sharing (copay, deductible, coinsurance) on a service. A cumulative 5% of family income cap on all cost sharing applies to all FPL levels.

Bibliography

Albrega, Jeremy. *Wisconsin's BadgerCare Program Offers Innovative Approach for Family Coverage.* Washington, D.C.: Academy for Health Systems Research and Health Policy, 2001.

Alcalde, Gabriela. *Section 1115 Demonstration Waivers Under the State Children's Health Insurance Program.* Washington, D.C.: The National Conference of State Legislatures, 2001.

American Academy of Pediatrics, *2001 RBRVS: What Is It and How Does It Affect Pediatrics?* (brochure). Online. Available: http://www.aap.org/visit/ 2001RBRVS.pdf. Accessed: February 1, 2002.

———, *2002 RBRVS: What Is It and How Does It Affect Pediatrics?* (brochure). Online. Available: http://www.aap.org/visit/ pedrbrvs.htm. Accessed: February 1, 2002.

———. *Medicaid Reimbursement Survey, 2001: 50 States and the District of Columbia.* Online. Available: http://www.aap.org. Accessed: February 1, 2002.

American Medical Association. *News Releases and Statements: January 28, 2002—States Look to Cigarette Taxes to Reduce Smoking, Help Cure Ailing Budgets.* Online. Available: http://www.ama-assn.org/ama/pub/article/3880-5846.html. Accessed: March 2, 2002.

———. *Physician Socioeconomic Statistics.* Chicago, IL, Center for Health Policy Research, 2000-2002.

American Obesity Association. *Report on AOA Cost Study,* 1999. Online. Available: http://www.obesity.org/cost_report.htm. Accessed: January 31, 2002.

Analytical Perspectives. *Budget of the United States Government, Fiscal Year 2001.* Washington, D.C.: US Government Printing Office, Table 14-4.

Arkansas Department of Finance and Administration. *Miscellaneous Tax Section.* Online. Available: http://www.state.ar.us/dfa/taxes/misc_tax/index.html. Accessed: November 19, 2001.

Arkansas Department of Human Services, *Nursing Home Rate Study* (July 2001). Online. Available: http://www.medicaid.state.ar.us/arkansasmedicaid/nhstudy. overvw.htm. Accessed: November 20, 2001.

Association of Academic Health Centers. *Academics for Access to Health Care Initiative.* Online. Available: http://www.ahcnet.org/pdf/aahci.pdf. Accessed: April 10, 2002.

Bennefield, Robert L. U.S. Census Bureau. *Current Population Reports, Health Insurance Coverage.* (1997). Online. Available: http://www.opic.state.tx.us/Healthinfo.html. Accessed: January 2, 2002.

Berndt, Trey. Special Assistant for Medicaid/CHIP Operations, Texas Health and Human Services Commission, Austin, Texas. Interview by Leah Kegler and Lisa Ewart, February 15, 2002.

Bielefeldt, M. Ralph. New York Children Health Plus. "Full Cost Buy-In Option." Email to Jie Zhou, January 14, 2002.

Birnbaum, Michael. *Expanding Coverage to Parents through Medicaid Section 1931.* Washington, D.C.: The Robert Wood Johnson Foundation, 2000.

————. *Full-Cost Buy-Ins: An Overview of State Experience.* Washington D.C.: State Coverage Initiatives, August 2001.

Blaisi, Jana. Deputy Director, Texas Association of Community Health Centers, Austin, Texas. Interviewed by Jennifer Eldridge, January 17, 2002.

Blue Cross Blue Shield of Texas. "Total Enrollment by Month." *Board of Directors and Committee Meetings—Briefing Book.* Austin, Tex., Texas Health Insurance Risk Pool, January 2000.

Boff, John. President/CEO, Texas Organization of Rural and Community Hospitals and Kevin Reed, Legal Counsel, Texas Organization of Rural and Community Hospitals. Interview by Jamie Dudensing, Kristie Kimbell, and Dr. David Warner, February 20, 2002.

Borges, Walt. "Managing Medicaid: Medicaid Managed Care Leaves Physicians, Patients, and Legislators Frustrated." *Texas Medicine*, vol. 11, no.96 (1996), pp. 34-41.

Bovberg, Randall R., Frank Ullman, Alison Evans, John Holahan, and Susan Flanagan. *Health Policy for Low-Income People in New Jersey.* Washington D.C.: The Urban Institute, 1998.

Browning, Steven. Executive Director, Texas Health Insurance Risk Pool. E-mail, "RE: Pool Project," to Jed Perry, January 25, 2002.

————. Executive Director, Texas Health Insurance Risk Pool. E-mail, "RE: One last piece of information," to Jed Perry, April 8, 2002.

————. Executive Director, Texas Health Insurance Risk Pool, Austin, Texas. Interviewed by Jed Perry, November 15, 2001.

————. "Health Insurance Premiums Reporting Form: Amounts Reported for Health Insurance Premiums for Texas Residents." *Board of Director and*

Committee Meetings – Briefing Book. Austin, Tex.: Texas Health Insurance Risk Pool, July 1999.

Bruen, Brian, and John Holahan. *Medicaid Enrollment and Spending Trends.* Washington, D.C.: The Kaiser Commission on the Uninsured, February 2001.

Bryant, Terry. Alabama Medicaid Director, Alabama Medicaid Agency. Email, "Re: Healthcare Finance Questions," to Kristi Kimble, February 12, 2002.

Bullock, Bob. Lieutenant Governor, State of Texas. Letter to The Honorable Judith Zaffirini, State Senator, March 15, 1994.

Bureau of National Affairs. "Arkansas: House Passes Bill to Levy 'Bed Tax" On Nursing Homes to Raise Medicaid Funds." *State News,* vol. 9, no. 6, Washington, D.C.: Health Care Policy Report, February 12, 2001. Online. Available: http://pubs.bna.com/ip/BNA/HCP.NSF/a21f6d0cc387645256743006db37c/d1976c858f09ce1a852569ee0079cfda?OpenDocument. Accessed: November 7, 2001.

————. "Utah: Legislature Approves Bill to Provide Matching Funds for Children's Health." *State News,* vol. 6, no. 10, Washington, D.C.: Health Care Policy Report, March 9, 1998. Online. Available: http://pubs.bna.com/ip/BNA/HCP.NSF/a21f0cc38764582574300db37c/2156d566eb172c11853565bf00785edf?OpenDocument. Accessed: November 11, 2001

————. "West Virginia, Legislature Passes Tobacco Tax Measure Bill to Eliminate Health Care Provider Tax." *State News,* vol. 9, Washington D.C.: Health Care Policy Report, April 23, 2001. Online. Available: http://pubs.bna.com/ip/BNA.NSF/a21f6df0cc387645256743006db37c/0e9098e8031a885256a3400833386?opendocument. Accessed: November 11, 2001.

Bureau of TennCare. *Daily Health Policy Report.* Online. Available: http://www.state.tn.us/tenncare/whatis.html. Accessed: November 9, 2001.

Bush, George W. "Radio Address of the President to the Nation: August 4, 2001." Online. Available at http://www.whitehouse.gov/news/releases/2001/08/20010804.html. Accessed: August 6, 2001.

Butler, Patricia A. "ERISA and State Health Care Access Initiatives: Opportunities and Obstacles." Washington, D.C.: The Commonwealth Fund. October 2000. Online. Available: http://www.cmwf.org/programs/insurance/butler_erisa_411.pdf. Accessed: March 3, 2002

California Department of Health Services, Projects and Initiatives. *California's Healthy Families SCHIP 1115 Demonstration Project.* Online. Available: http://www.dhs.cahwnet.gov/HFHeadline/California%20has%20Proposed%. Accessed: January 23, 2002.

California Major Risk Medical Insurance Program. *Area 3 Rates*. Online. Available: http://www.mrmib.ca.gov/MRMIB/MRMIP.html. Accessed: March 3, 2002

———. *Description of Plans and Benefit Highlights.* Online. Available: http://www.mrmib.ca.gov/MRMIB/MRMIP.html. Accessed: March 3, 2002.

Campaign for Tobacco-Free Kids. *Higher Cigarette Taxes Reduce Smoking Save Lives Save Money.* Online. Available: http://tobaccofreekids.org/reports/prices/. Accessed: January 29, 2002.

Capps, Randy. The Urban Institute. *Hardship among Children of Immigrants: Findings from the 1999 National Survey of America's Families*. Online. Available: http://newfederalism.urban.org/html/series_b/b29/b29.html. Accessed: November 8, 2001.

Center for Medicaid and Medicare Services, Department of Health and Human Services. *Enrolling and Retaining Low-Income Families in Health Care Coverage.* Washington, D.C., 2001.

———. *Health Insurance and Flexibility and Accountability Demonstration Initiative.* Washington, D.C.: Department of Health and Human Service, July 25, 2001.

———. *Managed Care Entities* (2000). Online. Available: http://www.hcfa.gov. Accessed: November 13, 2001.

———. *The State Children's Health Insurance Program Annual Enrollment Report.* February 6, 2002. Online. Available: http://www.hcfa.gov/init/schip01.pdf. Accessed: March 20, 2002.

Center for Public Policy Priorities. *CHIP and Children Who Are Not U.S. Citizens.* Online. Available: http://www.cppp.org/products/policyanalysis/briefingpapers/brpchip3.pdf. Accessed: January 11, 2002.

———. *Every Child Equal.* Austin, Tex: The Texas CHIP Coalition, September 2000.

———. *Inclusion of Undocumented Persons by Texas Indigent Health Care Providers.* Online. Available: http://www.cppp.org/products/policyanalysis/briefingpapers/brpHC1100.html. Accessed: January 10, 2002.

———. *Texas Taxes.* April 1999. Online. Available: http://internationalbudget.org/cdrom/papers/tax/TexasTaxes.htm. Accessed: September 12, 2001

———. *Where Will the Money Go?: A Revenue Preview,* May 9, 2001. Online. Available: www.cppp.org/products/policypages/111-130/111-130html/PP129.html. Accessed: September 12, 2001.

———————. *Why Isn't There Enough Money?* March 14, 2001. Online. Available: http://www.cppp.org/products/policypages/111-130/111-130html/PP117.html. Accessed: September 12, 2001

Center for Science in the Public Interest. "Soft Drinks Undermining Americans' Health." October 21, 1998 (press release). Online. Available: http://www.cspinet.org/new/ soda_10_21_98.htm. Accessed: November 20, 2001.

Center for Studying Health System Change. *Community Tracking Survey*. Online. Available: http://www.hschange.com/index.cgi?data=01. Accessed: April 24, 2002.

Centers for Disease Control and Prevention. National Center for Health Statistics. *National Health Interview Survey*. Online. Available. http://www.cdc.gov/nchs/nhis.htm. Accessed: April 24, 2002.

Christman, Evan, Scott Atnip, Laura Koenig, and Senator Chet Brooks. Lyndon B. Johnson School of Public Affairs. "Indigent Health Care in Texas." November 2001 (unpublished policy brief).

Christman, Evan. Research Assistant and PRP Student, Lyndon B. Johnson School of Public Affairs. Class Presentation, Lyndon B. Johnson School of Public Affairs, Austin, Texas, September 11, 2001.

Citizens' Council on Health Care. *Distribution, Utilization and Impact of the Minnesota Provider Tax*. January2000. Online. Available: http:// www.cchconline.org/ publication/providertaxsumm.php3. Accessed: November 20, 2001.

Clayton, Archie. Texas Department of Insurance. E-mail, "Texas Health Reinsurance System," to Jed Perry, March 8, 2002.

Cleveland Public Power. *Texas CHIP Fast Facts*. Online. Available: http://www.cppp.org/products/fastfacts/CHIP.html. Accessed: January 14, 2002.

Cleverley, William O. *Essentials of Health Care Finance, 4th Edition*. Gaithersberg, MD: Aspen Publishers, 1997.

Clifton, Guy, M.D. Hermann Hospital. "Addressing Houston's Emergency Room Crisis." Houston, Tex., October 30, 2001 (draft paper).

Colberg, Edli. Demographer/Program Specialist, Research and Forecasting, Texas Health and Human Services Commission. Class presentation, Lyndon B. Johnson School of Public Affairs, Austin, Texas, November 13, 2001.

Comer, Teresa. Texas Comptroller's Office. Email, "Re: Texas Franchise Tax", to Kate Brodsky, February 14, 2002.

Connecticut Department of Social Services. *Connecticut State Health Plan Under Title XXI of the Social Security Act.* By Linda J. Mead. Hartford, Conn., 1998.

——————. *Framework for Annual Report of State Children's Health Insurance Plans.* By Adele Kusnitz, and James Gaito. Hartford, Conn., 2000.

——————. *Framework for State Evaluation of Children's Health Insurance Plans Under Title XXI of the Social Security Act.* By Linda J. Mead. Hartford, Conn., 2000.

Connecticut's Attorney Generals Office. *Attorney General's Statement Regarding Increasing Cigarette Tax By $.61* January 24, 2002. Online. Available: http://www.cslib.org/attygenl/mainlinks/tabindex4.htm. Accessed: February 1, 2002.

Consumer Health Education Council. *Consumer Health Education Council.* Online. Available: http://www.healthchec.org. Accessed: November 7, 2001.

——————. *Getting and Keeping Coverage.* Online. Available: http://www.healthchec.org/consumer/getkeep.html. Accessed: November 7, 2001.

Consumers Union. *Consumer Gains Clouded by Long-Term Effect of Industry Subsidies.* (June 2, 1999). Online. Available: http://www.consumersunion.org/other/sesstx699.htm. Accessed: January 25, 2002.

Conviser, Richard. The Office for Oregon Health Policy and Research. *A Brief History of the Oregon Health Plan and its Features.* Online. Available: http://www.ohppr.state.or.us/docs/pdf/histofplan.pdf. Accessed: January 21, 2002.

Conwell, Leslie, and Ashley Short. *Premium Subsidies for Employer-Sponsored Health Coverage.* Washington, D.C.: The Center for Studying Health System Change, December 2001.

Cook, Eric, and Michael Vlaisavljevich. "Implications of Health Reform for State and Local Fiscal Policy." *National Tax Journal*, vol. 47, no. 3 (1994), pp. 639-654. Online. Available: http://www.ntj/tax.org. Accessed: January 30, 2002.

Cooke, Jason. "CHIP and Medicaid: Status Report." Presentation at conference on "Working Together for a Healthy Texas: Expanding Health Insurance Coverage for Texans," Texas State Planning Grant Conference, Austin, Texas, January 31-February 1, 2002.

——————. Presentation to Health and Human Services Commission at the CHIP Coaliton Meeting, Austin, Texas, September 20, 2000.

Cottrell, Terry. Project Director, Texas HIPP Program, Health and Human Services Commission, Austin, Texas. Interview by Lisa Ewart, November 14, 2001.

————. "Health Insurance Premium Payment Program (HIPP)." Austin, Tex.: Health and Human Services Commission, March 2001.

Coughlin, Teresa, and David Liska,. *The Medicaid Disproportionate Share Hospital Payment Program: Background and Issues.* Washington, D.C.: The Urban Institute, October 1997. Online. Available: http://newfederalism.urban.org/html/anf14/html#tab1. Accessed: November 20, 2001.

Coughlin, Teresa A., Joshua M. Wiener, Jill A. Marstellar, David G. Stevenson, and Susan Wallin. *Health Policy for Low-Income People in Wisconsin.* Washington D.C.: The Urban Institute, 1998.

Coughlin, Teresa, Leighton Ku, and Johnny Kim. *Reforming the Medicaid Disproportionate Share Hospital Program in the 1990s.* Washington, D.C.: The Urban Institute, January 2000.

Coughlin, Teresa A., Shruti Rajan, Stephen Zuckerman, and Jill A. Marsteller. *Health Policy for Low-Income People in Minnesota.* Washington D.C.: The Urban Institute, 1997.

CoverColorado. *PPO Rate Bulletin.* Online. Available: http://www.cuhip.com/main/index.html. Accessed: March 3, 2002.

Covering Kids. *Project Alberto: Texas Outreach Initiative.* Online. Available: http://www.coveringkids.org/projects/state.php3?StateID=TX. Accessed: November 5, 2001.

Cunningham, Peter J., Elizabeth Schaefer, and Christopher Hogan. *Who Declines Employer-Sponsored Health Insurance and is Uninsured.* Washington D.C.: Health System Change, 1999.

Davidoff, Amy, and Genevieve Kenney, Lisa Dubay, and Alshadye Yemane. *Patterns of Child-Parent Insurance Coverage: Implications for Coverage Expansions.* Washington, D.C.: The Urban Institute, 2001.

Davis, Jim. Director, Public Information Office, Texas Department of Insurance. "Information Request/Verification." Personal email to Scott Atnip, March 25, 2002.

Davis, Kimberly. Director of Medicaid and CHIP Outreach, Texas Health and Human Services Commission, Austin, Texas. Interviewed by Daniel Starr, January 18, 2002.

————. Director of Medicaid and SCHIP Outreach. "TexCare Partnership Outreach Workplan 2002-2003—Revised," Personal email to Daniel Starr, February 26, 2002.

DeFranxesco, Leanne, Christina Folz, Madeleine Konig, and Carole Lee. *State of the States*. State Coverage Initiatives, January 2002. Online. Available: http://www.statecoverage.net/pdf/stateofstates2002.pdf. Accessed: January 20, 2002.

Denton, Lynn. Communications Director, Texas Department of Health, Austin, Texas. Interviewed by Daniel Starr, November 8, 2001.

Doderer, Dennis. Deputy Assistant Director, Premium Support Program, Division of Medical Assistance and Health, New Jersey Department of Human Services, Trenton, NJ. Telephone Interview by Lisa Ewart, January 15, 2002.

Dorsey, Candace, CHIP Outreach Program Manager, Harris County Department of Health and Environmental Services, Houston, Texas; Helen Stagg, CHIP/Health Coordinator, Families Under Urban and Social Attack, Houston, Texas; Carolyn Franks, CHIP/TexCare Program Manager, Institute of Religion, Texas Medical Center, Houston, Texas; Heather Kanenberg, Public Policy Analyst, Children At Risk, Houston, Texas; Anita Garvey, CHIP Regional CBO Contract Manager/Health Plan Liaison, Region 6/5, Houston, Texas; and Sheryl Guilbeaux, CHIP Regional CBO Contract Manager/Health Plan Liaison, Region 6/5, Houston, Texas. Interviewed by Daniel Starr and Scott Atnip, February 8, 2002.

Dubay, Lisa, and Genevieve Kenney. *Covering Parents through Medicaid and SCHIP: Potential Benefits to Low-Income Parents and Children.* Washington, D.C.: The Urban Institute, 2002.

————. *The Effects of Family Coverage on Children's Health Insurance Status.* Washington, D.C.: The Urban Institute, 2001.

Dunkelberg, Anne. Senior Policy Analyst, Center for Public Policy Priorities, Austin, Texas. "Immigrants' Access to Benefits in Texas: Five Things to Remember." Presented to the 25th Annual Texas State National Association of Social Workers (NASW) Conference, Austin, Tex., October 12, 2001.

————. Senior Policy Analyst, Center for Public Policy Priorities, Austin, Texas. Interviewed by Jennifer Eldridge, November 15, 2001.

————. Senior Policy Analyst, Center for Public Policy Priorities, Austin, Texas. Interview by Michelle Harper and Leah Kegler, March 5, 2001.

————. Senior Policy Analyst, Center for Public Policy Priorities. Class Presentation, Lyndon B. Johnson School of Public Affairs, Austin, Texas, November 13, 2001.

Dunkelberg, Anne, and Cathy Schechter. *Children's Medicaid Eligibility Simplification Bill, SB 43, Sent to the Governor.* Austin, TEX: Center for Public Policy Priorities, 2002.

———. *Every Child Equal: What Texas Parents Want from Children's Medicaid.* Center for Public Policy Priorities, Austin, TEX, September 2000.

Dunn, Roy. Utah Department of Health. Email, "Using Tax Revenues for Medicaid," to Jamie Dudensing, January 24, 2002.

El Buen Samaritano. *Mid-Year Report, Project Year 2001-2002.* Austin, Texas, 2001.

Ellsworth, Ken. "State income tax resurfaces." *Abilene Reporter New.* May 8, 2001. Online. Available: http://www.texnews.com/1998/2001/local/tax0508.html. Accessed: November 21, 2001.

Ellwood, Marilyn. *The Medicaid Eligibility Maze: Coverage Expands, But Enrollment Problems Persist.* Washington, D.C.: The Urban Institute, 2000.

Employer Quality Partnership. *Looking for Value: An Employer's Guide to Evaluating Quality Health Plans.* Online. Available: http://www.eqp.org/page2.html. Accessed: November 4, 2001.

Evans, Selia. Healthy Kids Now! Program Director, Washington Department of Social and Health Services, Olympia, Washington. Telephone interview by Daniel Starr, January 16, 2002.

Falkenberg, Lisa. "Lawmakers: Prosperity of state depends on overhauling tax structure," *Abilene Reporter News* (April 9, 2001). Online. Available: http://www.reporternews.com/2001/texas/tax0409.html. Accessed: November 20, 2001.

Families USA. *Career Opportunities.* Online. Available: http://www.familiesusa.org/html.jobs/jobs.htm. Accessed: February 2, 2002.

———. *Consumer Health Assistance Programs: Report on a National Survey.* Washington, D.C., June 2001. Online. Available: http://www.familiesusa.org/media/pubs/index.htm. Accessed: February 1, 2002.

———. *Deep in the Heart of Texas: Uninsured in the Lone Star State.* Washington, D.C., 2000.

———. *Designing a Consumer Health Assistance Program.* Washington, D.C. (Pamphlet).

———. *Expanding Coverage for Low Income Parents: An Action Kit for State Advocates.* Washington, D.C., 2001.

———. *Five Good Reasons for States to Expand Coverage.* April 2000. Online. Available: http://www.familiesusa.org/index6.htm. Accessed: April 15, 2001.

———. *More than 725,000 Laid-Off Workers Have Lost Health Coverage Since the Recession Began in March.* Washington, D.C.: Families USA, 2001.

———. *The Current Medicaid Federal-State Partnership: Already a Good Deal for the States.* Washington, D.C., August 2001.

———. *Uninsured Parents and Medicaid Information, State-by-State.* Washington, D.C.: Families USA Health Action Annual Conference, January, 2001.

Federation of Tax Administrators. *State Excise Tax Rates On Cigarettes.* Online. Available: http://www.taxadmin.org/fta/rate/cigarett.html. Accessed: January 23, 2002.

Fenz, Caton M. The Access Project. *Providing Health Care to the Uninsured in Texas.* Online. Available: http://www.accessproject.org/downloads/TEXAS.pdf. Accessed: January 15, 2002.

———. Legislative Director, Texas State Representative Garnet Coleman, Austin, Texas. Telephone interview by Kenneth Apfel, Jamie Dudensing, Kristie Kimbell, Laura Koenig, and Dr. David Warner, February 4, 2002.

———. *Providing Health Care to the Uninsured in Texas: A Guide for County Officials.* Boston, MA: The Access Project, August 9, 2000.

Fisch, Stanley, M.D. Physician, Harlingen Pediatrics Association, Harlingen, Texas. Interviewed by Jennifer Eldridge, January 31, 2002.

Fix, Michael E. and Karen Tumlin. The Urban Institute. *Welfare Reform and the Devolution of Immigrant Policy.* Online. Available: http://newfederalism.urban.org/html/anf_15.htm. Accessed: November 8, 2001.

Flores, Benjamin. Presentation to the 11th Annual Midwestern Farmworker Stream Forum, Austin, Texas. December 6, 2001.

Florida Healthy Kids. *Florida KidCare Program Evaluation Report, 2001.* Online. Available: http://www.healthykids.org/overview/annual_reports/2002/2002_annual_report.pdf. Accessed: December 16, 2001.

Focus Group of Multiple Stakeholders. Computerized Feedback at TexCare Partnership Regional Stakeholder Meeting, Austin, Texas, February 6, 2002.

Food and Drug Administration, National Institute of Health. *Healthy People 2010: Nutrition and Overweight,* vol. II (November 2000). Online. Available: http://www.health.gov/healthypeople/Document/HTML/Volume2/19Nutrition.htm#_Toc490383116. Accessed: January 31, 2002.

Friedholm, DeAnn. Executive Director, Children's Defense Fund of Texas. Class Presentation, Lyndon B. Johnson School of Public Affairs, Austin, Texas, November 6, 2001.

————. Presentation to "State Budget Crisis: Working Together to Finance a Fair Budget Conference." ProTex, Austin, Texas, November 9, 2001.

Fronstin, Paul. *Small Employers and Health Benefits: Findings from the 2000 Small Employer Health Benefits Survey*, SR 35. Washington, D.C.: Employee Benefit Research Institute, October 2000.

Garcia, Olga. Texas Health and Human Services Commission. Presentation to the Senate Bill1053/1299 Workgroup, Austin, Texas, November 15, 2001.

Garza, Armando. Supervisor of Billing, Hidalgo County Indigent Health Care Program. Telephone interview by Laura Koenig, Austin, Texas, September 28, 2001.

General Accounting Office. *Major Federal Expansion of Medicaid Eligibility and Services (1984-1993).* HEHS95-122. Washington, D.C., 1995.

Georgetown University, Institute for Health Care Research and Policy. *A Consumer's Guide to Getting and Keeping Health Insurance in Texas*. (January 1998). Online. Available: http://www.healthinsuranceinfo.net. Accessed: February 2, 2002.

Glover, Sue. Legislative Analyst, Texas Association of Counties, Austin, Texas. Interview by Jamie Dudensing and Kristie Kimbell, February 1, 2002.

Gomez, Paula. Executive Director, Brownsville Community Health Center, Brownsville, Texas. Interviewed by Jennifer Eldridge, January 31, 2002.

Guyer, Jocelyn. *Trends in CHIP Expenditures: State-by-State Data.* Washington, D.C.: The Kaiser Commission on Medicaid and the Uninsured, October 2001.

Guyer, Jocelyn, and Cindy Mann. *A New Opportunity to Provide Health Care Coverage for New York's Low-Income Families.* Washington, D.C.: The Commonwealth Fund, 1999.

————. *Taking the Next Step: States Can Now Expand Health Coverage to Low-Income Parents Through Medicaid.* Washington, D.C.: Center on Budget Policy Priorities, 1998.

Guyer, Jocelyn, Andy Schneider, and Michael Spivey. *Untangling DSH: A Guide for Community Groups to Using the Medicaid DSH Program to Promote Access to Care.* Boston, MA: The Access Project, 2000.

Hart, Sue. Milliman USA. "Options for Expanding Health Insurance in Texas—CHIP Full Cost Buy-In." Paper presented at the Texas State Planning Grant Conference, Houston, Texas, January 31-February 1, 2002.

Hart, Sue, and Esther Blount. "Options for Expanding Health Insurance in Texas—Small Employer Market." Paper presented at conference on "Working Together for a Healthy Texas: Expanding Health Insurance Coverage for Texans," Texas State Planning Grant Conference, Austin, Texas, January 31- February 1, 2002.

Health Care Financing Administration. *California's 1115 Medicaid Demonstration for Los Angeles County Fact Sheet.* Online. Available: http://www.hcfa.gov/medicaid/1115/lacnfact.htm. Accessed: November 29, 2001.

———. *Connecticut Title XXI State Plan Amendment Summary.* Online. Available: http://www.hcfa.gov/init/chpfsct.htm. Accessed: January 14, 2002.

———. *Florida Title XXI Program Fact Sheet.* Online. Available: http://www.hcfa.gov/init/chpfsfl.htm. Accessed: December 16, 2001.

———. *Health Insurance Flexibility and Accountability (HIFA) Initiative Fact Sheet.* Online. Available: http://www.hcfa.gov/medicaid/hifa/cafactsh.htm. Accessed: April 1, 2002.

———. *HIPAA Online: What is guaranteed availability of individual coverage?* Online. Available: http://www.hcfa.gov/medicaid//hipaa/online/230021.asp. Accessed: December 5, 2001.

———. *Minnesota Title XXI Program Fact Sheet.* Online. Available: http://www.hcfa.gov/init/chpfsmn.htm. Accessed: November 14, 2001.

———. *New Jersey Title XXI Demonstration Fact Sheet.* Online. Available: http://www.hcfa.gov/init/1115nj.htm. Accessed: November 14, 2001.

———. *New York Title XXI Program Fact Sheet.* Online. Available: http://www.hcfa.gov/init/chpfsny.htm. Accessed: January 14, 2002.

———. *North Carolina Title XXI Program Fact Sheet.* Online. Available: http://www.hcfa.gov/init/chpfsnc.htm. Accessed: January 14, 2002.

———. *The State Children's Health Insurance Program: Preliminary Highlights of Implementation and Expansion.* Washington, D.C., July 2000.

Health Insurance Association of America. *Guide To Health Insurance.* Online. Available: http://www.hiaa.org/consumer/guidehi.cfm. Accessed: November 8, 2001.

———. *The Insurance Guide for Business Owners.* Online. Available: http://www.hiaa.org/consumer/guidebo.cfm. Accessed: November 8, 2001.

Health Policy Tracking Service. *Florida State SCHIP Plan Summary.* Online. Available: http://state-serve.hpts.org/hpts2000. Accessed: December 20, 2001.

Hearne, Jean. *Medicaid Disproportionate Share Payments*. Washington, D.C.: Congressional Research Service, 2001.

Henry J. Kaiser Family Foundation. *Medicaid: A Primer.* Washington, D.C., 1999.

———. *State Health Facts Online.* Online. Available: http://www.statehealthfacts.kff.org. Accessed: November 16, 2001.

Hiller, King. Director, Legislative Relations, Harris County, Houston, Texas. Telephone interview by Kristie Kimbell, Austin, Texas, February 4, 2002.

Holahan, John, and Niall Brennan. *Who are the Adult Uninsured?* Washington, D.C.: The Urban Institute, 2000.

Holahan, John, Suresh Rangarajan, and Matthew Schirmer. *Medicaid Managed Care Payment Methods and Capitation Rates: Results of a National Survey.* (Washington, D.C.: Urban Institute, 1999). Online. Available: http://newfederalism.urba.org/html/occa26.html. Accessed: October 29, 2001.

Hopper, Leigh, "Lottery Winners' loss is poor patients' gain: Area Hospitals get $46 Million in Unclaimed Funds." *Houston Chronicle* (April 5, 2002). Online. Available: http:www.chron.com/cs/CDA/prinstory.hts/topstory2/1343438. Accessed: April 5,2002.

House Research Organization. *The Tax System and Public School Financing in Texas.* March 24, 1997. Online. Available: http://www.capitol.state.tx.us/hrofr/ focus/taxes.pdf. Accessed: November 10, 2001.

Huff, Charlotte, and Kelly Melhart. "Tobacco Fund Loss Troubles Hospitals." *Fort Worth Star Telegram* (February 25, 2002). Online. Available: http://www.dfw.com/mld/startelegram. Accessed: February 30,2002.

Hunt, Sandra, Susan Maerki, Doug Porter, Janice Fang, PriceWaterhouseCoopers. *Applying RBRVS to Medi-Cal: Case Studies in Seven States.* Oakland, CA: Medi-Cal Policy Institute, June 2001. Online. Available: http://admin.chcf.org/ documents/mcpi/. Accessed: January 31, 2002.

Hunt, Sandra, Susan Maerki, Rob Tompkins, PriceWaterhouseCoopers. *Comparing CPT Code Payments for Medi-Cal and Other California Payers*. Oakland, CA: Medi-Cal Policy Institute, June 2001. Online. Available: http://admin.chcf.org/ documents/mcpi/ComparingCPTCodePaymentsForMedi-CalAndOtherPayers.pdf. Accessed: January 31, 2001.

Hutzler, Shirly. Lobbyist, Texas Association of Health Underwriters. "Question." Personal email to Scott Atnip, January 26, 2002.

———. Lobbyist, Texas Association of Health Underwriters. "Question." Personal email to Scott Atnip, March 5, 2002.

———. Lobbyist, Texas Association of Health Underwriters, Austin, Texas. Telephone interview by Scott Atnip, February 14, 2002.

Institute for Child Health Policy. *Crowd Out: Evidence From the Florida Healthy Kids Program.* Online. Available: http://www.ichp.edu/Publications/default.htm. Accessed: April 23, 2002.

———. *Florida KidCare Program Evaluation Report, 2000.* Online. Available: http://www.ichp.edu/FloridaKidCare/1999Reports/FlaKCAppendices.pdf. Accessed: April 30, 2002.

Institute for Health Care Research and Policy, Georgetown University. "Chapter 3. Your Protections When Buying Health Insurance." *A Consumer's Guide to Getting and Keeping Health Insurance in Texas.* Online. Available: http://www.healthinsuranceinfo.net/tx03.html. Accessed: March 3, 2002

Institute for Health Policy Solutions. *Coordinating State Children's Health Insurance Programs with Employer-Based Coverage: Design and Implementation of Premium Assistance Programs.* Washington, D.C.: Institute for Health Policy Solutions, 1999.

Insure.com. *Health Plan Comparison Worksheet* (November 9, 2001). Online. Available: http://www.insure.com/health/plancomparison.html. Accessed: November 18, 2001.

———. *Tips for Buying Health Coverage* (February 22, 2001). Online. Available: http://www.insure.com/health/individual.html. Accessed: November 18, 2001.

Jacobson, Michael F., and Kelly D. Brownell. "Small Taxes on Soft Drinks and Snack Foods to Promote Health." *American Journal of Public Health*, vol. 90, no.6 (June 2000), pp. 854-857.

Japonica Partners. *Free Cash Flow: A Better Value Indicator?.* Online. Available: http://www.japonica.com/network/freecashflow.html. Accessed: January 31, 2002.

Jennings, Patty. Chairwoman, New Mexico Comprehensive Health Insurance Pool, Roswell, New Mexico. Telephone interview by Jed Perry, March 1, 2002.

Kaiser Commission on Medicaid and the Uninsured. *Daily Health Policy Report.* Online. Available: http://kaisernetwork.org/daily_reports/rep_index.cfm?DR_ID=8006. Accessed: November 13, 2001.

———. *Issues Related to Unspent S-CHIP Money.* Washington, D.C.: The Henry J. Kaiser Family Foundation, 2001.

Kaiser Family Foundation. *State Health Facts Online*. Online. Available: http://www.statehealthfacts.kff.org. Accessed: November 9, 2001.

Kegler, Leah. "Utilizing Federal Waiver Flexibility: Expanding Through Section 1931." Professional Report. Lyndon B Johnson School of Public Affairs, The University at Texas at Austin, 2002.

Kinney, Donna. Manager of Regulatory Advocacy, Texas Medical Association, Austin, Texas. Interview by Sarah Stout, December 6, 2001.

Krebs-Carter, Melora, and John Holahan. *State Strategies for Covering Uninsured Adults*. Washington, D.C.: The Urban Institute, 2000.

Ku, Leighton, and Matt Broaddus. *How to Review Cost Estimates for Family Coverage Expansions*. Washington, D.C.: The Center on Budget and Policy Priorities, 2001.

———. *The Importance of Family-Based Insurance Expansions: New Research Findings about State Health Reforms*. Washington, D.C.: Center on Budget and Policy Priorities, September 2000.

Ku, Leighton, and Shannon Blaney. Center on Budget and Policy Priorities. *Health Coverage for Legal Immigrant Children: New Census Data Highlight Importance of Restoring Medicaid and SCHIP Coverage*. Online. Available: http://www.cbpp.org/10-4-00health.htm. Accessed: January 3, 2002.

Lambrew, Jeanne. *Health Insurance: A Family Affair*. Washington, D.C.: The Commonwealth Fund, May 2001.

———. *Section 1115 Waivers in Medicaid and the State Children's Health Insurance Program: An Overview*. Washington, D.C.: The Kaiser Commission on Medicaid and the Uninsured, July 2001.

Lavine, Dick. Senior Fiscal Analyst, Center for Public Policy Priorities, Austin, Texas. Telephone interview by Laura Koenig, January 29, 2002.

Lee, Richard. Director of Public Education, Texas Department of Insurance, Austin, Texas. Telephone interview by Jacqueline Angel, Scott Atnip, Karla Buitrago, and Kristen Lindberg, February 1, 2002.

Lessem, Ann, James Dyer, Steve Borders, and Jason Vendel. "Uninsured Texans: Attitudes Toward Coverage." Paper presented at conference on "Working Together for a Healthy Texas: Expanding Health Insurance Coverage for Texans," Texas State Planning Grant Conference, Austin, Texas, January 31-February 1, 2002.

Levinson, Cynthia. Vice President, Texas Health Education Assistance Resources and Training (HEART). "Help with Policy Research Project." Personal email to Kristen Lindberg, February 05, 2002.

Levit, Katharine, Cynthia Smith, Cathy Cowan, Helen Lazenby, and Anne Martin. "Inflation Spurs Health Spending in 2000." *Health Affairs,* 21(1): 172-181.

Lewis, Valerie. *Medicaid Waivers: California's Use of a Federal Option.* Oakland, Calif.: Medi-Cal Policy Institute, March 2000.

Linan, Rose Marie. Team Leader, Indigent Health Care Division, Texas Department of Health, Austin, Texas. Telephone interview by Evan Christman, September 19, 2001.

Longley, Diane. "Concurrent Breakout Session on Consumer Education and Outreach: Making Private Insurance Work." Conference on "Investing in Texas: Financing Health Coverage Expansion," Austin, Texas, March 22, 2002.

Lori Achman and Deborah Chollet, "Insuring the Uninsurable: An Overview of State High-Risk Health Insurance Pools." Washington, D.C.: The Commonwealth Fund, August 2001. Online. Available: http://www.cmwf.org/programs/insurance/achman_uninsurable_472.pdf. Accessed: March 3, 2002.

Louisiana Health Plan. *High Risk Health Pool Rates Table.* Online. Available: http://www.lahealthplan.org. Accessed: March 3, 2002.

Louisiana Revised Statutes. Title 22. Insurance, Chapter 1. Insurance Code. Part VI-A. Louisiana Health Plan. La. R.S. 22:239 (2001), § 239.

Ludwig, David S., Karen E. Peterson, and Steven L. Gortmaker, "Relation Between Consumption of Sugar-Sweetened Drinks and Childhood Obesity: A Prospective, Observational Analysis." *The Lancet*, vol. 357, no. 9255, February 17, 2001, pp. 505-508. Online. Available: http://www.thelancet.com/search/search.isa. Accessed: January 31, 2002.

Lyndon B. Johnson School of Public Affairs, *Expansion through Waivers,* Policy Research Project Report Working Paper, Austin, Tex., 2002. (draft)

————. *Expanding Health Care Coverage for the Uninsured in Texas.* Policy Research Report Series, no. 141. Austin, Tex., 2001.

Malcolm, Jan. "The Minnesotacare provider tax debate." *The Medical Journal of Allina,* vol. 6, no.3 (1997), pp. 1-5. Online. Available: http:// www.allina.com/Allina_Journal/Summer1997/malcolm.html. Accessed: November 20, 2001.

Man, Anthony. "State's Medicaid funding, or fingers in the dike." *Illinois Issues,* vol. XVIII, no. 6, August/September 1991. Online. Available: http://www.lib.niu.edu/ipo/ii910833.html. Accessed: February 1, 2001.

Management Sciences for Health. *Home Page*. Online. Available: http://www.msh.org. Accessed: February, 15, 2002.

Mann, Cindy. *The New Medicaid and CHIP Waiver Initiatives.* Washington, D.C.: The Kaiser Commission on the Uninsured, 2002.

Marchon, Terri. Public Affairs Associate, New York Department of Insurance, New York, NY. Interview by Jed Perry, October 9, 2001.

Marin, Elena, M.D. Executive Director, Su Clinica Familiar, Harlingen, Texas. Interviewed by Jennifer Eldridge, February 1, 2002.

Marrero, Jose. President, JAM Creative. Class presentation, Lyndon B. Johnson School of Public Affairs, Austin, Texas, November 6, 2001.

Maternal and Child Health Bureau. *MCHB Mission.* Online. Available: http://mchb.hrsa.gov. Accessed: January 4, 2002.

Matherlee, Karen. *Issue Brief: the Federal-State Medicaid Match: An ongoing Tug-of War over Practice and Policy.* Washington, D.C.: National Health Policy Forum, George Washington University, December 2001,pp. 1-10. Online. Available: http://www.nhpf.org/pdfs/8-760+(web).pdf. Accessed: November 20,2001.

McNeely, Dave, "Income tax on verge of Texas Horizon," *Abilene Reporter News.* April 15, 2001. Online. Available: http://www.reporternews.com/2001/opinion/tax0415.html. Accessed: November 18, 2001.

Menges, Joel, Chris Park, Jennifer Babcock, Lisa Chimento, Randall Haught, Silver Ho, The Lewin Group. *Comparing Physician and Dentist Fees Among Medicaid Programs.* Oakland, CA: Medi-Cal Policy Institute, June 2001. Online. Available: http://admin.chcf.org/documents/mcpi/ComparingPhysicianAndDentistFees.pdf. Accessed: January 31, 2002.

Merlis, Mark. *Medicaid: Program and Demonstration Waivers.* Washington, D.C.: Congressional Research Service, 1994.

Meyer, Jack A., and Lise S. Rybowski. The Commonwealth Fund. "Business Initiatives to Expand Health Coverage for Workers in Small Firms." (October 2001). Online. Available: http://www.cmwf.org. Accessed: November 4, 2001.

Milby, June. Coordinator, NC Health Choice for Children. "Full Cost Buy-In Option," Email to Jie Zhou, January 15, 2002.

Miller, Michael. "Community Catalyst/ Health Care for All." Presentation at Families USA Conference, Washington D.C., January 17, 2002.

Milligan, Charles. *Section 1115 Waivers and Budget Neutrality: Using Medicaid Funds to Expand Coverage.* Washington, D.C.: State Coverage Initiatives of the Robert Wood Johnson Foundation, 2001.

Minnesota Department of Revenue. *Tax Reform Assessment Phase Health Care Tax Background.* Online. Available: http://www.taxes.state.mn.us/reform/stdygr/healbkgnd.html. Accessed: January 27, 2002.

———————. *Minnesota Revenue Notice Number 00-07,MinnestoaCare Tax- Hospital Gross Revenues.* Online. Available: http://www.taxes.state.mn.us/rnotices/00_07.html. Accessed: November 20, 2001

———————. *Reforming the tax system: Health Care Tax Reform Team.* Online. Available: http://www.taxes.state.mn.us/reform/stdygr/healarch.html. Accessed: January 30, 2002.

Minnesota Statutes 2001. *Table of Chapters, Table of contents for Chapter 295.* Online. Available: www.revisor.leg.state.mn.us/stats/295/52.html. Accessed: November 23, 2001.

Mullan, Fitzhugh, M.D. "Tin-Cup Medicine." Health Affairs, vol. 20, no. 6 (November/December 2001), pp. 216-221.

Murdock, T. Michael. Huntingtonnews.net. *Provider Coalition Formed to Phase Out Healthcare Services Tax* (January 10,2001). Online. Available: http://www.huntingtonnews.net/state/ProviderCoalition1.html. Accessed: November 23,2001.

Murray, Bruce. Executive Vice President, UHA Hospitals and Health Systems Association. Email, "Utah Medicaid Tax," to Jaime Dudensing, November 26, 2001.

National Association of Community Health Centers. *Conference Committee Approves Record Increase for Health Center Program.* Online. Available: http://www.nachc.com/Federal_Affairs/2002/Conference_Passage.htm. Accessed: January 4, 2001.

National Association of Insurance Commissioners. *2001 Small Employer Health Benefits Premium Comparison Survey.* Online. Available: http://www.naic.org. Accessed: December 17, 2001.

———————. *Basic Health Benefits Plan (Plan A/50).* Online. Available: http://www.naic.org. Accessed: December 17, 2001.

———————. *New Jersey Health Insurance Bureau* (March 8, 2001). Online. Available: http://www.naic.org. Accessed: December 17, 2001.

———. *New Jersey Health Reform Insurance Information* (September 13, 2001). Online. Available: http://www.naic.org. Accessed: December 17, 2001.

———. *New Jersey Individual Health Care Program Carriers.* Online. Available: http://www.naic.org. Accessed: December 17, 2001.

———. *New Jersey Individual Health Coverage Program Rates.* Online. Available: http://www.naic.org. Accessed: December 17, 2001.

———. *New Jersey Managed Care Bureau.* Online. Available: http://www.naic.org. Accessed: December 17, 2001.

———. *New Jersey Office of Life and Health Insurance* (June 11, 2001). Online. Available: http://www.naic.org. Accessed: December 17, 2001.

———. *New Jersey Small Employer Health Benefits Parity.* Online. Available: http://www.naic.org. Accessed: December 28, 2001.

———. *New Jersey Small Employer Health Benefits Buyer's Guide.* Online. Available: http://www.naic.org. Accessed: December 17, 2001.

———. *New Jersey Small Employer HMO Chart.* Online. Available: http://www.naic.org. Accessed: December 28, 2001.

———. *New Jersey Small Employer Standard Health Benefits Plan Summary.* Online. Available: http://www.naic.org. Accessed: December 28, 2001.

———. *New Jersey Small Employer Carriers.* Online. Available: http://www.naic.org. Accessed: December 17, 2001.

———. *Snapshot Of Standard Health Benefits Plans.* Online. Available: http://www.naic.org. Accessed: December 28, 2001.

———. *The New Jersey Individual Health Coverage Program, Buyer's Guide* (1998). Online. Available: http://www.naic.org. Accessed: December 17, 2001.

———. *What Is New Jersey Health Insurance Reform?* Online. Available: http://www.naic.org/nj/ihc_she.htm. Accessed: December 17, 2001.

National Association of State Medicaid Directors. *Medicaid 1115 Waivers.* Online. Available: http://medicaid.aphsa.org/waivers/1115waivers.htm. Accessed: January 8, 2001.

National Center for Chronic Disease Control and Prevention and Health Promotion. *Obesity and Overweight: A Public Health Epidemic* (September 12, 2001). Online. Available: http://www.cdc.gov/nccdphp/dnpa/obesity/epidemic.htm. Accessed: January 31, 2002.

National Federation of Independent Business. *Association Health Plans (AHP), Talking Points*. Washington, D.C. (pamphlet).

———————. *The NFIB Small-Business Growth Agenda for the 107th Congress.* Washington, D.C. (pamphlet).

National Governor's Association. *Health Insurance Coverage and Financing*. Online. Available: http://www.nga.org/center/topics/1,1188,D_355,00.html. Accessed: November 15, 2001.

National Immigration Law Center. *Texas AG Issues Opinion that County Hospitals Not Allowed to Serve "Not Qualified" Immigrants*. Online. Available: http://www.nilc.org/immspbs/health/health012.htm. Accessed: January 22, 2002.

Nestle, Marion. *Soft Drink "Pouring Rights": Marketing Empty Calories.* Department of Nutrition and Food Studies, New York University, 2000. Online. Available: http://www.asu.edu/educ/epsl/Archives/CERU%20Archives/cace-00-03/cace-00-03.htm. Accessed: January 31, 2002.

New Jersey Department of Banking and Insurance. *Department of Banking and Insurance*. Online. Available: http://www.njdobi.org. Accessed: December 17, 2001.

———————. *Enforcement and Consumer Protection* (August 8, 2000). Online. Available: http://www.njdobi.org/enfcon.htm. Accessed: January 8, 2002.

New Mexico Comprehensive Health Insurance Pool. *New Mexico Comprehensive Health Insurance Pool.* Online. Available: http://www.aidsinfonet.org/322-chip.html#anchor21641. Accessed: March 3, 2002.

New York State Department of Health. *New York Child Health Plus Promotion*. Online. Available: http://www.health.state.ny.us/nysdoh/chplus/brochure.htm. Accessible: January 9, 2002.

———————. *New York Child Health Plus*. Online. Available: http://www.health.state.ny.us. Accessed: January 9, 2002.

———————. *State Child Health Plan Under Title XXI of the Social Security Act: New York State*. By Dennis P. Whalen. New York, NY, 1998.

Norton, Stephen. *Recent Trends in Medicaid Physician Fees, 1993-1998.* Discussion paper no. 99-12. Washington, D.C.: Urban Institute, September 1999. Online. Available: newfederalism.urban.org/html/discussion99-12.html. Accessed: November 15, 2001.

Novartis. *Texas Summary 2000,* Online. Available: http://www.novartisvin.com/content/Statefacts/state_result.asp?State=TX&date=2000. Accessed: February 22,2002.

Office for Oregon Health Plan Policy and Research. *The Oregon Health Plan and Oregon's Health Care Market, A Report to the 71st Legislative Assembly.* Salem, Ore., August 2000.

__________. *The OHP 2 Waiver Application.* Online. Available: http://www.ohppr.state.or.us/Waiver_Application/index_waiver.htm. Accessed: February 4, 2002.

Office of Public Insurance Counsel. *A Review of Health Insurance Underwriting Guidelines Used in Texas.* Online. Available: http://www.opic.state.tx.us/health1.html. Accessed: January 26, 2002.

__________. *Annual HMO Reports Now Available.* Online. Available: http://www.opic.state.tx.us/PRHMO2001.htm. Accessed: January 2, 2002.

__________. *Comparing Texas HMOs* (2000). Online. Available: http://www.opic.state.tx.us/counties2000.html. Accessed: October 30, 2001.

__________. *Current Bill of Rights.* Online. Available: http://www.opic.state.tx.us/BOR_intro.htm. Accessed: January 2, 2002.

__________. *Health Insurance Coverage in Texas: Context and Demographics.* Online. Available: http://www.opic.state.tx.us/Healthykids.html. Accessed: January 2, 2002.

__________. *Health Insurance Information.* Online. Available: http://www.opic.state.tx.us/Healthinfo.html. Accessed: January 24, 2002.

__________. *Office of Public Insurance Counsel.* Online. Available: http://www.opic.state.tx.us/whatis.html. Accessed: January 24, 2002.

Office of State and National Partnerships, Bureau of Primary Health Care. *Current Approaches to Medicaid Reciprocity and Portability.* Online. Available: http://bphc.hrsa.gov/osnp/Medicaid2.htm. Accessed: January 15, 2002.

Office of the Secretary of Health and Human Services. "Medicaid Program: Demonstration Proposals Pursuant to Section 1115(a) of the Social Security Act: Policies and Procedures." *Federal Register,* 59(186). Washington, D.C., September 27, 1994.

Office of the Surgeon General. *Overweight and Obesity: At A Glance.* Online. Available: http://www.surgeongeneral.gov/topics/obesity/calltoaction/fact_glance.htm. Accessed: January 31, 2001.

Oregon Revised Statutes. Title 56. Insurance. Chapter 735. Alternative Insurance. Medical Insurance Pool. ORS § 735.614,1999. Assessments for expenses of pool.

Palmer, David. Director of Actuarial Analysis, Texas Health and Human Services Commission. "RE: Medicaid Question." Email to Leah Kegler, December 17, 2001.

People's Community Clinic. *About Us*. Online. Available: http://www.pcclinic.org/about.html. Accessed: March 24, 2002.

————. *2000 Services Report*. Online. Available: http://www.pcclinic.org/report.html. Accessed: March 24, 2002.

Pogue, Anita. Director of Information Assistance, Consumer Protection Division Texas Department of Insurance, Austin, Texas. Telephone interview by Jacqueline Angel, Scott Atnip, Karla Buitrago, and Kristen Lindberg, February 1, 2002.

Pool Administrators Inc. "Reinsurance Rates Effective August 1, 2001." Memorandum to All Reinsuring Carriers in Texas. *Texas Health Reinsurance System*, July 27, 2001.

Robert Wood Johnson Foundation. "Full-Cost Buy-Ins: An Overview of State Experience." State Coverage Initiative Issue Brief. Washington, D.C., August 2001.

Rowland, Diane. *Health Insurance for Unemployed Workers.* Washington, D.C.: The Kaiser Commission of the Uninsured, 2001.

Rundle, Rhonda. "Obesity Tops Smoking for Medical Costs." *The Wall Street Journal* (March 12, 2002), p. B7.

Ryan, Jennifer M. "Health Insurance Family Style: Public Approaches to Reaching the Uninsured." *Issue Brief No. 767.* Washington, D.C.: National Health Policy Forum, September 24, 2001.

Rylander, Carole Keeton. *Texas Health Care Spending.* Austin, Tex.:, Texas Comptroller of Public Accounts, March 2001.

Salo, Matt. *Briefing on President Bush's Medicaid Flexibility Initiative Medicaid Flexibility for the Uninsured*? Washington, D.C.: Alliance for Health Reform, August 2001.

Scarborough, Steve. Partner, Health Data Partners, L.L.P., Austin, Texas. Interview by Jamie Dudensing and Kristie Kimbell, February 28, 2002.

Schneider, Andy, and Rachel Garfield. *Medicaid Benefits.* Washington, D.C.: The Kaiser Commission on Medicaid and the Uninsured, 2000.

Scully, Thomas. *Briefing on President Bush's Medicaid Flexibility Initiative Medicaid Flexibility for the Uninsured*? Washington, D.C.: Alliance for Health Reform, August 28, 2001.

Selden, Audrey. Consumer Protection Division, Texas Department of Insurance. "FY 2002-2003 Business Plan." Personal email to Jacqueline Angel, February 14, 2002.

Senate Bill 1053 Workgroup. *Preliminary Report to the Texas Legislature.* Austin, Tex., 2001.

Senate Bill 1299 Workgroup. *Border Rate Workgroup on Medicaid and SCHIP Final Report.* Austin, Tex., 2001.

Sexton, Jennifer. *Overview of the Iowa Health Insurance Premium Payment (HIPP) Program.* Washington, D.C: Institute for Health Policy Solutions, February 2000.

Shenkman, Elizabeth and Jana Col. *Children's Health Insurance Program in Texas: The New Enrollee Survey Report.* Gainesville, Florida: Institute for Child Health Policy, January 2001.

Silow-Carrol, Sharon, Stephanie E. Anthony, and Jack A. Meyer. *State and Local Initiatives to Enhance Health Coverage for the Working Uninsured.* New York, NY: The Commonwealth Fund, November 2000.

Smith, Anita. Manager, Health Insurance Purchasing Unit, Iowa Department of Human Services. Presentation, Effective Coverage Expansions for Uninsured Kids and Their Working Parents: Links to Job-Based Coverage Conference, Washington D.C., May 18, 2001.

Social Security Act, ch.19, sec 1903, parts (w)(3)(A), (w)(3)(C), (w)(3)(D), (w)(3)(E), (w)(3)(4), and (w)(7)(A).

State Bar of Texas Health Law Section. *Medicaid Legislation, Rural Community Health Systems* (SB 1246, 1997). Online. Available: http://www.texhealthlaw.org/Public/archive/s7medicaid.pdf. Accessed: April 15, 2002.

State Coverage Initiatives. *State Coverage Matrix.* Online. Available: http://www.statecoverage.net/matrix.htm. Accessed: April 23, 2002.

——————. *State of the States.* Washington, D.C.: Academy for Health Care Services Research and Health Policy, 2002.

——————. *State-Only High-Risk Pool.* Online. Available: http://www.statecoverage.net/highrisk.htm. Accessed: March 3, 2002.

State of Arkansas. *Soft Drink Tax.* Online. Available: http://arkleg.state.ar.us/data/TAXBOOK/TAXES/SOFTDR~1.htm. Accessed: November 19, 2001.

State of Illinois, Department of Insurance. *Complaints*. Online. Available: http://www.state.il.us/ins/Complaints/Complaints.htm. Accessed: November 11, 2001.

————. *Contact the Illinois Department of Insurance*. Online. Available: http://www.state.il.us/ins/Contact_us.htm. Accessed: November 11, 2001.

————. *Department Overview*. Online. Available: http://www.state.il.us/ins/overview.htm. Accessed: November 11, 2001.

————. *Health Insurance*. Online. Available: http://www.state.il.us/ins/healthInsurance/healthInsurance.htm. Accessed: November 11, 2001.

————. *I Want to File a Complaint*. Online. Available: http://www.state.il.us/ins/Complaints/file_complaint.htm. Accessed: November 11, 2001.

————. *Illinois Department of Insurance: 66th Annual Report and Summary of Annual Statements*. Springfield, Ill., 2000. Online. Available: http://www.state.il.us/ins/AnnualReportLinks.htm. Accessed: November 18, 2001.

————. *Office of Consumer Health Insurance*. Online. Available: http://www.state.il.us/ins/OCHI/office_consumer_health_ins.htm. Accessed: November 11, 2001.

State of New Hampshire Department of Revenue Administration, *NH State Tax Form—2 2002*. Online. Available: http://webster.state.nh.us/revenue/forms/index.htm. Accessed: December 16, 2001.

State of New Jersey. *New Jersey People—Be Healthy*. Online. Available: http://www.state.nj.us/njpeople/healthy.html. Accessed: December 17, 2001.

State of West Virginia. *Excise Taxes*. Online. Available: http://www.state.wv.us/taxrev/97taxlaws/9761_excise.pdf. Accessed: November 19, 2001.

State Office of Administrative Hearings. *Welcome to SOAH*. Online. Available: http://www.soah.state.tx.us/Backgrnd/SOAH.htm. Accessed: January 26, 2002.

Statewide Health Coordinating Council, Texas Department of Health. *2001-2002 Texas State Health Plan Update: Ensuring a Quality Health Care Workforce for Texas, Appendix H Ad Hoc Committee on Consumer Information*. Online. Available: http://www.tdh.state.tx.us/stateplan01/default.htm. Accessed: January 24, 2002.

Sutton, Donna Fay. *Office of Health Care Ombudsman, Annual Report 2000*. Burlington, Vermont: Vermont Office of Health Care Ombudsman.

Texas A & M University System Health Science Center. *Health Insurance Statistics, 2000.* Online. Available: http://srph.brc.tamus.edu/srphis. Accessed: February 13, 2001.

Texas Academy of Family Physicians. *77th Legislative Compendium: Managed Care.* Online. Available: http://www.tafp.org/Departments/Leg/lc-managedcare.htm. Accessed: January 25, 2002.

Texas Association of Community Health Centers. *What is an FQHC?* Online. Available: http://www.tachc.org. Accessed: November 14, 2001.

———. "Robert Wood Johnson Foundation Grant Narrative." Austin, Tex., 2001.

———. "Texas Association of Community Health Centers Membership Directory." Austin, Tex., 2000.

———. "Texas Statewide Strategic Plan Prepared for BPHC and NACHC." Austin, Tex., August 22, 2001 (draft proposal).

———. *Project Alberto Report* (Austin, Tex., 2000).

———. *Project Alberto/Covering Kids Initiative.* Online. Available: http://www.tachc.org/o_pa_main.htm. Accessed: January 2, 2002.

Texas Association of Counties. "Tobacco Reimbursement Funds will be Distributed Later this Month." *TACNews*, vol. 9, no. 54 (April 6, 2001). Online: Available: http://www.county.org/resources/TACnews/news04061.html. Accessed: January 31, 2002.

Texas Association of Public and Nonprofit Hospitals, Austin, Texas Interview with selected staffers and one member by Jamie Dudensing, Kristie Kimbell, and Dr. David Warner, February 6, 2002.

Texas Blue Ribbon Task Force on the Uninsured. *Report to the 77th Legislature.* Austin, Texas, February 2001.

Texas CHIP Coalition. *What is this new CHIP program?* Online. Available: http://www.main.org/txchip/page3.html. Accessed: October 20, 2001.

Texas Comptroller of Public Accounts. *2002-2003 Biannual Revenue Estimate.* Online. Available: http://www.window.state.tx.us/taxbud/bre0203/tablea3.html. Accessed February 1, 2002.

———. *Comptroller Rylander Certifies Budget; Warns of Potential $5 Billion Shortfall Next Session*, June 6, 2001. Online. Available: http://www.window.state.tx.us/news/1060bud.html. Accessed: October 2, 2001.

———. *Franchise Tax.* Online. Available: http://www.window.state.tx.us/taxinfo/frantax.html. Accessed: November 14, 2001.

———. *Hospital District Taxes.* Austin, Tex., 2000 (Excel file).

———. *Tax Exemptions and Tax Incidence Report.* January 2001. Online. Available: http://www.window.state.tx.us/taxinfo/incidence/table19.html. Accessed: November 20, 2001.

———. *Texas Health Care Spending* (March 2001). Online. Available: http://www.window.state.tx.us/specialrpt/hcs/intro.html. Accessed: February 1, 2002.

———. *Texas Health Care Spending* (March 2001). Online. Available: http://www.window.state.tx.us/specialrpt/hcs/pg33.html. Accessed: November 15, 2001.

Texas Department of Health and Texas Health Quality Alliance. *January 2000 Provider Satisfaction Survey for Medicaid Managed Care: Final Technical Report.* Austin, Tex., July 27, 2000.

Texas Department of Health, Indigent Health Care Division. *Summary, Indigent Health Care Program, August 2000.* Austin, Tex., October 3, 2000.

———, Office of Policy and Planning. *Agreement Regarding the Disposition of Tobacco Settlement Proceeds.* June 8, 1999. Online. Available: http://www.tdh.state.tx.us/dpa/tobsett.htm. Accessed: January 31, 2002.

———. *Indigent Health Care Division.* Online. Available: http://www.tdh.state.tx.us/hcf/ihcp/default.htm. Accessed: January 28, 2002.

———. *County Directory.* Online. Available: www.tdh.state.tx.us/hcf/ihcp. Accessed: April 8,2002

———. *HMO Rate Setting Methodology FY 2002.* Austin, Texas, 2001.

———. *Hospital Survey Data on Diskette.* Austin, Tex.: Office Of Health Information and Analysis, 1999 (Database on disk).

Texas Department of Health. *January 2000 Provider Satisfaction for Medicaid Managed Care: Final Executive Summary.* Austin, Tex., July 27, 2001.

———. *Participating Plans.* Online. Available: http://www.tdh.state.tx.us/hcf/mc/plans/particip.htm. Accessed: November 16, 2001.

———. *Summary of Disproportionate Share Hospital Payments.* Austin, Tex.,2000. (Excel file on disk).

———. *Summary of Indigent Healthcare Program Matching Grants*. Online. Available: http://www.tdh.state.tx.us/hcf/ihcp. Accessed October 15, 2001.

———. *Texas Medicaid Managed Care Update: July 24, 2001*. Online. Available: http://www.tdh.state.tx.us/hdf/mc/reports. Accessed: January 3, 2002.

———. *Texas STAR Medicaid Managed Care Report: Second Edition, Fiscal Year 1998*. Austin, Tex., May 2000.

———. *The Health Insurance Premium Payment (HIPP) Reimbursement Program for Texas Medicaid Recipients and Family*. Online. Available: http://www.tdh.state.tx.us/cshcn/hipp.htm. Accessed: November 19, 2001.

———. *Women's Health in Texas*. Online. Available: http://www.tdh.state.tx.us/women/famsrc.stm. Accessed: January 10, 2002.

Texas Department of Human Services. *Budget and Statistics: SCHIP Program*. Online. Available: http://www.bms.dhs.state.tx.us/SCHIP.htm. Accessed: December 13, 2001.

———. *Colonias Factbook*. Online. Available: http://chud.tamu.edu/colonias/factbook.html#health. Accessed: February 1, 2002.

———. *Reference Guide 2000*. Online. Available: http://www.dhs.state.tx.us/publications/refguide/2000/StateRankings.html. Accessed: April 10, 2002.

———. *Title XIX Expenditure History List*. Austin, Tex, November 2000.

Texas Department of Insurance, State Planning Grant Division. *Grant Proposal, Project Abstract*. Online. Available: http://spg.tdi.state.tx.us/grant/abstract.htm. Accessed: January 25, 2002.

———. *Texas State Planning Grant Interim Report* (Austin, Tex., October 2001). Online. Available: http://spg.tdi.state.tx.us/pubs/interim. Accessed: January 26, 2002.

Texas Department of Insurance. "Characteristics of Texans With and Without Health Insurance." Paper presented at a conference on "Working Together for a Healthy Texas: Expanding Health Insurance Coverage for Texans," Texas State Planning Grant Conference, Austin, Tex., January 31- February 1, 2002.

———. "Concurrent Breakout Sessions to Discuss Options for Expanding Health Insurance." Conference on "Working Together for a Healthy Texas: Expanding Health Insurance Coverage for Texans," Texas State Planning Grant Conference, Austin, Texas, January 31- February 1, 2002.

———. "Policy Options Under Review by SPG." Paper presented at a conference on "Working Together for a Healthy Texas: Expanding Health Insurance Coverage for Texans," Texas State Planning Grant Conference, Austin, Texas, January 31- February 1, 2002.

———. "Sample Texas Small Employer Rate Guide." Paper presented at a conference on "Working Together for a Healthy Texas: Expanding Health Insurance Coverage for Texans," Texas State Planning Grant Conference, Austin, Texas, January 31- February 1, 2002.

———. "Small Employer Health Insurance Survey Results." Paper presented at a conference on "Working Together for a Healthy Texas: Expanding Health Insurance Coverage for Texans," Texas State Planning Grant Conference, Austin, Texas, January 31- February 1, 2002.

———. *2000 Accident and Health Complaint Index.* Online. Available: http://www.tdi.state.tx.us. Accessed: January 2, 2002.

———. *2001 Annual Report* (November 2001). Online. Available: http://www.tdi.state.tx.us/commish/annual01.html. Accessed: January 2, 2002.

———. *2001-2002 Automobile Insurance Rate Guide* (revised September 2001). Online. Available: http://www.tdi.state.tx.us. Accessed: January 2, 2002.

———. *2001-2002 Homeowners Insurance Rate Guide* (revised September 2001). Online. Available: http://www.tdi.state.tx.us. Accessed: January 2, 2002.

———. *2001-2002 Texas Long-Term Care Rate Guide* (revised May 2001). Online. Available: http://www.tdi.state.tx.us/consumer/ltcrgintro.html. Accessed: January 2, 2002.

———. *77th Legislature Enacts More Than 80 Insurance Bills.* Online. Available: http://www.tdi.state.tx.us/commish/lege80.html. Accessed: January 25, 2002.

———. *A Word from the Commissioner: Help Us Fight Insurance Fraud.* Online. Available: www.tdi.state.tx.us/commish/help.html. Accessed: January 26, 2002.

———. *Assistance for Providers* (revised April 2001). Online. Available: http://www.tdi.state.tx.us/consumer/cbo52.html. Accessed: January 2, 2002.

———. *Continuing Education: Agents, Adjusters, Providers.* Online. Available: http://www.tdi.state.tx.us/agent/agcehome.html. Accessed: January 26, 2002.

———. *Glossary—Common Insurance Terms.* Online. Available: http://www.tdi.state.tx.us/consumer/glossary.html. Accessed: January 26, 2002.

———. *Health Care Coverage for Texas Children* (revised May 2001). Online. Available: http://www.tdi.state.tx.us/consumer/cbo72.html. Accessed: November 11, 2001.

———. *Health Maintenance Organizations* (revised December 2000). Online. Available: http://www.tdi.state.tx.us. Accessed: January 2, 2002.

———. *Helping You With Your Insurance Complaint* (revised April 2000). Online. Available: http://www.tdi.state.tx.us/consumer/consum83.html. Accessed: January 2, 2002.

———. *HICAP Highlights—Private Fee-for-Service Plans.* Online. Available: http://www.tdi.state.tx.us/consumer/hicap/hicapnews200.html. Accessed: January 26, 2002.

———. *HMO Resource.* Online. Available: http://www.tdi.state.tx.us. Accessed: January 2, 2002.

———. *If My Insurance Company Fails* (revised September 2000). Online. Available: http://www.tdi.state.tx.us/consumer/cbo6.html. Accessed: January 2, 2002.

———. *Independent Review Organizations* (revised January 2000). Online. Available: http://www.tdi.state.tx.us/consumer/iro.html. Accessed: January 26, 2002.

———. *Insurance for Texans with Disabilities.* Online. Available: http://www.tdi.state.tx.us/consumer/cbo39.html. Accessed: January 26, 2002.

———. *Insurance Fraud* (revised April 2001). Online. Available: http://www.tdi.state.tx.us/consumer/cbo44.html. Accessed: January 26, 2002.

———. *Insurance on the Internet: Shopping Tips and Dangers* (revised February 2000). Online. Available: http://www.tdi.state.tx.us. Accessed: January 2, 2002.

———. *Insurance Resource for Small Businesses.* Online. Available: http://www.tdi.state.tx.us/commish/smbiz.html. Accessed: November 11, 2001.

———. *Jose Montemayor: Texas Commissioner of Insurance.* Online. Available: http://www.tdi.state.tx.us/commish/jose.html. Accessed: January 2, 2002.

———. *Listing of Companies Offering Small Employer Accident and Health Coverage.* Online. Available: http://www.tdi.state.tx.us/company/lhsmallemp.html. Accessed January 25, 2002.

———. *Long-Term Care Insurance.* Online. Available: http://www.tdi.state.tx.us/consumer/cbo32.html. Accessed: January 26, 2002.

———. *Major Texas Insurers*. Online. Available: http://www.tdi.state.tx.us/company/top40.html. Accessed: January 2, 2002.

———. *Medicare Supplement Insurance Handbook and Rate Guide* (revised September 2001). Online. Available: http://www.tdi.state.tx.us. Accessed: January 2, 2002.

———. *Medicare+Choice Options for Medicare Beneficiaries*. Online. Available: http://www.tdi.state.tx.us/consumer/cbo36.html. Accessed: January 26, 2002.

———. *Mission Statement*. Online. Available: http://www.tdi.state.tx.us. Accessed: January 24, 2002.

———. *Senior Issues*. Online. Available: http://www.tdi.state.tx.us. Accessed: January 2, 2002.

———. *Small Employers Health Insurance: Questions and Answers* (revised January 2001). Online. Available: http://www.tdi.state.tx.us/consumer/cbo40.htm. Accessed: November 11, 2001, and February 21, 2002.

———. *Speakers Bureau Calendar of Events*. Online. Available: http://www.tdi.state.tx.us/consumer.speak.html. Accessed: January 26, 2002.

———. *Summary of Health Care Coverage Options for Texas Children* (revised September 2001). Online. Available: http://www.tdi.state.tx.us. Accessed: January 2, 2002.

———. *Texas Department of Insurance*. Online. Available: http://www.tdi.state.tx.us. Accessed: January 2, 2002.

———. *Texas State Planning Grant*. Online. Available: http://spg.tdi.state.tx.us. Accessed: January 26, 2002.

———. *Texas Workers' Compensation Rate Guide* (December 5, 2001). Online. Available: http://www.tdi.state.tx.us/company/rcomp.html. Accessed: January 2, 2002.

———. *Trabajando Para Usted Un Guía para el Consumidor* (revised June 2001). Online. Available: http://www.tdi.state.tx.us/consumer/news3s.html. Accessed: January 2, 2002.

———. *What is the Speakers Bureau?* Online. Available: http://www.tdi.state.tx.us. Accessed: January 2, 2002.

———. *Your Health Care Coverage* (revised June 2001). Online. Available: http://www.tdi.state.tx.us/consumer/cbo05.html. Accessed: November 11, 2001.

Texas Education Agency. "Building Bridges to Healthy Kids and Better Students: Strengthening School-Based Outreach and Enrollment for Health Insurance." Austin, Tex., February 2002.

Texas Government Code Annotated, ch. 466, sec. 466.408.

Texas Health and Human Service Commission. SB 1053 Workgroup. Workgroup presentation, Austin, Texas, October 26, 2001.

————. *1995 Texas Medicaid Legislation.* 74th Texas Legislature, regular session. March 25, 1999. Online. Available: http://www.hhsc.state.tx.us/medicaid/med_info/medleg_74.html. Accessed: April 15, 2002.

————. *Advisory Committee for Senate Bill 1053 and Senate Bill 1299* (Austin, Tex., October 26, 2001).

————. *Budget Brief: November 2001.* Austin, Texas, November 2001.

————. *Budget Brief: October 2001.* Austin, Texas, October 2001.

————. *Children's Medicaid Simplification-Senate Bill 43 Proposed Implementation Outline.* Online. Available: http://www.hhsc.state.tx.us/chip/SB43/SB43_Simplification_Intro.html. Accessed: January 27, 2002.

————. *CHIP Cost-sharing Change Scenarios.* Online. Available: http://www.hhsc.state.tx.us/chip/cnews/prgmdsgnscen071801.htm. Accessed: April 5, 2002.

————. *CHIP Program Design Issues.* Online. Available:http://www.hhsc.state.tx.us/ chip/cnews/PrgmDsgnIssues071801.html. Accessed: November 1, 2001.

————. *Cumulative Application, Enrollment and Eligibility Determination Activity for 11/5/01.* Online. Available: http://www.hhsc.state.tx.us/CHIP/ WeeklySumRpt.htm. Accessed: November 17, 2001.

————. *Cumulative Application, Enrollment and Eligibility Determination Activity for 12/31/01.* Online. Available: http://www.hhsc.state.tx.us/CHIP/ WeeklySumRpt.htm. Accessed: January 10, 2002.

————. *Cumulative Application, Enrollment, and Eligibility Determination Activity for 1-14-02.* Online. Available: http://www.hhsc.texas.gov/SCHIP/weeklysumrpt.htm. Accessed: January 31, 2002.

———. *Demographic Profile of Texans Without Health Insurance Coverage* (2000). Online. Available: http://www.hhsc.state. tx.us/budget/cons_bud/dssi/brt/brtchchap3.pdf. Assessed: January 05, 2002.

———. *Medicaid Managed Care Rate Setting*. Austin, Texas, 2000.

———. *Medicaid Managed Care Report* (November 1, 2000). Online. Available: http://www.hhsc.state.tx.us/Medicaid/ MMCR_Main/MMCR_html_frontpage.htm. Accessed: January 10, 2002.

———. *Medicaid Managed CareReport, Chapter13 – Medicaid Managed Care in Rural Areas*. Online. Available: http://www.hhsc.state.tx.us/medicaid/ mmc_htm/c13_rural_managed_care.htm. Accessed: April 15, 2002.

———. *Medicaid/Texas Health Steps Health Care Orientation* (November 2001). Online. Available: http://www.hhsc.state.tx.us/CHIP/SB43/SB43_script.pdf. Accessed: November 13, 2001.

———. *Proposed CHIP Cost-sharing Changes, Request for Public Comment.* Online. Available: http://www.hhsc.state.tx.us/ chip/cnews/chip_cost_sharing.html. Accessed: April 5, 2002.

———. Research and Forecasting. *Demographic Profile of the Texas Population Without Health Insurance in 2000* (October 2001). Online. Available: http://www.hhsc.state.tx.us/budget/cons_bud/dssi/ TXUNIN2000.html. Accessed: May 6, 2002.

———. Research Department. *Baseline Projection of Otherwise Uninsured Texas Children Under 19 by Poverty Income Status: Years 2000-2006*. Austin, Tex., January 2001. (Computer printout.)

———. *Texas Medicaid 1115 Summary*. Austin, Tex, 1995.

———. *Texas Medicaid in Perspective* (Austin, Tex., February 1999).

Texas Health Care Information Council. *About THCIC*. Online. Available: http://www.thcic.state.tx.us/AboutTHCIC.htm. Accessed: January 24, 2002.

———. *Straight Talk on Texas HMOs: A Purchaser's Guide* (November 2001). Online. Available: http://www.thcic.state.tx.us/Publications.htm. Accessed: November 4, 2001.

———. *Your HMO Quality Check-up: A Consumer's Guide to Texas Commercial HMOs* (August 2001). Online. Available: http://www.thcic.state.tx.us/Publications.htm. Accessed: November 4, 2001.

Texas Health Education Assistance Resources and Training. *Medicaid STARLink* (January 2001). Online. Available: http://www.txheart.org/starlink.html. Accessed: April 3, 2002.

Texas Health Insurance Risk Pool. *Frequently Asked Questions*. Online. Available: http://www.txhealthpool.com/faq.html. Accessed: March 3, 2002

———. *Health Insurance Premiums Reporting Form: Amounts Reported for Health Insurance Premiums for Texas Residents*, (Austin, TX, 2000).

———. *Health Pool Benefits,* Online. Available: http://www.txhealthpool.com/benefits.html. Accessed: March 3, 2002.

———. *Health Pool Eligibility*. Online. Available: http://www.txhealthpool.com/eligibil.html. Accessed: March 3, 2002

———. *Premium Rate Table*, (January 1, 2002). Online. Available: http://www.txhealthpool.com/010102%20Rate%20table.pdf. Accessed: March 3, 2002.

———. *Premium Rates for Health Pool Coverage*. Online. Available: http://www.txhealthpool.com/rates.html#Tables. Accessed: March 3, 2002.

———. *The 2000 Annual Report of the Texas Health Insurance Risk Pool*. Austin, Texas: June 1, 2001.

Texas House Bill 2498, 77th Legislature (2001).

Texas House Bill 3038, 77th Texas Legislature, regular session (2001).

Texas House of Representatives, House Research Organization. *SB 1839*. May 22, 2001.Online. Available: http://www.capitol.state.tx.us/hrofr/frame2.htm. Accessed: November 4, 2001.

———. *House Bill 2430: House Committee Report—Fiscal Note*. Online. Available: http://www.capitol.state.tx.us/tlo/billnbr.htm. Accessed: January 24, 2002.

Texas Institute for Health Policy Research. *The Uninsured in Texas, Policy Brief* (September 29, 2000). Online. Available: http://www.healthpolicyinstitute.org/publications/policy_briefs/uninsured_paper_policy_brief.pdf. Accessed: November 11, 2001.

Texas Insurance Code, Annotated, ch. 3, art. 3.77

———, ch. 26, art. 21. *Small Employer Health Benefit Plans; Employer Election*. Online. Available: http://www.capitol.state.tx.us/statutes/intoc.html. Accessed: January 26, 2002.

———, ch. 26, art. 32. *Index Rates*. Online. Available: http://www.capitol.state.tx.us/statutes/intoc.html. Accessed: January 26, 2002.

———, ch. 26, art. 42. *Small Employer Health Benefit Plans*. Online. Available: http://www.capitol.state.tx.us/statutes/intoc.html. Accessed: January 26, 2002.

———, ch. 26, art. 73. *Agents*. Online. Available: http://www.capitol.state.tx.us/statutes/intoc.html. Accessed: January 26, 2002.

Texas Legislative Budget Board. *House Bill 2430: Enrolled Version, Bill Analysis*. Online. Available: http://www.capitol.state.tx.us/tlo/billnbr.htm. Accessed: January 24, 2002.

———. *House Bill 2430, House Committee Report—Fiscal Note* (April 25, 2001). Online. Available: http://tlo2.tlc.state.tx.us. Accessed: January 24, 2002.

———*House Bill 2430: Introduced Version, Bill Analysis.* Online. Available: http://www.capitol.state.tx.us/tlo/billnbr.htm. Accessed: January 24, 2002.

———. *House Bill 471: Enrolled Version, Bill Analysis.* Online. Available: http://www.capitol.state.tx.us/tlo/billnbr.htm. Accessed March 7, 2002.

———. *House Bill 949: Enrolled Version, Bill Analysis.* Online. Available: http://www.capitol.state.tx.us/tlo/billnbr.htm. Accessed March 7, 2002.

———. *SP 43 Enrolled Version Fiscal Note,* 77th Regular Session. May 22, 2001. Online. Available: http://www.capitol.state.tx/tlo/ 77rfiscal/SB00043.htm. Accessed: September 30, 2001.

———. "Spotlight: Health Insurance Flexibility and Accountability (HIFA) Demonstration Initiative." *Federal Fund Watch.* Austin, Tex., Volume 7(4), October 2001.

———. *Summary of Conference Committee Report on Senate Bill 1.* May 23, 2001. Online. Available: http://www.lbb.state.tx.us/Publish_AppBills_LBEs.htm. Accessed: September 18, 2001.

———. *Text of Conference Committee Report, Senate Bill. 1.* May 23, 2001. Online. Available: http://www.lbb.state.tx.us/Publish_AppBills_LBEs.htm. Accessed: October 4, 2001.

Texas Legislature. *Bill History: HB 2430.* Online. Available: http://www.capitol. state.tx.us/tlo/billnbr.htm. Accessed: January 26, 2002.

———. *Bill History: SB 771.* Online. Available: http://www.capitol.state.tx.us/ tlo/billnbr.htm. Accessed: February 22, 2002.

———————. *Senate Bill 771: Proposed Version*. Online. Available: http://www.capitol.state.tx.us/tlo/billnbr.htm. Accessed: February 22, 2002.

Texas Medical Association. *Status Report: Rural Community Health Systems*. Online. Available: http://www.texmed.org/pmt/pay/rhh/ruralleg.asp. Accessed: April 15, 2002.

Texas Office of House Bill Analysis. *SB 1839 Bill Analysis.* 77th Texas Legislature, Regular Session, Austin, Tex., May 16, 2001. Online. Available: http://tlo2.tlc.state.tx.us/cgi-bin/tlo/textframe.cmd?LEG=77&SESS=R&CHAMBER=S&BILLTYPE=B&BILLSUFFIX=01839&VERSION=3&TYPE=A. Accessed: November 4, 2001.

Texas Organization of Rural and Community Hospitals. *TORCHNet: Frontline*. Online. Available: http://www.torchnet.org/fl11-08.html. Accessed: April 15, 2002.

Texas Senate Bill 1, 77th Texas Legislature, Regular Session (2001).

Texas Senate Bill 10, 75th Texas Legislature, Regular Session (1995). Online. Available: http://tlo2.tlc.state.tx.us/cgi-bin/tlo/textframe.cmd?LEG=74&SESS=R&CHAMBER=S&BILLTYPE=B&BILLSUFFIX=00010&VERSION=5&TYPE=B Accessed: April 15, 2002.

Texas Senate Bill 1156, 77th Texas Legislature, Regular Session (2001). Online. Available: http://tlo2.tlc.state.tx.us/cgi-bin/tlo/textframe.cmd?LEG=77&SESS=R&CHAMBER=S&BILLTYPE=B&BILLSUFFIX=01156&VERSION=5&TYPE=B. Accessed: April 15, 2002.

Texas Senate Bill 1246, 75th Texas Legislature, Regular Session (1999). Online. Available: http://tlo2.tlc.state.tx.us/cgi-bin/tlo/textframe.cmd?LEG=75&SESS=R&CHAMBER=S&BILLTYPE=B&BILLSUFFIX=01246&VERSION=5&TYPE=B. Accessed: April 15, 2002.

Texas Senate Research Center. *HB 710, Bill Analysis*, 75th Legislative Session. Texas State Legislature. March 19, 1997. Online. Available: http://www.capitol.state.tx.us/cgi-bin/tlo/textframe.cmd?LEG=75&SESS=R&CHAMBER=H&BILLTYPE=B&BILLSUFFIX=00710&VERSION=4&TYPE=A. Accessed: April 28, 2002

Texas State Board of Medical Examiners. *Physicians In and Out of State*. January 2002. Online. Available: http://www.tsbme.state.tx.us/demo/docs/d2002/0102/inout.htm. Accessed: February 22,2002.

TexCare Partnership. *Cumulative, Application, Eligibility Determination, and Enrollment Activity for 2-18-02*. Online. Available: http://www.hhsc.state.Tex.us/chip/WeeklySumRpt.pdf. Accessed: February 22, 2001.

———. *CBO Best Practices* (2000). Online. Available: http://www.texcarepartnership.com/Documents/CBO Best Practices.doc. Accessed November 8, 2001.

———. *Children's Health Insurance Program 2000 Annual Report.* Austin, Tex., 2000.

———. *CHIP Start Up Comparisons.* Online. Available: http://www.texcarepartnership.com/CHIP-Comparison-Stats-Page.htm. Accessed: March 7, 2001.

———. *TexCare Partnership Outreach Work Plan: Children's Medicaid and the Children's Health Insurance Program January 2002-August 2003* (draft). Austin, Tex., January 2002.

———. *TexCare Partnership Outreach: Guidance for Community-Based Organizations' Outreach Projects 2002-2003 Strategic Work Plan.* Austin, Tex., January 2002.

———. *TexCare Partnership Statewide Outreach Initiatives, September 2000-August 2001* (June 2001). Online. Available: http://www.hhsc.state.tx.us/CHIP/cnews/TCP_Initiatives.pdf. Accessed: November 17, 2001.

The Independent Institute. *Book Summary Taxing Choice: The Predatory Politics of Fiscal Discrimination.* Online. Available: http://www.independent.org/tii/content/briefs/BriefTaxingChoice.html. Accessed: January 29,2002.

The Migrant Clinicians Network. *Farmworker Health Issues.* Online. Available: http://www.migrantclinician.org/. Accessed: January 20, 2002.

———. *Farmworker Migration Patterns.* Online. Available: http://www.migrantclinician.org. Accessed: January 20, 2002.

———. *The Farmworker Population: Background.* Online. Available: http://www.migrantclinician.org. Accessed: January 20, 2002.

The Texas Health Access Project. "Random Access: Holes in the Texas Health Care Safety Net: Reports from the Communities." Austin, Tex., 2001.

The Texas Legislature Online. *The Texas Constitution, Article 8 - Taxation And Revenue, Section 24 - Personal Income Tax; Dedication Of Proceeds.* Online. Available: http://www.capitol.state.tx.us/txconst/sections/cn000800-002400.html. Accessed: November 16, 2001.

The University of Texas Health Science Center at San Antonio. "Regional Academic Health Center." Online. Available: http://rahc.uthscsa.edu. Accessed: April 10, 2002.

Thomas, Paul, and Lynne Hudson. "The Texas Children's Health Insurance Program (CHIP) One Year Later—Where Do We Go From Here?" *Texas Journal of Rural Health,* vol. IXI (2001), p. 44.

Tollen, Laura. *Purchasing Private Health Insurance through Government Health Care Programs: A Guide for States.* Washington D.C.: Institute for Health Policy Solutions, Inc., June 1999.

"Transition to the Market." Focus Group at "Investing in Texas: Financing Health Coverage Expansions" Conference, Lyndon B. Johnson School of Public Affairs, Austin, Texas, March 22, 2002.

U.S Census Bureau. *Census 2000 Supplemental Survey.* Online. Available: http://factfinder.census.gov/home/en/c2ss.html. Accessed: April 4, 2002.

————. *Quick Facts, Profile of Selected Characteristics.* Online. Available: http://factfinder.census.gov/servlet/BasicFactsServlet. Accessed: April 4, 2002.

————. *Survey of Income and Program Participation.* Online. Available: http://www.bls.census.gov/sipp. Accessed: May 6, 2002.

————. *United States Census 2000.* Online. Available: http://www.census.gov/main/www/cen2000.html. Accessed: April 8, 2002.

————. *U.S. Bureau of the Census, Texas Metropolitan Statistical Area Population Estimates: 1900 to 2000* . Online. Available: http://www.cpa.tx.us/ecodata/popdata/msa1 . Accessed: January 31,2002.

U.S. Department of Health and Human Services. Agency for Healthcare Research and Quality. *Medical Expenditure Panel Survey.* Online. Available: http://www.meps.ahrq.gov. Accessed: April 24, 2002.

————. *Children's Health Insurance Expansions: State Experiences in Developing Benefit Packages and Cost-Sharing Arrangements.* February 17,1998. Online. Available: http://aspe.os.dhhs.gov/health/reports/benefits/state_approaches_to_costsharing.htm. Accessed: November 20, 2001.

————. *Cost Sharing.* Online. Available: http://aspe.os.dhhs.gov/health/reports/benefits/state_approaches_to_costsharing.htm. Accessed: November 20, 2001.

————. *Examining Substitution: State Strategies to Limit Crowd out in the era of Children's Health Insurance,* January 10, 2001. Online. Available: http://aspe.os.dhhs.gov/health/reports/hinsubst/XSubstit.htm. Accessed: November 20, 2001.

———. Office of the Assistant Secretary for Planning and Evaluation. *Understanding Estimates of the Uninsured: Putting the Differences in Context* (January 2001) Online. Available: http://aspe.hhs.gov/health/reports/hiestimates.htm#7 Accessed: January 28, 2002.

———. "State Child Health; Revisions to the Regulations Implementing the State Children's Health Insurance Program; Final Rule." *Federal Register*, vol. 66, no. 122, June 25, 2001, pp. 33810-33824. Online. Available: http://www.hcfa.gov/init/hcfa2006.pdf. Accessed: April 5, 2002.

U.S. Department of Health, Education and Welfare, Welfare Administration, Bureau of Family Services. "Medical Assistance Programs Under Title XIX of the Social Security Act." *Handbook of Public Assistance Administration, Supplement D.* Washington, D.C., 1966.

U.S. Department of Labor, Bureau of Labor Statistics. *1999 March Current Population Survey*. Online. Available: http://www.bls.census.gov/cps/cpsmain.htm. Accessed: April 8, 2002.

———. *2000 March Current Population Survey*. Online. Available: http://www.bls.census.gov/cps/cpsmain.htm. Accessed: April 8, 2002.

———. *2001 March Current Population Survey*. Online. Available: http://www.bls.census.gov/cps/cpsmain.htm. Accessed: April 8, 2002.

Umphress, John. Staff, Texas Association of Public and Nonprofit Hospitals, Austin, Texas. Interviewed by Jamie Dudensing and Kristie Kimbell, February 28, 2002.

University of Houston Law Center, Health Law and Policy Institute. *Small Employers Guide to Health Care Plans*. Online. Available: http://www.lawlib.uh.edu/healthlaw/tccempl.html. Accessed: November 18, 2001.

Urban Institute. *National Survey of America's Families*. Online. Available: http://www.urban.org/Content/Research/NewFederalism/NSAF/Overview/NSAF Overview.htm. Accessed: April 24, 2002.

Verdier, James M. "State Provider Assessments to Fund Medicaid." *National Tax Journal,* vol. 46, no. 3 (1993), pp. 377-383. Online. Available: http://www.ntj/tax.org. Accessed: January 8,2002.

Vermont Legal Aid, Inc. "Proposal for Health Care Ombudsman." Presentation at the "Families USA Health Action 2002" conference, Washington, D.C., January 2002.

Waldman, Beth. Acting Director of Program Implementation, Massachusetts Division of Medical Assistance. Presentation, Effective Coverage Expansions for Uninsured

Kids and Their Working Parents: Links to Job-Based Coverage Conference, Washington D.C., May 18, 2001.

Walker, Nancy. State Legislative Aid, City of Austin, Austin, Texas. Telephone interview by Scott Atnip, January 24, 2002.

Warner, David. Professor, Lyndon B. Johnson School of Public Affairs, Austin, Texas. "Standard Adjustment Amount for Texas Hospitals." Personal email to Sarah Stout, January 24, 2002.

Washington Department of Social and Health Services. *DSHS Children's Campaign Wins National 'Best of the Best' Award* (June 2001). Online. Available: http://www.wa.gov/dshs/mediareleases/pr01152.shtml. Accessed: January 8, 2002.

Welles, Henry. Program Specialist, Texas Department of Health. "RE: Data you Requested," Email to Sara Stout, February 25, 2002.

———————. Program Specialist, Texas Department of Health, Austin, Texas. Interview by Sarah Stout, January 30, 2002.

Westmoreland, Tim. *Briefing on President Bush's Medicaid Flexibility Initiative Medicaid Flexibility for the Uninsured*? Washington, D.C.: Alliance for Health Reform, August 28, 2001.

———————. Health Care Financing Administration, Department of Health and Human Services. Letter to State Health Officials, July 31, 2000.

Wilkes, David. SCHIP Actuary, Birch and Davis. Presentation to the Senate Bill 1053/1299 Workgroup, Austin, Texas, November 15, 2001.

Wisconsin Council on Families and Children. *Wisconsin's BadgerCare Program.* Online. Available: http://www.wccf.org/BadgerCare.pdf. Accessed: February 3, 2002.

Wollam, Allison. "Financial Aches Dog Houston HMOs." *The Houston Business Journal* (April 6, 2001). Online. Available: http://houston.bcentral.com/jouston/stories/ 2001/04/09/story1.html. Accessed: November 25, 2001.

Zuckerman, Stephen, Jennifer Haley, and John Holahan. *Health Insurance, Access, and Health Status of Nonelderly Adults.* Washington, D.C.: Urban Institute, 2001.

Zuckerman, Stephen, Teresa Coughlin, Len Nichols, David Liska, Barbara Ormond, Alicia Berkowitz, Meghan Dunleavy, Jodi Korb, and Nelda McCall. *Health Policy for Low-Income People in California.* Washington D.C.: The Urban Institute, 1998.